AF675724

A History of

YALE'S SCHOOL OF MEDICINE

A History of

YALE'S SCHOOL OF MEDICINE

Passing Torches to Others

GERARD N. BURROW, M.D.

1701 YALE UNIVERSITY TERCENTENNIAL 2001

YALE UNIVERSITY PRESS / NEW HAVEN & LONDON

Copyright © 2002 by Yale University. All rights reserved.
This book may not be reproduced, in whole or in part, including illustrations, in any form (beyond that copying permitted by Sections 107 and 108 of the U.S. Copyright Law and except by reviewers for the public press), without written permission from the publishers.

Designed by Mary Valencia.
Set in Minion type by Achorn Graphic Services, Worcester, Massachusetts.
Printed in the United States of America by Edwards Brothers, Ann Arbor, Michigan.

Library of Congress Cataloging-in-Publication Data

Burrow, Gerard N. 1933–
A History of Yale's School of Medicine : passing torches to others / Gerard N. Burrow.
p. cm.
Includes bibliographical references and index.
ISBN 0-300-09207-5 (alk. paper)
1. Medical colleges—Connecticut—History. 2. Medical education—Connecticut—History. I. Title.
[DNLM: 1. Yale University. School of Medicine. 2. Schools, Medical—history—Connecticut. 3. Education, Medical—history—Connecticut. W 19 B972y 2002]
R747.Y27 B87 2002
610.71′1746′8—dc21
2002016800

A catalogue record for this book is available from the British Library.

The paper in this book meets the guidelines for permanence and durability of the Committee on Production Guidelines for Book Longevity of the Council on Library Resources.

10 9 8 7 6 5 4 3 2 1

To

Karlton G. Percy, M.D., Yale College '07
Who removed my tonsils and stimulated my interest in medicine

and

Thomas R. Forbes, Ph.D., M.A. (Hon.), Yale University
Who admitted me to Yale and stimulated my interest in academic medicine

ΛΑΜΠΑΔΙΑ ΕΧΟΝΤΕΣ ΙΑΔΩΣΟΥΣΙΝ ΑΛΛΗΛΟ

"Those having torches will pass them on to one another"
—Plato, *The Republic*

Inscription above the entrance to the Sterling Hall of Medicine

CONTENTS

PREFACE

My life at Yale began in October 1953, when Thomas R. Forbes, the assistant dean, accepted me into the School of Medicine. I remained at Yale for the next twenty-two years, two of which were spent with the Yale contingent at the Atomic Bomb Casualty Commission in Nagasaki.

I slept in a garret and lived in the Medical Library during my first year of medical school. Saturated with studying, I would roam the library stacks. While browsing one day, I came across a copy of *Arrowsmith* with an inscription on the inside cover to the father of neurosurgery—" 'To Harvey Cushing, and if he isn't the best doctor in the world, I would like to know who is,' Sinclair Lewis, Litt. D., fairly Hon."

I joined the Nathan Smith Club, named for the school's founding professor, where medical students presented papers to each other and to interested faculty. John F. Fulton, a distinguished physiologist and medical historian who had spent time at Oxford, was the host for my presentation. He and my subject, Thomas Dover, had both been members of Magdalen College, whose name I unfortunately mispronounced, and from his volcanic response I was convinced that my medical career had ended prematurely.

During college years, final examinations had signaled the end of studying a particular subject. The "Yale system" of medical education, where no specific reading was assigned and no particular books were recommended, was at first frustrating. But I and my fellow students eventually picked up a book out of boredom or desperation and began studying. As there was no one to say "Time's up!" we were left with an ingrained feeling that studying is never quite finished. This lifelong desire or need to learn has been the great gift of the Yale system. The apparent intellectual freedom was not desirable for everyone. Classmates who required a more disciplined curriculum were distinctly uncomfortable in the free-floating environment of Yale. For the majority, however, medical-school years were a happy time, free from the rigid, "Look on either side of you, one of you won't be here next year!" atmosphere. Students who sought that freedom tended to gravitate to Yale. An inordinate number of my classmates were embryonic psychoanalysts, more interested in Sigmund Freud than in *Gray's Anatomy.*

After graduation, I remained at Yale on the medical house staff, rising to the exalted position of chief resident eleven years after entering medical school. Asked to join the medical faculty by Paul Beeson, I stayed in New Haven for a further eleven years. I was involved in a number of activities outside the Department of Medicine and replaced Tom Forbes as chairman of the medical school's admissions committee. When I decided to accept a position as chief of endocrinology at the University of Toronto, I wondered aloud whether there was "life after Yale."

I eventually became chairman of the Department of Medicine at the University of Toronto, and my benchmark for success was always the Department of Medicine at Yale. In 1988, I went to the University of California at San Diego as vice-chancellor of health sciences and dean of the School of Medicine. Averill Liebow, my pathology professor at Yale, had moved to San Diego when the medical school was founded and had instituted a modified form of the Yale system, including a research-thesis requirement. When Leon Rosenberg stepped down as dean at Yale, I returned to New Haven to meet with the search committee to lobby for the preservation of the Yale system. I soon left sunny California to become the fourteenth dean of the Yale University School of Medicine.

I returned to Yale in 1992 after being away for sixteen years, having practiced both in the universal health-care system of Canada and in the entrepreneurial West Coast research atmosphere of San Diego. The University of California at San Diego was a young school, and almost anything a dean did established a tradition. Yale was almost three hundred years old, and anything a dean did tended to interfere with an extant tradition. Medical students at UCSD were every bit as bright as Yale students but lacked the wide diversity of backgrounds. Yale medical students often had substantial careers before entering medical school and brought a richness of experience to the class. Yale students were much more involved in extracurricular community activities and in matters of international health, perhaps because of faculty interest both in the Department of Epidemiology and Public Health and in the School of Medicine.

The depth of faculty strength at Yale was truly impressive. The faculty and departmental chairmen at Yale viewed themselves as much more independent than did their counterparts at either San Diego or Toronto. The medical-school culture at Yale was much closer to the Faculty of Arts and Sciences than was the case at the other institutions. A number of the clinical chairmen at Yale religiously took triennial leave, which left the departments with acting chairmen for six months every three years.

Relations with the university administration at Yale were complicated by the fact that I had been recruited by one president and interacted with two more, as well as with three provosts, during my five-year tenure as dean. Interaction with the Yale administration was more guarded, perhaps reflecting the differences between public and private universities. Research funding and clinical income at the medical school accounted for almost half of Yale University's operating budget. Half of the university's full-time faculty members were located in the medical school but were financially covered by only 8 percent of the university's endowment. Recent decreases in clinical revenues have increased the administration's anxieties about its ultimate financial responsibility for the medical school.

Despite valiant efforts, the rich history of the Yale University School of Medicine has never been chronicled. The three-hundredth anniversary of Yale College in 2001 provided an occasion to record the history of the medical school. Having spent a total of thirty-one years at Yale and ten years as a dean at Yale and UCSD, I was particularly interested in both the history of Yale's medical school and its relationship with the parent university and the major affiliated hospital. Relationships among the three institutions are perhaps the main issues facing deans of medical schools and university presidents today. I had been interested in medical history since my student days in the Nathan Smith Club and later as a faculty member in the Beaumont

Medical Club. I was also available to write the history, having just stepped aside as dean.

I have interjected personal comments on historical events in relation to present-day issues where appropriate. Not surprisingly, the same problems that I faced as a dean were faced by my predecessors all the way back to Charles Hooker, the first dean, in 1845. I hope that the lessons of history will be of some assistance to future Yale deans. But as every dean learns, some problems have no solution.

I decided to end the book with the appointment of Robert Berliner as dean in 1972. Much of the reference material after that date is restricted and too recent to be examined dispassionately. Nevertheless, an understanding of the present state of the medical school is necessary fully to appreciate its past. The Yale University School of Medicine is generally viewed as one of the world's great medical schools, but it is difficult to document why. Based on past history and the present state of the school, what does the future hold for medicine in general and for Yale in particular?

A medical school is often described as a three-legged school with responsibility for teaching, research, and patient care. What distinguishes medical schools from research institutes and clinics is the educational component. But although education is central to a school's mission, it is often given lip service, and faculty members are actually promoted or paid for their research or practice attainments. Nevertheless, the title of this book illustrates that centrality. *Yale's School of Medicine: Passing Torches to Others* is based on a Greek inscription from Plato's *Republic* located above the entrance to the rotunda of the Sterling Hall of Medicine. The inscription was chosen by Grover Atterbury, the architect for the addition of the Institute of Human Relations to the Sterling Hall of Medicine. When Dean Milton C. Winternitz asked Professor Austin M. Harmon about the translation, Harmon commented, "The torch has come to be almost synonymous with the transmission of learning from one generation to another" (L. M. Davey, "Sharing Light," *Yale Medicine* [Fall–Winter 1996]: 60–61).

ACKNOWLEDGMENTS

One of the most difficult issues for a fledgling historian is how to begin. I am indebted to Frank Turner for informing me during lunch at Mory's, after I had spent six months wandering aimlessly in the forest of Manuscripts and Archives at Sterling Memorial Library, that the way to write history is to start writing. I began writing about Abraham Flexner's 1910 report to the Carnegie Foundation for the Advancement of Teaching and subsequently moved forward and backward in time from that point. I am indebted to Gaddis Smith, who exclaimed over his shoulder while we were kayaking, "The book is more important than the date!" That exclamation lifted a great burden from my shoulders. Toby Appel, the Medical Library historian, continually reminded me that this would be the first published history of the medical school. She and Mona Florea were enormously helpful in supplying source references. Naomi Rogers, who had written a history of Hahnemann Medical College, provided useful guidance. James Hanley, Mary Yearl, Christiane Nockels, Kari McLeod, and Kari Theobald were invaluable research assistants.

I am deeply indebted to the late Elizabeth Thomson, along with her co-authors, Herbert Thoms, Levin Waters, Averill Liebow, and Fred Kilgour, who made a good start on a history of the medical school. Arthur Viseltear wrote a number of articles dealing with the Department of Epidemiology and Public Health in particular, which were enormously helpful. I am also indebted to Wendy Nan Jacobson, who wrote her Wesleyan undergraduate honors thesis on the history of the medical school at Yale. I owe a particular debt of gratitude to Kenneth M. Ludmerer. His books *Learning to Heal* and *Time to Heal* provide a bench mark for studies on American medical education.

Without access to the appropriate source material, no history can be written. Manuscripts and Archives at Sterling Memorial Library was everything that would be expected from one of the world's preeminent libraries. After the staff had trained me thoroughly in the mores and folkways of M&A, they went out of their way to be helpful, as did Toby Appel in the Historical Medical Library. Linda Lorimer, secretary of the university, allowed me access to restricted files and the minutes of the corporation up to 1952. The staffs of the Rockefeller Archive Center, the Library of Congress, and the Johns Hopkins University School of Medicine were also helpful. The Yale–New Haven Hospital and the Hospital of Saint Raphael kindly opened their archives for my research. I am particularly indebted to Stephen Cohen and Konstantine Sofer of Howard Hughes Medical Institute for help with figures 41 and 42. All photographs are from the Yale University Harvey Cushing/John Hay Whitney Medical Library, Medical Historical Library.

A number of individuals accessed their institutional memories to validate or correct impressions I had gained. Arthur Ebbert was extremely helpful throughout the preparation of the manuscript. Paul Beeson, Philip Bondy, Fritz Redlich, and Robert McCollum were also helpful, as were numerous others. Ultimate responsibility for accuracy is of course mine.

John Ryden, director of Yale University Press, read the manuscript in its early stages. Jean Thomson Black, senior editor, Otto Bohlmann, and Margaret Otzel provided firm direction. Toby Appel read several iterations. Finally, I would like to thank the Esther A. and Joseph Klingenstein Fund and the Greentree Foundation for their financial support, which made this project possible.

1

INTRODUCTION

Several important themes have tended to recur throughout the rich history of the Yale University School of Medicine since it was chartered as the Medical Institution of Yale College nearly two hundred years ago, in 1810. First and foremost among these themes has been the close relationship between the university and the medical school from its inception. Most medical schools in the United States were founded as private proprietary schools, which were subsequently subsumed by a university; Cooper Medical College, for example, became the Stanford University School of Medicine. The Medical Institution, in contrast, was founded by the Yale Corporation. As a result, the culture of Yale College fashioned the ethos of the medical school. Success in science was fostered from the beginning. Benjamin Silliman, who was appointed professor of chemistry and natural history in 1802, played a key role in the founding of the Medical Institution. Russell Chittenden, director of the Sheffield Scientific School, played a similarly influential role in the medical school seventy-five years later. Partly as a result of this basic emphasis on science, clinical medicine has never assumed the importance at Yale that it did at other medical schools.

The religious origins of Yale College have played a special role in its relationship with the medical school. Education was basic to the Puritan outlook. The desire for a university with lectures in medicine and law, first put forward at Yale by President Ezra Stiles in 1778, was a clear expression of Puritanism. Cotton Mather, one of the leading Puritan divines in New England, talked of the need to heal the body as well as the soul. Persistence of what Mather called the "Angelical Conjunction" is a plausible explanation for why the Yale Corporation has rescued the medical school on a number of occasions from a "near-death experience," when the prudent course of action would have been to let it expire.

Another legacy of university influence on the medical school at Yale has been an unswerving commitment to excellence on the part of the medical faculty. During the latter part of the nineteenth century, medicine had entered a dark period. The public rightly distrusted doctors and medical practice. Alternative medicine was flourishing, and enrollment in legitimate medical schools was decreasing as proprietary schools churned out inadequately trained doctors. In the midst of this turmoil, the faculty of the Medical Institution of Yale College continued to raise standards, with a resulting drop in medical-student enrollment. Because faculty salaries depended on fees from students, the more the faculty members elevated standards, the less remuneration they received.

Chronic underfunding has been the major reason for the recurrent threat of medical-school extinction. During the early years of the medical school, Yale College had financial problems, and available funds were committed to the undergraduate experience. Although the close relationship with the university played an important role in the success of the medical school, Yale College was clearly the center of attention. Not until the 1960s, with increased research funding and clinical income, did the medical school become a revenue-generating institution. Money has always played an important role in the life of the school, as it has at every academic institution. In the course of the medical school's history, there have been good medical-school deans and bad ones, good university presidents and bad ones, but if funds were plentiful, a lot of problems were either solved or covered over.

National events also played an important role in the success of the medical school. Abraham Flexner was commissioned to review the nation's medical schools. Flexner's assessment in 1910 that Yale and Harvard were the only two medical schools in New England worth keeping was instrumental in continuing the Yale Corporation's support of the medical school. Similarly, the federal decision to support research at universities after World War II helped the medical school eliminate a chronic deficit that threatened its future.

In addition to national influences, local influences played an important role in shaping the medical school. The Medical Institution of Yale College was founded as a joint effort of the college and the Connecticut Medical Society, which may have helped prevent the kind of proliferation of medical schools in Connecticut that occurred in neighboring states. The State Hospital was founded in New Haven by local physicians and Yale's medical faculty. Implementation of the full-time clinical system in return for Rockefeller Foundation support estranged the community physicians and led to the flourishing of the Hospital of Saint Raphael and the Grace Hospital in New Haven. Later, the presence of well-trained community physicians also contributed to the lack of emphasis on clinical areas within the medical school.

The "Yale system" of medical education, which does not assign or recommend particular texts but emphasizes intellectual freedom and has a research-thesis requirement, has been a recurrent theme for the past seventy-five years. Yale medical students do not in fact have more free time than students at other schools and may even have less than some. The perception, however, that faculty members are interested in students having more freedom results in most, although not all, medical students seeming less stressed. Critics have remarked that treating the medical students like graduate students may be a response to a lack of clinical material in New Haven rather than a new educational thrust. Be that as it may, Yale medical students continue to enjoy the Yale system.

The Medical Institution of Yale College opened its doors in 1813. To appreciate the impact of the Medical Institution, however, we need to bear in mind the effect of the founding of Yale College in 1701 on medical care in the colonies. The fact that the charter to grant M.D. degrees in addition to licensing physicians had been given to the Connecticut Medical Society meant that the university had to share control of the medical school. Hence, the use of the word *institution* rather than *department*, which would have implied total university control. The importance of a strong beginning for the medical school was recognized by Yale College, and the recruitment of Nathan Smith as the founding professor, paired with Benjamin Silliman, guaranteed that strength.

Nathan Smith's death in 1829, the opening of competing medical schools, and a general disillusionment with medicine resulted in a dark period of Yale medicine until the 1880s. The college was almost totally disengaged from the medical school and did not deign even to answer faculty pleas for help. Toward the latter part of the nineteenth century, science began to flourish on the Yale College campus after the formation of the Sheffield Scientific School in 1861. Some of this scientific excellence began to permeate the medical school, but something more had to happen or the school would fade from the scene.

And something did happen. In 1910 the Carnegie Foundation for the Advancement of Teaching commissioned Abraham Flexner to review medical education in the United States. After completing the Carnegie report, Flexner joined the Rockefeller Foundation to implement improvements in medical education in the United States. Convinced that full-time clinical practice was the solution, he offered financial support to Yale if it would move to a full-time clinical system. Such a move required academic control of the New Haven Hospital, and the new dean, George Blumer, set out to accomplish the task, which involved raising funds for the hospital. The faculty members were willing to support the change, but the community physicians were adamantly opposed to it.

Dean Blumer made several key appointments during his decade-long tenure, including his successor, Milton C. Winternitz, as professor of pathology and C.-E. A. Winslow as professor of public health. Winternitz, a product of Johns Hopkins, succeeded Blumer as dean with incredible energy. Scientific medicine was introduced with his recruitment of Francis Blake and John Peters to the Department of Medicine. He championed the Yale system and fostered the concept of social medicine with the formation of the Institute of Human Relations. Capitalizing on the base that Blumer built, Winternitz was able to garner university funds for buildings and professorships. A complex personality who was either loved or hated, he was involved in everything. But after fifteen years, the department chairmen had had enough, and Winternitz's term as dean was not renewed.

The next fifteen years were quiet ones for the school, although not for the world. During the height of the Depression, the medical school tried to grapple with social responsibility, led by John Peters, a forceful proponent. The Depression ended with World War II, which involved the medical school more completely than did any other war. The majority of the students were in military programs, and medical education was accelerated—to no one's satisfaction. The five years following the war were spent reintegrating students, graduates, and faculty into a normal medical-school routine. Finances were again a problem. The school was running a chronic deficit, and President Charles Seymour warned that the university could not continue to support the medical school forever.

A federal decision to support basic research in universities did much to restore financial health to the medical school. The appointment of Vernon Lippard in 1952 as the first full-time dean with connections to foundations was also important for the medical school's success. Funds became available to recruit outstanding individuals like Paul Beeson as chairman of the Department of Medicine, who in turn recruited excellent young faculty. This was the period during which the medical school rose to international prominence.

Facilities were expanded to keep pace with the growth in faculty size. One of the most important additions had already occurred in 1939 with the construction of the Medical Library. The Medical Library at Yale is not merely a place that houses books and journals but is truly the soul of the medical school. It offers a supportive ambience of scholarship that embraces the individual.

Vernon Lippard stepped aside in 1967, just in time to escape the rising social unrest that pervaded the country, the city, the university, and the medical school. Success of the Yale system depended on teachers teaching and students studying. The turmoil caused by anti–Vietnam War sentiment and the civil rights movement severely threatened the integrity of the program. Medical students and faculty were going in different directions. The community made its unhappiness with the medical school and hospital forcefully known. Nevertheless, the institution held together.

The medical school is composed of departments, which act relatively independently. The Department of Medicine is the largest department, with research funding equal to that of all the basic science departments together. Starting with Nathan Smith, the department consisted of a single professor until the 1920s, when Francis Gilman Blake was appointed chairman in 1921. He brought with him John Punnett Peters, a giant in American medicine who made laboratory medicine clinically relevant. The appointment of Paul Beeson in the 1950s, and the faculty he recruited, brought the department national prominence.

In a similar vein, the appointment of C.-E. A. Winslow in 1915 had heralded the beginning of a major concentration on public health. His determination to make public health a part of the medical school has persisted, but with difficulty. The department is named Epidemiology and Public Health, reflecting the conflict between Winslow and John Peters, who was in favor of studying disease rather than promoting health, a conflict that continues to this day.

This overview of the medical school's history will I hope set the scene for a more careful look at the events that formed the Yale University School of Medicine and its relationship to its parent university. We shall also need to bear in mind the role that Yale College played in the practice of medicine in Connecticut before the founding of the Medical Institution of Yale College in 1810.

2

THE FOUNDING YEARS

More than one hundred years passed between the Connecticut Legislature's act of 1701 establishing a Collegiate School where "youth may be instructed in the Arts and Sciences" and the act creating the Medical Institution of Yale College, approved by the General Assembly at its October session in 1810.[1] Graduates of Yale College, however, had been involved in the practice of medicine long before the founding of the medical school.[2] At least 224 Yale graduates, or about 10 percent of those awarded bachelor of arts degrees, practiced medicine during the eighteenth century. These rates are comparable to the proportion of Yale graduates practicing medicine in the nineteenth century and are not dissimilar to twentieth-century proportions.[3]

The Yale College curriculum was designed primarily for the education of clergymen. During the first half-century of the college's existence, nearly one-fourth of Yale graduates were ordained as ministers. The curriculum provided a classical education, which was also necessary to read the medical texts written in Latin. President Ezra Stiles occasionally lectured on medicine, and the college did possess a human skeleton.[4] In 1901 William Welch, dean of the Johns Hopkins University School of Medicine and a Yale alumnus, commented that Yale College provided its graduates with "a training of mind and character adapted to the circumstances of time and place, and fitting them for the work of life in any field."[5]

During the eighteenth century, the majority of the distinguished medical practitioners in Connecticut were clergymen who had graduated from Yale College. Cotton Mather of Massachusetts, one of the leading clergymen and Puritan theologians of his time, characterized the combination of ministry and medicine as an "Angelical Conjunction," which "administered unto the souls of the people the more effectually, for being able to administer to their bodies."[6] Mather introduced variolation as a way to inoculate against smallpox, a technique he had learned from his slave.[7] Collaborating with the physician Zabdiel Boylston, Mather began variolation in the colonies before its public introduction in England. Reports of the clinical trial had a powerful effect on British opinion and therapeutic practice.[8] Mather's interest in medicine was such that he reportedly participated in an autopsy on his son. Although a member of the Harvard Corporation, Mather was disenchanted with growing liberal tendencies and urged Boston-born Elihu Yale to support the Collegiate School in New Haven, suggesting that it might be named Yale College, which it was in 1718.[9] A Yale trustee even suggested to Mather that he assume its presidency.

The earliest of the Yale-educated clerical physicians, Phineas Fiske, graduated in 1704 from the Collegiate School, which at that time operated at both Killingworth and Saybrook before moving to New Haven in 1716. Jared Eliot (figure 1), a clerical physician and the son of a clerical physician, graduated in 1706. Eliot's classmate Jonathan Dickinson, the first president of Princeton College, also practiced medicine. His paper *Observations on That Terrible Disease, Vulgarly Called the Throat-Distemper*, published in 1740, was the first medical publication by a Yale graduate.[10]

Jared Eliot, an ordained minister, never missed a Sunday sermon, despite a busy medical practice. Considered the most outstanding physician in Connecticut, he was consulted more than any other physician in New England for chronic complaints.[11] He was always on the go. "Idleness was his abhorrence, but every portion of time was filled with action by him." Whenever Benjamin Franklin traveled from New York to Boston, he would visit Eliot, who was renowned as an easy conversationalist and charming company. El-

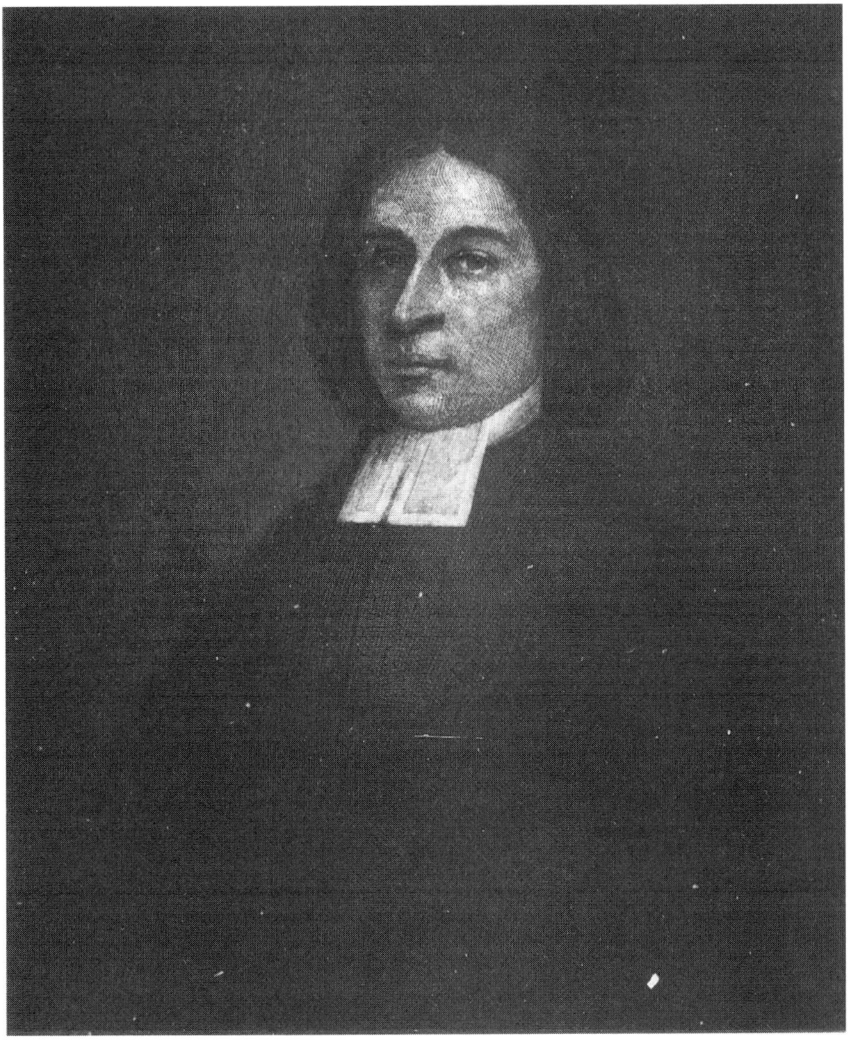

Figure 1. Jared Eliot

iot was elected a trustee of Yale College in 1730 and remained in the position until his death in 1763. In the course of his distinguished medical career, he trained perhaps as many as fifty physicians. Medical education in that era consisted of an apprenticeship for three or four years. The curriculum was made up of "books on the shelf, the skeleton in the closet, the pestle and the pill-slab in the back room, roaming the forests and fields for roots and herbs and, following astride of the colt he was breaking, the horse which was honored with the saddlebags."[12]

John Griswold, Class of 1721, was the earliest graduate of Yale College to devote himself exclusively to the profession of medicine.[13] Graduates of the college whose principal or sole professional occupation was the practice of medicine included some of the most influential medical men of the time.[14] Leverett Hubbard was a corporator, or founder, and first president of both the New Haven County Medical Society and the Connecticut Medical Society. Eneas Munson was the first name listed on the faculty of Yale's Medical Institution, and Eli Todd was the first superintendent of the Retreat for the Insane in Hartford.

The American Revolution engaged many Yale-educated medical practitioners, some serving as line officers. Twenty-three Yale practitioners served as surgeons or surgeon's mates, and six other Yale physicians served as officers in the army. Joshua Babcock, the first graduate of Yale College to study medicine in Europe, was a major general in the Rhode Island militia. Among the veterans returning after the Treaty of Paris was signed in 1783 and the army disbanded were a large number of former surgeon's mates who possessed some medical knowledge and were looking for a career. To the dismay of the Yale College graduates, the absence of restrictions on entering the medical profession resulted in a large influx of so-called medical practitioners, which provided the impetus for the establishment of the New Haven County Medical Society in order to define standards of medical practice.

When Ezra Stiles, Yale Class of 1746, received notice that he had been appointed president of Yale College in 1778, he was reluctant to leave his ministry in Portsmouth, New Hampshire. Asked by the Yale Corporation to draft a plan for a university that would include lectures in medicine and law, Stiles suggested a series of practical teaching experiences in law and medicine, followed by an apprenticeship. The concept of a medical school at Yale had its roots in the 1806 deliberations of the Yale Corporation and a committee of the Connecticut General Assembly to consider "enlarging and extending a plan of education in Yale College."[15] Connecticut was a theocracy, and education was an integral part of Puritan belief. The corporation submitted Stiles's plan to the General Assembly, which instituted a lay board elected by the General Assembly that would control the disbursement of state grants for the university's professorships. It took a further sixteen years to bring about the founding of the Medical Institution of Yale College.

Timothy Dwight, Yale Class of 1769, who was a grandson of Jonathan Edwards, succeeded Ezra Stiles as president of Yale in 1795. He had been a tutor at the college, a chaplain in the army during the Revolution, and a member of the Massachusetts Legislature. For twelve years prior to becoming president of Yale, he had served as pastor in Greenfield, Connecticut. President Dwight was finally able to convince the Connecticut Legislature that a larger Yale College was important for Connecticut, and that more professorships were needed, particularly in science.

Of fundamental importance to the founding of the medical school was the establishment of a professorship in chemistry in 1802. Benjamin Silliman (figure 2), a Yale College graduate, was studying law while serving as a tutor at the college. He was unhappy with law and was offered a job in Georgia. President Dwight had taken a parental interest in him. Convinced that the study of chemistry and geology would be increasingly important as the natural resources of the country were developed, Dwight appointed Silliman to the chair of chemistry and natural history. Silliman, who lacked a scientific background, set out to learn chemistry, which would be important for the medical school Dwight was planning.

The Yale Corporation, acting on the recommendation of the General Assembly, passed a resolution in 1806 to establish a medical professorship. Professor Benjamin Silliman and the Reverend Nathan Strong of Hartford were appointed to implement the resolution.[16] As the Connecticut Medical Society controlled medical education in the state by virtue of its charter of 1792, negotiations ensued between the Yale Corporation and the Connecticut Medical Society, with President Dwight chairing the joint committee. The Connecticut Medical Society (which became the Connecticut State Medical Society in 1905) was empowered to confer medical degrees as well as act as an examining and licensing body, and from the beginning had actively exercised these prerogatives. The charter of the society stated that the M.D. degrees were honorary, and they appear to have been awarded to physicians who had been in practice for a prolonged period. Two Yale graduates, Mason Fitch Cogswell, Class of 1780, and Eli Ives, Class of 1799, were strong medical-school supporters within the society, and all but one member of the committee appointed by the society were Yale College graduates. Nevertheless, negotiations between the college and the society dragged on for the next three years.[17] Whether Yale College could have awarded M.D. degrees without the consent of the society is unclear.

Negotiations with the Connecticut Medical Society delayed the opening of the medical school but did ensure the school's acceptance by the Connecticut medical community. The society required a one-year medical course to obtain a license, which was good for Yale, and one student from each county was allowed to attend the medical-school course without charge, which was good for the Connecticut Medical Society. Furthermore, no other medical

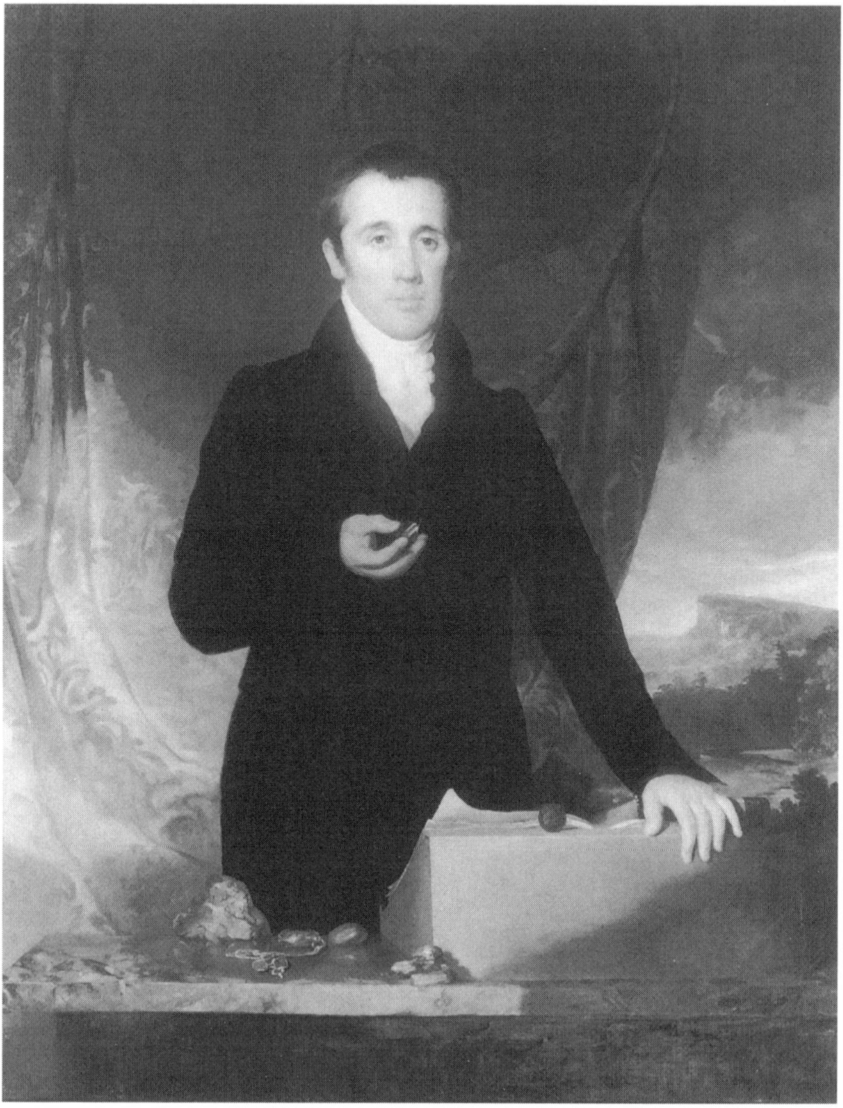

Figure 2. Benjamin Silliman Sr.

schools received a charter in Connecticut during the nineteenth century, despite the proliferation of medical schools in other states.

A medical society had been formed in Litchfield in 1779, with Yale graduates playing an important role. In 1763, two years before the second state medical society in the country was founded in Philadelphia, an attempt to organize a state medical society in Connecticut had failed. In 1783, a week after George Washington said farewell to his troops in Fraunces' Tavern in New York, Eneas Munson and Leverett Hubbard, brother-in-law of Yale president Ezra Stiles, convened a small group of physicians in a New Haven coffeehouse to form the New Haven County Medical Society.[18] Professional improvement and camaraderie were strong reasons for founding it, as was the desire to combine with other societies to form a state medical society that would be chartered by the legislature and would regulate the practice of medicine. The state society would pass regulations that would "prevent the world from the horrid imposition of quacks, medicasters and vain pretenders, with which it is now infested."[19]

Although the General Assembly had insinuated that the real purpose of the New Haven County Medical Society was to increase physicians' incomes, the society played an important educational role in disseminating medical knowledge by corresponding with other societies elsewhere in America and in Europe. In 1788, New Haven physicians published a pamphlet entitled "Cases and Observations by the Medical Society of New Haven County in the State of Connecticut," which contained twenty-eight articles. This was the first volume of medical transactions ever published in the United States. The most significant published contribution to medicine by a Yale graduate in this era came from the country's first epidemiologist, Noah Webster, Class of 1778. Although not a physician, he published an important two-volume work in 1799 entitled *A Brief History of Epidemic and Pestilential Diseases.*[20]

The lay public was interested in health care even then. Every educated person knew something about medicine, and newspapers were full of medical information. President Stiles had the Yale seniors debate "Whether it is safe to grant the proposed charter for medical Societies in Connecticut."[21] The General Assembly granted a charter to the Connecticut Medical Society in 1792, giving the society authority to issue licenses for the practice of medicine as well as to confer "honorary degrees" in medicine.

Some seventy years earlier, Yale College had awarded the first M.D. degree in North America in 1723 to Daniel Turner, a London physician. Turner's dermatological treatise *De morbis cutaneis,* first published in 1714, went through five editions in English and was also translated into French and German.[22] Licensed by the surgeon's guild after a seven-year apprenticeship, Turner became interested in medicine and purchased his release from the guild for fifty pounds. He was then accepted as a licentiate of the Royal College of Physicians in London.[23] Turner hoped also to be admitted to the Fellowship of the Royal College. This required a university degree, and anyone who was not a graduate of Oxford or Cambridge commonly purchased a M.D. degree in Scotland. Turner, however, had offended the Glasgow medical faculty by describing this practice in unfavorable terms in his book *The Modern Quack.* After being told by Jeremiah Dummer, the London agent for Connecticut who had been instrumental in obtaining Elihu Yale's gift, that the new college in New Haven had a desperate need for books, Turner sent a collection of twenty-five volumes "robbed" from his own library to Yale College.[24] Along with his gift he sent a letter (in Latin, of course) seeking a doctoral degree.

> Viris vere literatis. . . .
>
> To the Truly Learned Gentlemen, President and College of Yale Academy, in the Connecticut Colony, in New England Province, Daniel Turner, Licenciate of the Royal College of Physicians of London, gives and declares his greetings and good wishes.
>
> Most Erudite Lords—
>
> I have recently received a letter from Your most deserving friend, Lord Jeremiah Dummer, in which he imparted to me the history of Your Academy, founded not many years ago by Lord Yale. I rejoice to hear that truly fine Literature as well as liberal Arts and Sciences flourish among You, at the very place where in the past century they were hidden, and instead crude Inertia and Ignorance were abundant. However, the good man urgently complained to me about the infantile state of Your Library, and together with several other Professors, both of Medicine as well as of Natural Philosophy, gently requested that we contribute our works to this same place: therefore, in order to further, wherever and as much as I am able to, the cause of literary affairs, I send you, most brilliant Gentlemen, several books which I published some time ago, along with the System of the Art of Surgery, in two volumes, as soon as transmitted from the press: aside from these, I have deprived my little collection of a most precious tome, the Great Anatomy—is it not so?—by our Cowper which, as far as I know, no one now possesses, so that it might adorn Yours: Do accept those, I beg you, as proof of my friendship toward Your University, and believe the donor to remain always, to the utmost of his ability, most excellent Gentlemen,
>
> Your Sincere Friend,
D. Turner.

> Postscriptum.
>
> If Your Lordships judge me worthy of the Degree of Doctor of the Yale Academy, and care to transmit to me a Diploma, I shall accept it not only as a token of Your Gratitude, but shall consider it an honor as great as if it had been conferred by another, even more renowned University.[25]

Daniel Turner was awarded an honorary degree of doctor of medicine at the Yale Commencement on September 11, 1723, but to no avail. Although Dummer thought the Yale diploma first rate, the Royal College of Physicians had resolved to discourage such practices and to recognize only degrees from Oxford and Cambridge.[26] In 1721, the Royal College sent a letter to Oxford and Cambridge asking the universities to be "cautious in admitting Drs. in Physick."[27] At their meeting on November 5, 1725, the Royal College Registrars' Committees, petitioned by Daniel Turner, again deliberated the matter of Yale College "and whether they had any Legal Authority for conferring Degrees . . . and the consideration of Mr. Turner's Title and Certificate from thence."[28] As there was insufficient information as to the "Constitution and Settlement of Yale College in the Province of Connecticut," the committees deferred their decision until "next Censors' Day." On December 3, "the Treasurer having procured a copy of the Charter of Harvard College in New England . . . it did appear from thence, that they had no Authority of conferring Degrees." By extension, Yale College, too, was deemed to "have no power to confer Degrees in Physick."[29] The unfortunate Mr. Turner appeared to have his Yale diploma rejected solely on the basis of the Harvard charter!

With the granting of its original charter in 1810, the Medical Institution of Yale College became the sixth medical school in the United States, preceded by the Medical Department of the University of Pennsylvania in 1765, the College of Physicians and Surgeons in New York in 1807 (originally in 1768 as King's College), and the medical departments of Harvard in 1783, Dartmouth in 1797, and the University of Maryland in 1807. In 1811, the Yale Corporation appointed a committee to meet with the Connecticut Medical Society to bring the medical school into being, a process that was to take two years.

Benjamin Silliman had prepared himself for the opening of the Medical Institution of Yale College and played a key role in the initial appointments. He had attended lectures by professors in the medical school at the University of Pennsylvania, where his fellow students were aspiring young physicians who exposed him to medical subjects in addition to chemistry. Silliman was aware that the idea of a medical school at Yale had been contemplated at the time of his appointment in 1802. It seems that he expected from the first to be ultimately connected with a medical school at Yale College.[30] After completing his studies at Pennsylvania without receiving a degree, a not uncommon occurrence, Silliman went on to Edinburgh in 1805, where he mostly attended medical lectures.[31]

In a series of letters to Jonathan Knight, who was studying medicine in Pennsylvania, Silliman indicated the likelihood of Knight's appointment to Yale but requested that this information be kept confidential although Knight might tell his father.[32] Jonathan Knight, who had been studying medicine in Philadelphia, sought his father's permission to bring his anatomical specimens home and place them in the new medical institution without mentioning his appointment.[33] Correspondence between father and son suggests that young Jonathan had had little interaction with the professors in Philadelphia.[34] Knight was not appointed as an assistant professor until 1812, perhaps because the Connecticut Medical Society met only once a year.

Mason Fitch Cogswell, a prominent Connecticut physician, was invited to become professor of surgery and anatomy, but he was reluctant to leave Hartford and declined the appointment. Strong leadership was needed to get the school started. Jonathan Knight was too young to provide that leadership, and the corporation extended its search beyond Connecticut. Yale College graduates who were medical students at Dartmouth were enthusiastic about Nathan Smith (figure 3), the founder of the Dartmouth school, who, along with John Warren of Boston, was considered the most outstanding physician in New England.[35] Timothy A. Gridley, Yale M.A. 1808, wrote to his classmate Knight about a discussion he had had with Smith concerning the prospects of a medical institution at Yale. In the course of the discussion Smith had stated that Yale would in a few years surpass any school this side of Philadelphia: Yale College was the finest institution in the United States, had the ablest professors, and was under the best regulations.[36] If offered a position at Yale, said Smith, he would accept it without the least hesitation.

A poor boy from a small village in Vermont, Smith had received an exceptional medical education for his time, even more so because of his origins. After training with country practitioners, he went on to obtain a medical degree from Harvard, the only student in a class of four to receive the degree of bachelor of medicine. Not content, he made the transatlantic voyage and studied medicine for a year in Edinburgh and London. By 1813 he had accumulated two decades of experience as a physician. Fifty-one years old, with an outstanding reputation as a surgeon, teacher, and organizer, Smith was

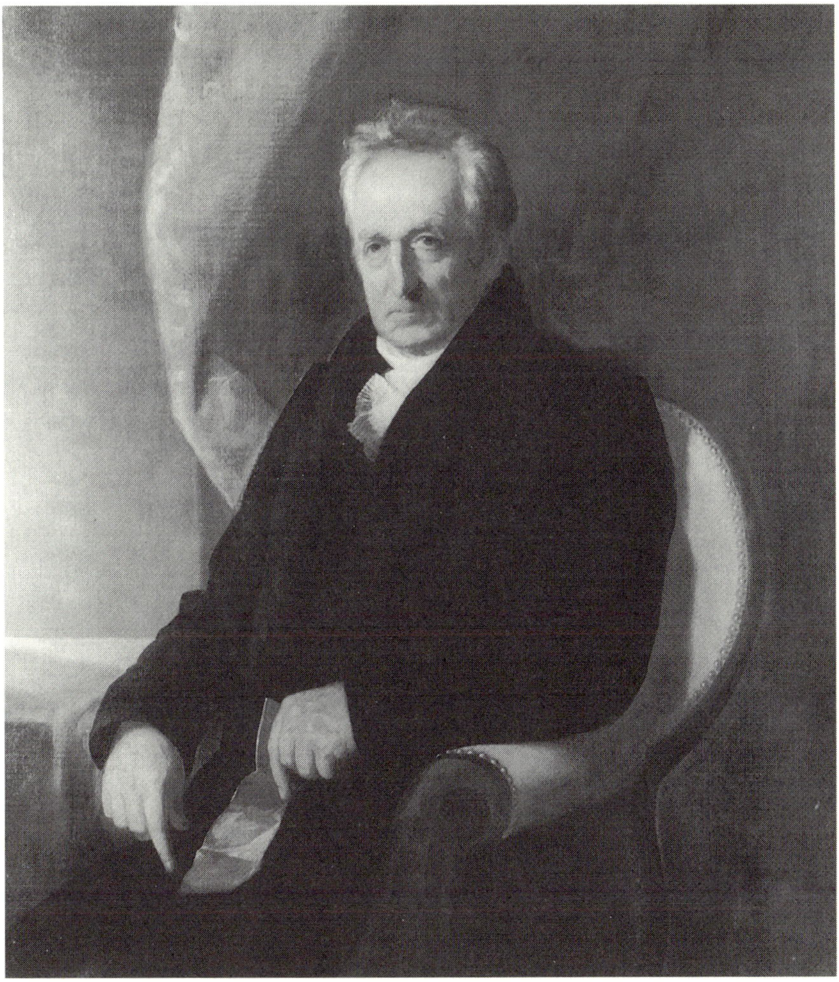

Figure 3. Nathan Smith

tired of giving lectures in chemistry, anatomy, and surgery as well as teaching "theory and practice of physic" at Dartmouth. He was also tired of struggling with the New Hampshire Legislature about obtaining bodies for anatomical dissection. Smith feared that the legislature might enact laws that "will inflict corporal punishment on any person who is concerned in digging or dissecting." He commented, "I have at length determined to leave Hanover, but at present have not concluded on any certain place of future residence."[37]

The presence of Benjamin Silliman at Yale was a strong attraction. Smith had early on appreciated the effect that chemistry would have on the practice of medicine. He was "pursuing with ardor the modern analysis so different from the ancient, . . . operating in a hospital consecrated to experiments of that kind, on liquids and organs altered by disease before and after death; by experiments tried with prudence after the notions formed by preceding data."[38]

Nathan Smith was considered the perfect appointment for Yale so far as his professional qualifications were concerned. He was, however, reported to have expressed unorthodox views about divine revelation and other tenets of Calvinistic Christianity in his lectures from time to time, influenced perhaps by his Anglican wife and father-in-law.[39] Smith did, it seems, have an influence on prayer at Dartmouth; President Wheelock reputedly came from Dr. Smith's lecture room to evening prayers in the old chapel and gave thanks more or less as follows: "O, Lord! We thank Thee for the Oxygen gas; we thank Thee for the Hydrogen gas; and for all the gases. We thank Thee for the Cerebrum; we thank Thee for the cerebellum, and for the Medulla Oblongata."[40]

At that time Yale was the embodiment of a conservative college based on Calvinist principles. President Dwight and the corporation considered Smith a religious "infidel and flatly opposed Smith's election as Professor."[41] Smith, however, vehemently denied that he had ever entertained "heretical" views. As he was considered too honorable to be duplicitous, Dwight eventually relented, and Smith never gave anyone reason to question his religious orthodoxy in his lectures. He arrived in New Haven in 1813 accompanied by his two sons, who were to enroll in the Medical Institution and Yale College, respectively. His wife and seven other children remained behind in New Hampshire, as he had been unable to sell his house. The entire family eventually moved into the building on Elm Street that now houses the Graduate Club.

The Medical Institution opened in the fall of 1813 with a faculty nominated by the Yale Corporation and the Connecticut Medical Society. The faculty consisted of Eneas Munson as professor of materia medica and botany, Nathan Smith as professor of the theory and practice of physic, surgery, and obstetrics, Benjamin Silliman as professor of chemistry and pharmacy, Eli Ives as adjunct professor of materia medica and botany, and Jonathan Knight as professor of anatomy. Silliman continued to play an important role in guiding the institution. In letters to Knight, he defined the role of the various faculty members and counseled Knight not to be concerned about the appointment of Smith.[42] Knight could learn from Smith, said Silliman, and would eventually succeed Smith in surgery; meanwhile, anatomy would offer an excellent entry to the medical faculty. Smith soon became so busy that he transferred responsibility for teaching obstetrics to Knight.

Nathan Smith and Benjamin Silliman represented as strong an academic medical combination of basic science and clinical medicine as could be found in any of the country's six medical schools. Smith received a salary of $1,000 a year, excluding fees. At that time full professors at Yale College were being paid $1,100 annually. Smith and Silliman were the only salaried members of the medical faculty. The rest of the faculty supported themselves from student fees and from clinical practice. Clinical fees had been set by the Connecticut Medical Society, with a usual fee of fifty cents for a house call with a prescription and a fee of five dollars for surgery.[43]

The Medical Institution of Yale College (figure 4) opened in November 1813 without fanfare or mention in the local papers. It boasted thirty-seven students, including seventeen from Connecticut, eight of whom were from the greater New Haven area.[44] The Yale Corporation provided the institution with the facilities necessary to start a medical school, directing "that the Prudential Committee be authorized to procure a bell for the Medical Institution, and tables and seats for the lecture rooms and dining hall—also to enlarge the laboratory, and to do any other things which appear of indispensable necessity to the organization of the Medical Institution."[45] Classrooms and living quarters were on the edge of town, at the corner of Grove and Prospect streets, across from the Grove Street cemetery. This building, owned by James Hillhouse, was originally designed to be a hotel and included a lecture hall on the top floor, a dining room, space for an anatomy lab in the basement, and student rooms scattered throughout. The building, which eventually became South Sheffield Hall, was purchased in 1814 with a grant of $20,000 from the Connecticut Legislature. The medical school remained at this location until 1860, when it moved to a site at 150 York Street, closer to the hospital.

In addition to the medical course, every medical student had to spend three years as an "apprentice" to a practicing physician (or two years if he had also attended college). The course was designed to complement the apprenticeship. Each entering student was handed a copy of "The By-Laws of the Medical Institution of Yale College," which informed the new matriculant that his life would be as strictly regulated as that of an undergraduate. This included where he could eat and when he could leave his room (not on Saturday night or on Sunday, "except for prayer and worship").[46] The medical students "during their residence in the institution are subject to the

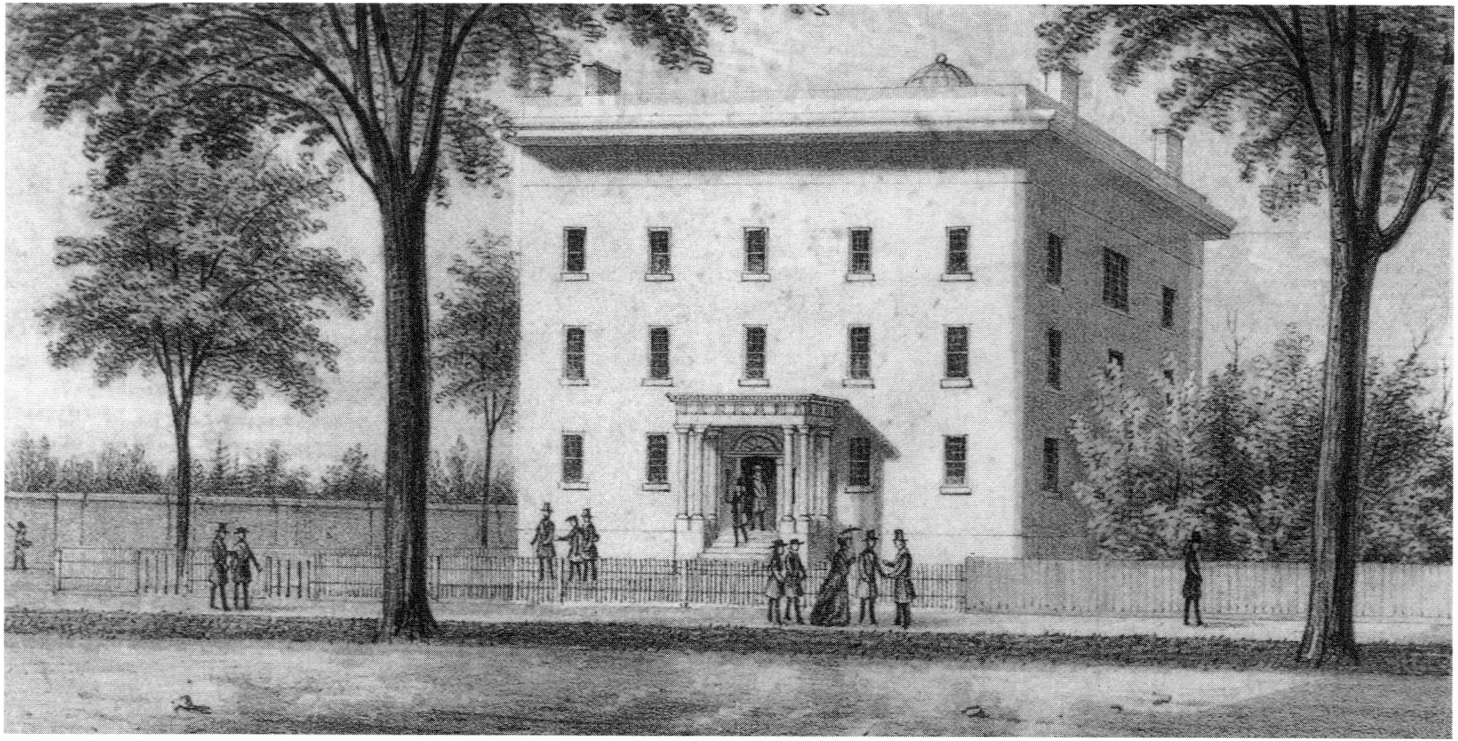

Figure 4. The Medical Institution of Yale College

same moral and religious restraints as those of the Academical College."[47] Strict curfews were initially in place for the medical students but were abandoned when it became apparent that the regulations were unenforceable.

The medical school benefited greatly from the presence of Nathan Smith, who did much of his significant work in New Haven. His small-town rural background had endowed him with common sense, onto which his education had grafted knowledge, originality, and keen observation. In 1824 he published a classic description of typhoid fever entitled *A Practical Essay on Typhous Fever.*[48] One of his last publications was an excellent description of osteomyelitis under the general title of "Necrosis."[49] In 1813 Smith's expertise in osteomyelitis was reputed to have saved the leg of a five-year-old boy in Hanover and in doing so to have unwittingly contributed to the founding of a religion.[50] The boy had been seen by a number of physicians from Hanover, including Smith, with the majority recommending amputation. Smith thought that he could excise the diseased bone fragments and save the leg, which he successfully did. Thirteen years later the boy, Joseph Smith, who had moved to Palmyra, New York, experienced a vision of an angel. That date is viewed by the Elders of the Church of Jesus Christ of Latter-Day Saints as the inaugural date of the Mormon religion.

Nathan Smith was an accomplished surgeon, and in 1822 he described the operation for ovariotomy, unaware that in 1809 Ephraim McDowell already had performed the first such operation, in a log cabin in Danville, Kentucky.[51] Smith performed the first amputation of the knee joint in America in 1824. In the midst of these accomplishments, he managed to continue a relationship with Dartmouth until 1816, and in 1821 he founded the Medical School of Maine at Bowdoin College in Brunswick with a course of lectures. He was also affiliated with the new medical school in Burlington, Vermont, where his second son was professor of surgery and anatomy. His continuing involvement with other medical schools was in part due to the fact that he was unable to support his large family on his Yale salary and tuition fees alone.

With the exception of Benjamin Silliman, the other members of the faculty lacked Smith's lustrous reputation, although they did contribute to the school's growing esteem. Eli Ives (figure 5) was a highly respected physician and in 1829 succeeded to the professorship of the theory and practice of physic when Smith died.[52] Ives, a 1799 graduate of Yale College, accepted a position as headmaster of Hopkins Grammar School in New Haven immediately before graduation and at the same time began the study of medicine with his father and Eneas Munson. He also attended lectures at the Univer-

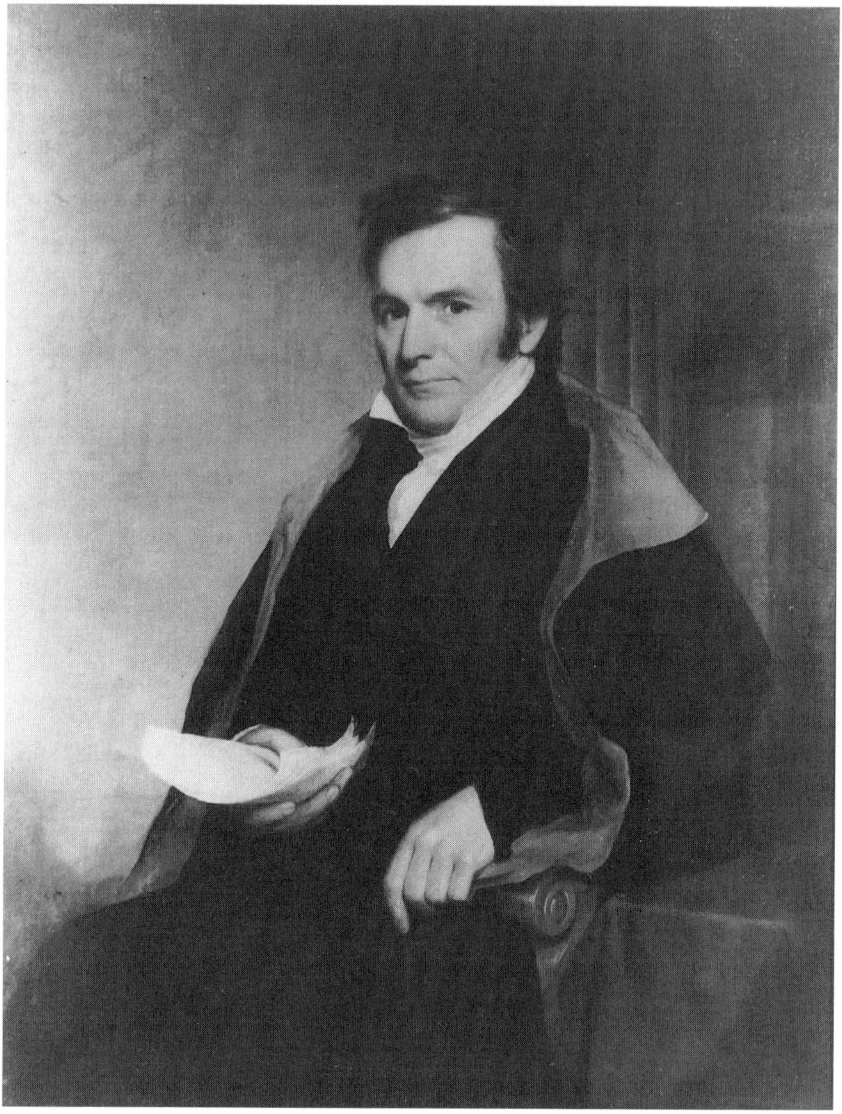

Figure 5. Eli Ives

sity of Pennsylvania. He was widely known as a botanist and established a botanical garden with a hothouse on the grounds of the medical-school building on Grove Street. "It was a pleasant sight—to see the good doctor lead a patient into this garden and dispense his medicine with a spade."[53] In 1820 Ives had succeeded Munson as professor of materia medica and botany as well as diseases of children. At the time, the care of infants was

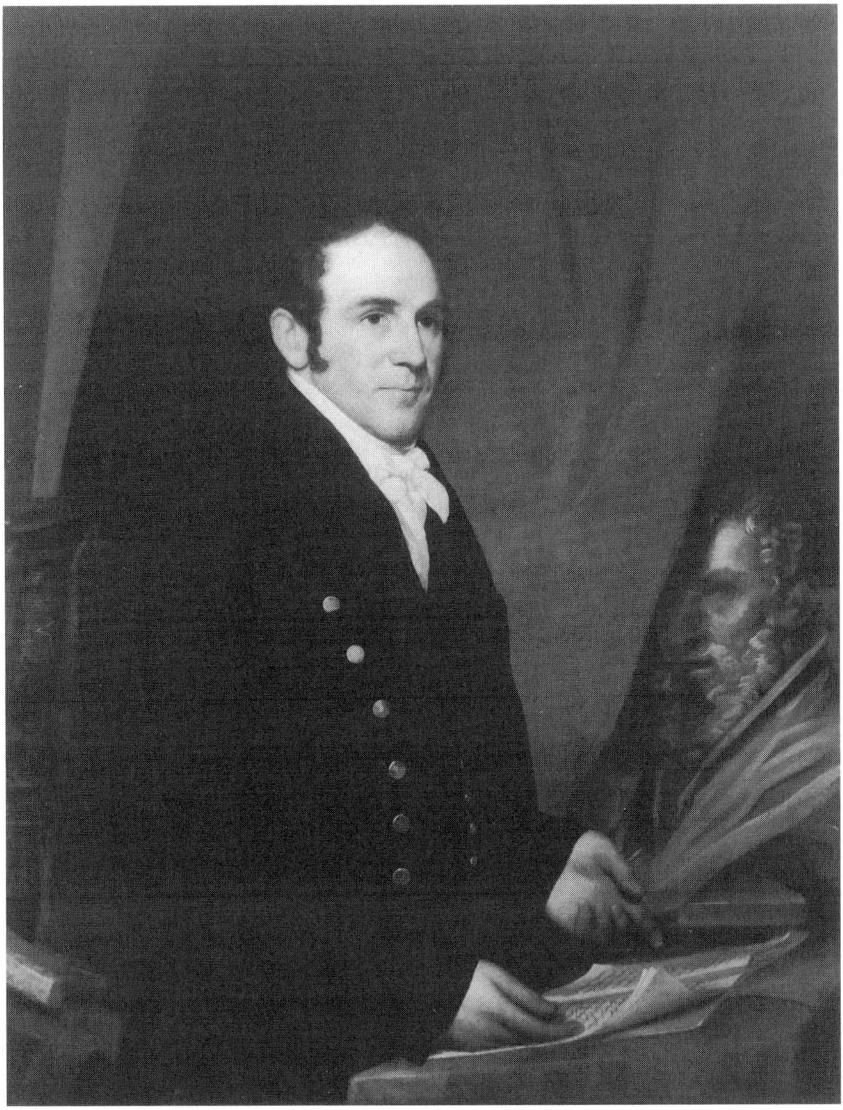

Figure 6. Jonathan Knight

for the most part relegated to nurses and midwives, as established physicians had little interest in the subject. Ives's lectures were designed to acquaint physicians with illness in children, and he has been called America's first academic pediatrician.[54]

Ives's colleague Jonathan Knight (figure 6) became one of the most influential members of the medical profession. A founder of the American

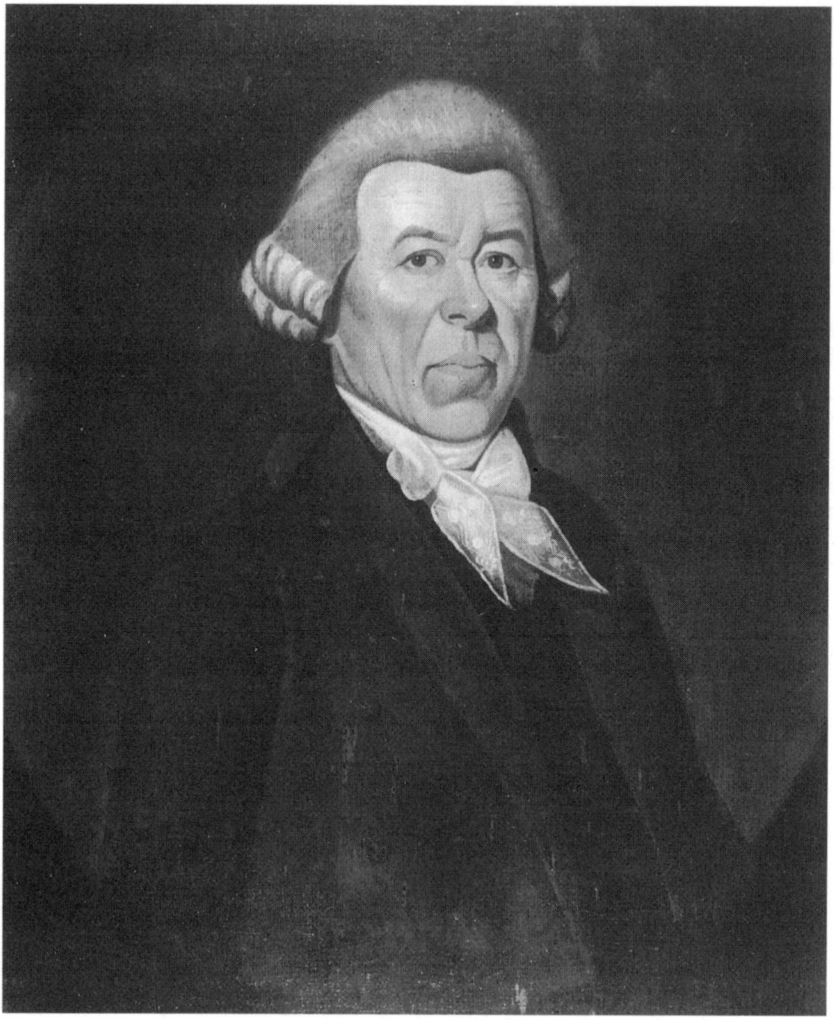

Figure 7. Eneas Munson

Medical Association, he presided in 1846 and 1847 over the convention that formed the AMA and in 1853 was elected president of the association. Like Nathan Smith, Knight was multidimensional, and in 1838 he transferred to the chair of surgery on the death of Thomas Hubbard. A superb lecturer, Knight was an active teacher in the medical school for fifty-one years.

Eneas Munson (figure 7), who was almost eighty when he was appointed to the chair in materia medica and therapeutics, never actually taught, and his appointment was largely ornamental. Munson had entered the ministry after graduation from Yale College in 1755.[55] He had an irreverent sense of humor, which may have been a factor in his decision to give up the ministry and study medicine under a preceptor. On one occasion during a sermon, he had read all the old notices he found in the pulpit! Munson clearly marched to the beat of a different drum. He believed in alchemy and carried out experiments on the transmutation of metals when he had finished his medical practice for the day.[56] Afraid of being struck by lightning, he would not venture out in thunderstorms. Despite these idiosyncracies, Eneas Munson was a caring, committed physician who developed a large practice in New Haven, undoubtedly aided by his good humor. He was awarded an M.D. by the Connecticut Medical Society in 1792 and was seventy-nine when he was appointed to the faculty of the Medical Institution. He died in 1826 at the age of ninety-two. This diverse and distinguished faculty provided a strong teaching base for the new medical school.

The course at the Medical Institution of Yale College was originally six months long but was shortened in 1815 or 1816 to five months and, with increasing competition from other schools, to four months, October through January. The length of study varied with the qualification desired.[57] If the individual wanted a license to practice medicine in Connecticut, one course of lectures was required. To be awarded a degree of doctor of medicine from Yale, the student was required to take two courses, one of which had to be at the Medical Institution. All candidates for licensure were examined at length by a joint board of the Connecticut Medical Society and the Medical Institution. Jonathan Knight reported in the 1820s that the joint board had examined fourteen candidates and was occupied for three full days.

The state charter required that the course be taught in the form of lectures, with little opportunity for recitation or discussion, and students were not divided into different classes. The courses included anatomy and physiology taught by Jonathan Knight, theory and practice of medicine, surgery, and obstetrics taught by Nathan Smith, and materia medica and botany, chemistry, and pharmacy taught by Benjamin Silliman. Students could also attend lectures in natural philosophy, mineralogy, and geology. "The students have access to the library of the Academical, as well as of the Medical Institution. There is a respectable Anatomical Museum, and every demonstration which is needed in that department is given."[58] The second-year course was a repetition of the first year, with the same material taught. This was true of all other medical schools at the time. Yale medical students had no opportunity to see patients until after the opening of the State Hospital in 1833, when weekly clinics were instituted.

American textbooks did not exist, so students had to rely on notes and on English textbooks. Both Smith and Silliman edited American editions of English texts, publishing their own works in 1824 and 1830, respectively. American textbooks did not become widely available until mid-century, and most of these emanated from the faculty of the University of Pennsylvania. In 1819 Silliman founded the *American Journal of Science* at Yale, which became the principal journal through which science was promoted in the United States.

The War of 1812 had little effect on the new Medical Institution of Yale College or on the college itself. The end of the war, however, marked the beginning of the transition of New Haven from a colonial town to an industrial city. In 1815 regular steamship service was initiated between New Haven and New York. The industrialization of New Haven was greatly aided by the mechanical genius of Eli Whitney, Yale College 1792, who invented the cotton gin in 1794 and was the first person to introduce the concept of interchangeable parts for guns. From his plant on Lake Whitney he delivered his first guns to the U.S. government in 1801. Whitney suffered from an enlarged prostate, and with Nathan Smith's help he devised urological instruments for his condition, to no avail. Nothing could be done but administer sedatives as he lay dying in 1825.[59]

The growing industrialization of the town did not immediately lead to easier access to cadavers needed for students to obtain practical experience in anatomy. People were still reluctant to donate their bodies, and the Medical Institution at Yale, like other medical schools, was suspected of grave robbing to obtain anatomical material for dissection. In January 1824, Laban Smith, a farmer from West Haven, discovered that the grave of his daughter Bathsheba, "a respectable young female of nineteen" who had been buried a few days before, had been opened and the body removed. The father and irate relatives suspected medical students and obtained a warrant to search the medical-school building. The warrant was presented to Jonathan Knight, the only faculty member present at the time, who accompanied the distraught father on a search of the building.[60] The body of the young woman was eventually found buried in the cellar.[61]

The body was removed from the cellar, cleaned, and placed in a wagon, which was then driven through the streets of New Haven. An increasingly emotional crowd gathered and eventually marched on the medical school. With cries of "Yale! Yale!" the medical students sought assistance from the Yale College students, who responded with "pistols, dirks and clubs" and gathered in front of the medical-school building.[62] Civil authorities summoned by the medical faculty commanded the mob to disperse, but without effect. Finally, the Governor's Foot Guard was called and marched to the Medical Institution, fully armed with guns and swords and accompanied by fife and drums. Despite the military presence, civil unrest continued for a week.

Subsequent investigation identified a medical student as being responsible. He was found guilty of the crime but had conveniently left the state. Ephraim Colburn, an assistant at the Medical Institution, was also charged and put on trial. The case of *The People v. Ephraim Colburn* ultimately engendered legislation that actually benefited medical education in Connecticut.[63] As a result of the incident, the legislature passed a new act that made the punishment for grave robbing more severe but also permitted the corpses of criminals to be made available for anatomical dissection. One of the reasons that Nathan Smith had left Dartmouth for Yale was pending legislation in New Hampshire that would have made postmortem dissection subject to corporal punishment.[64] The "anatomy riots" of 1824 in New Haven never recurred, but they did foster a town-gown suspicion that persisted.

If the medical school were to thrive, students would need access to patients, "because theory without practice in this, as well as everything else, is comparatively of little use."[65] On May 26, 1826, the legislature passed an act to establish the State Hospital (figure 8) in New Haven.[66] There were ten incorporators, nine of them physicians, including four on the faculty of the Medical Institution, and Benjamin Silliman, who did not practice medicine. The legislature, however, rejected an appeal for funds to finance the hospital. Undaunted, the incorporators appealed to the U.S. Treasury to use unspent tax money collected for the care of seamen in New Haven. But they were turned down and again appealed to the legislature, outlining the funds available, including the fact that the four medical-school professors had committed 10 percent of their income, or a minimum of $100, annually for the next five years to finance the hospital. The legislature agreed to provide the final $5,000 needed.

Just before the hospital was ready to open in 1833 on a site bounded by Cedar Street and Howard Avenue, a cholera epidemic broke out in New Haven in 1832, and the New Haven Board of Health wanted the new hospital to admit cholera patients. The hospital directors refused, stating that the hospital's charter prohibited it from admitting patients with communicable diseases. The townspeople were infuriated, which delayed popular acceptance of the hospital. As a result of this incident and the prevailing culture of caring for patients at home, the hospital was underutilized during its early years, and patient rooms were rented out to boarders.

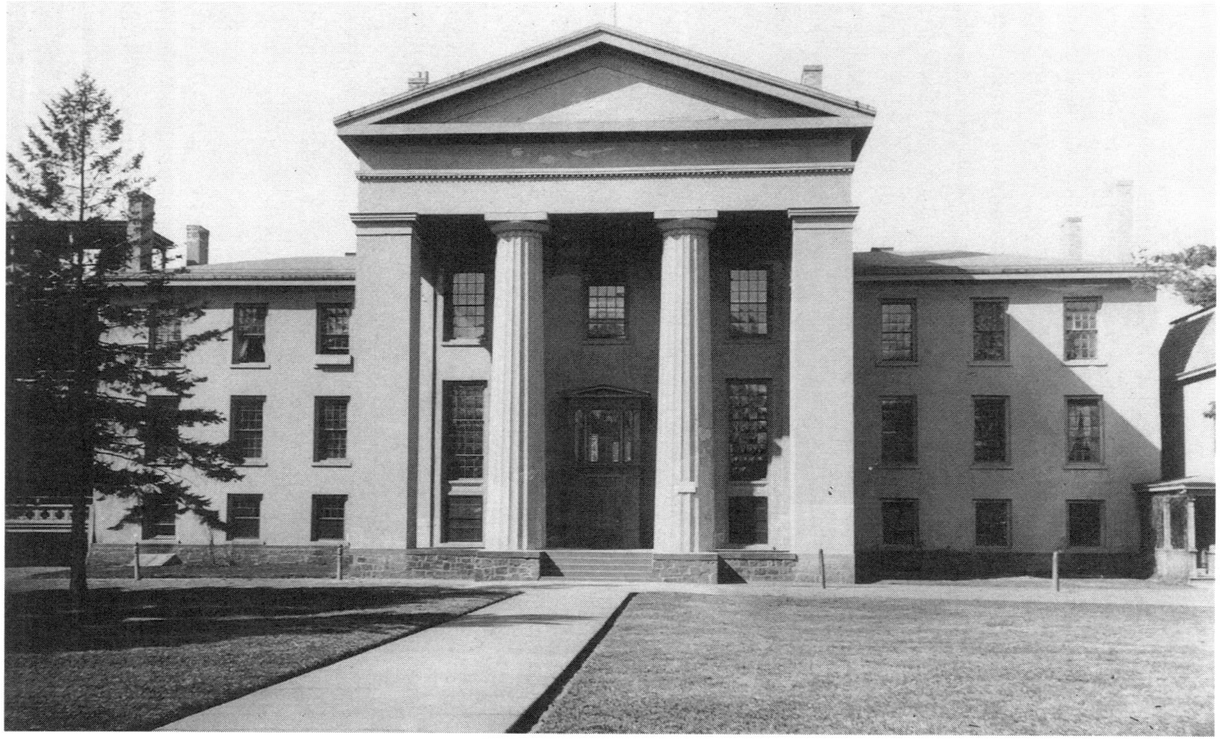

Figure 8. The State Hospital

Despite such difficulties and obstacles, the medical faculty constantly strove to raise academic standards. Already in 1818 the professors had recommended to their colleagues in the Connecticut Medical Society that two courses of medical instruction be required for licensure rather than one. But although the society was interested in keeping the standards of practice high in Connecticut, the recommendation was rejected as too stringent. In 1827, however, several New England medical schools and medical societies jointly agreed to raise both admission standards and the level of course work. The length of the medical course under a preceptor was increased to three years for college graduates and four years for others. Applicants to the Medical Institution of Yale College were expected to demonstrate "a competent knowledge of the Latin language, and some acquaintance with the principles of Natural Philosophy." In 1829 the Connecticut Legislature ratified the changes recommended in the agreement reached by the New England medical schools. One course of study remained the minimum for licensure. Yale duly set about raising educational standards and increased the number of professors at the Medical Institution from four to six.[67] Unfortunately, Yale was once again ahead of its time. The other medical schools did not follow suit to implement the agreed-upon changes, and Yale was forced to abandon the higher standards for economic reasons.

Even though the Connecticut Medical Society had the deciding vote in governing the medical school, the faculty members gradually assumed more control, because they were on site and knew the students and the curriculum. The legislature passed several amendments to the act, including the removal of the restriction on the number of professors appointed to the Medical Institution. These multiple amendments became so complicated that in 1834 two separate acts were passed, one for the Medical Institution of Yale College and one for the Connecticut Medical Society.

The unexpected death of Nathan Smith from a "febrile illness" in January 1829 dealt a severe blow to the medical school. Six months previously, Smith had developed a brief illness that left him weak and debilitated throughout the fall and early winter. He suffered a paralytic stroke and died two weeks after being attended by two of his distinguished pupils, George C. Shattuck of Boston and Ruben D. Mussey of Dartmouth. At the time of Smith's death, the medical school was thriving. A small positive financial balance existed, and student enrollment was the highest it would be until the 1890s. The school had produced three hundred and forty-nine graduates, of whom two hundred and seventy-four had received the M.D. degree and the others a license to practice.[68] Of the M.D. recipients, fifty-seven were college graduates as well, and all but fifteen came from Yale. Fifteen of the graduates became professors or presidents of the Connecticut or Ohio medical societies. The first matriculant, J. P. Kirtland, became professor of the theory and practice of medicine at Western Reserve University and president of the Ohio Medical Society.

The combination of the death of Nathan Smith and the elevation of academic standards resulted in enrollment dropping to fifty students. Contributing factors included the opening of other medical schools in New England. If students were prosperous, they tended to go to Philadelphia, New York, or Boston, where the faculties were better known, the facilities better, and the hospitals offered a wider variety of patients for study. Thomas Cooper, an Oxford-educated chemist who became president of South Carolina College in 1821, commented in an address to the Medical Board of South Carolina that "the Medical Schools of the United States are principally those of Philadelphia and New York. . . . I say nothing respecting those of New England, because they have furnished no manifest occasion for peculiar notice, nor have they risen above the level of mediocrity."[69]

Edmund Randolph Peaslee, a Dartmouth College graduate, set down his impressions of the Medical Institution in which he enrolled as a student in 1839 for an entire fee of $76 for the four-month term. Of the four professors, Ives was "an amusing fellow," Knight "a most splendid lecturer," Hooker "a smart young man," and William Tully "a very learned man." Peaslee had fifty classmates, of whom only three or four had a B.A. and two an M.A. There were enough cadavers for dissection, at a charge of $15 each, with six students sharing a cadaver. Peaslee commented that there was no hospital available to students but that during his first year this did not make any difference. Medical clinics were instituted weekly at the medical school in 1842 and subsequently increased to twice a week, alternating between the Medical Institution and the hospital. "The students are gratuitously admitted to the Connecticut Hospital whenever surgical operations or other cases of interest occur." Members of the Connecticut Medical Society addressed the medical students annually from 1840 to 1860, usually advising them to join a medical society and urging them to subscribe to medical journals. The student audience was also repeatedly admonished to attend church. One of the advantages of New Haven touted in the medical-school circular was the "freedom of the city from theaters, circuses, and other public places of amusements." But compared to Hanover, New Hampshire, where Peaslee had been an undergraduate, New Haven must have been exciting. He en-

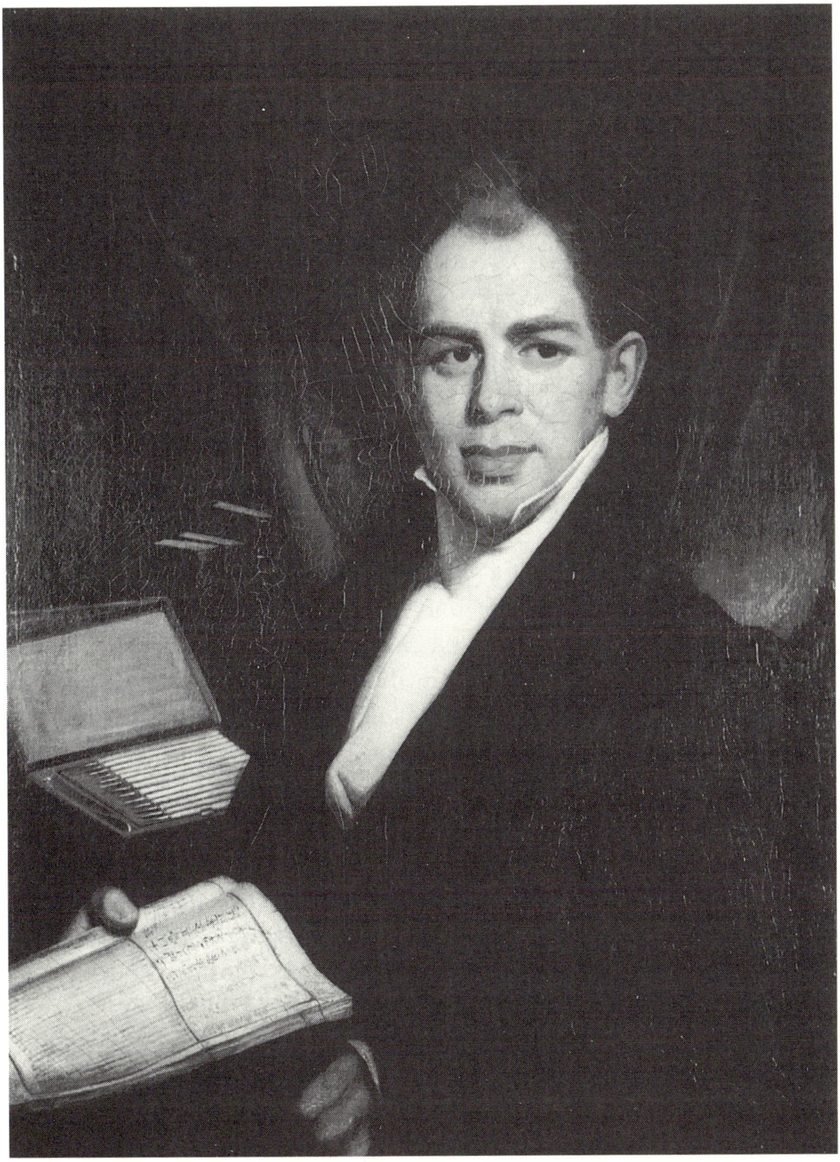

Figure 9. Peter Parker

joyed the social life of the town, although he wondered why so few "medical students are young men of literary taste or merit."[70]

Some exceptional students graduated from the Medical Institution during the early period. Among them was Peter Parker (figure 9), Yale College 1831, a prime representative of Cotton Mather's "Angelical Conjunction." Born in 1804 on a farm in Framingham, Massachusetts, to a deeply religious family of modest means, Parker wanted to become a minister and bring Christianity to foreign lands, which required a college education. He entered Amherst College at the age of twenty-three, having had to help his father on the farm. Disturbed by the lack of adequate library facilities, Parker decided to transfer to another college in his final year. Finding the theology at Harvard too liberal, he settled on Yale. He was elected to the Brothers in Unity club, which gave him the library access he had sought, and he could tell his mother and sister that "the studies of the present year have been truly elevating and ennobling to the mind."[71]

Parker decided that missionary work in China would offer him the opportunities he wanted. He was supported in his desire by the American Board of Commissioners for Foreign Missions but thought that he needed further study in divinity. The idea of also receiving a medical education seems to have been an afterthought. After embarking on his divinity studies, he realized that the qualifications for a missionary in China included "a very practical knowledge of medicine and surgery." He put together a three-year program, at the end of which he would be both an ordained minister and the recipient of the degree of doctor of medicine. His daily activities truly were an "Angelical Conjunction," as we see in a letter to his mother in 1831: "I arise at half-past five in the morning, and attend prayers in the Seminary. From this till breakfast, at half-past six, study Hebrew or Greek. From eight to ten, again study Hebrew or Greek. From ten to eleven, attend Dr. Ives' lecture on the theory and practice of medicine. From eleven to twelve, I am engaged in Miss Hotchkiss' school. From twelve to one, attend Dr. Knight's lecture on anatomy. From two to three p.m., a recitation to Professor Gibbs in Hebrew or Greek. From three to four I have a class in chemistry, or Paley's theology, then one hour for exercises, and the remainder of the day for study and attending meetings. This is a fair outline of every day's employment."[72]

Parker does not mention obtaining practical experience by seeing patients or working at the hospital, which makes his later accomplishments all the more impressive. He did have experience in visiting the sick, however. When cholera appeared in New Haven as part of a worldwide epidemic in July 1832, Parker was exposed to the disease while visiting afflicted patients. New Haven escaped relatively unscathed, with only sixty-six cases reported and twenty-six deaths—perhaps thanks to the good efforts of the New Haven Board of Health and Peter Parker. He apparently did contract what appeared to be tuberculosis and was advised by Eli Ives to take time off and rest, but he soon returned to his daily activities and experienced no further problems.

Parker's hard work was rewarded in March 1834 with the degree of doctor of medicine, after he had successfully appeared before the Board of Medical Examiners of the Connecticut Medical Society and the Medical Institution. Two months later, he was ordained a minister of the Presbyterian Church and on June 1, 1834, the American Board of Commissioners for Foreign Missions appointed him a missionary to China with the following admonishment: "The character of a physician, or of a man of science . . . you will never suffer to supersede or interfere with your character of a teacher of religion." The priorities of the "Angelical Conjunction" were clear, healing the soul before healing the body. Prior to sailing for Canton, Parker spent some time at the New York Eye and Ear Infirmary, because he had heard that ophthalmic problems were particularly common in China. He had written his Yale medical thesis on purulent ophthalmia.[73]

Canton was the only Chinese city open to foreigners, who were restricted to one area of the city, required to live in warehouses along the waterfront, and not allowed to have their families with them. Not permitted to practice medicine in Canton, Peter Parker moved to Singapore, where he learned Chinese and practiced some medicine. Returning to Canton after seven months with the help of a senior Chinese merchant named Houqua, Parker founded an ophthalmic hospital in a warehouse. The dispensary was a huge success. Two thousand patients were treated in the first year. In addition to caring for patients, Parker was interested in educating bright young Chinese students. The uncle of one of his talented students, Lam-Qua, painted nearly two hundred pictures of the hospital's tumor patients. Lam-Qua had studied with the English painter George Chinnery and was well known in China. Parker used the paintings during his lecture tours in the United States and Europe to illustrate the extent of medical problems in China. Many of the paintings are now housed at the Yale Historical Medical Library.

The realization that the West had something to offer the Middle Kingdom mitigated the restrictions that had been imposed on Parker's mission, but by 1840 the political climate had reached a point where Parker could no longer remain in China. He sailed for home, having treated 6,300 patients in the hospital during its five years of operation.[74] Parker sometimes performed as many as sixteen cataract operations a day. The eventual defeat of China in the opium war was inevitable, and Parker busied himself in the United States in the meantime raising funds for Chinese missionary hospitals.[75] He also sought to convince authorities that the United States should establish diplomatic relations with China when the war was over. Parker talked to President Martin Van Buren and Secretary of State–designate Daniel Webster, a Dartmouth graduate. He addressed a combined session of Congress on January 31, 1841, about China and recorded the event in his diary: "I have this morning preached to one of the most enlightened audiences of any age or nation—the Senate and House of Representatives—at the Capitol in Washington."[76] During his visit to Washington he also met Harriet Webster, the secretary's niece, and married her.

When Peter Parker returned to Canton in 1842, Mrs. Parker accompanied him and became one of the first foreign women to live in China. The hospital was relocated in a better and larger setting. The addition of more mission doctors and Chinese assistants resulted in three thousand patients being seen over the next year. The hospital continued to flourish, but Parker was increasingly drawn into the diplomatic relations between China and the United States. In 1855, at the age of forty-one, he was appointed Commissioner to China by President Franklin Pierce. In later years he reflected that he had preached the "gospel of salvation" to tens of thousands of Chinese and had cared for fifty-two thousand patients.[77] Peter Parker truly did represent the "Angelical Conjunction" and was the archetype of the "liberal arts" physician that Yale has fostered since its beginnings.

3

HARD TIMES

The Dark Years

Nathan Smith's death in 1829 meant a great loss to the young Medical Institution of Yale College. His reputation as a clinician in conjunction with Benjamin Silliman's reputation as a scientist had been responsible for much of the school's initial success. Silliman now replaced Smith as the driving force behind the Medical Institution. From a pragmatic point of view, Smith had represented one-fifth of the medical faculty, holding the chairs in both medicine and surgery. To replace him Eli Ives was appointed professor of the theory and practice of medicine and Thomas Hubbard, a rural practitioner, became professor of surgery. William Tully took over Ives's former professorship of materia medica. In 1838 Silliman recommended to President Jeremiah Day that for financial reasons Tully be made a lecturer in Yale College as well as professor of materia medica, which he had been appointed in 1829. The number of medical students was so small that Tully had received only $360 from student fees in 1837, and he lacked a private practice to sustain him financially.[1] Timothy Beers, a typical family doctor, was appointed professor of obstetrics.

With Thomas Hubbard's death in 1838, Jonathan Knight moved from the professorship of anatomy and physiology to assume the chair in surgery, an outcome Silliman had discussed with Knight as a long-term plan in 1812. Charles Hooker in turn was appointed to Knight's chair in anatomy. Physicians of the time were generalists who moved from discipline to discipline with relative ease. The medical faculty at Yale played musical chairs among the various disciplines within a close-knit group whose members were often related, directly or through marriage. "At one period three of the six professors were brothers-in-law, who seemed to regard the school as a kind of family association—to the understandable irritation of their colleagues."[2] Yale College in general tended to look among the "first families" of Connecticut for appointments to the faculty almost until the 1900s.

In 1845 the medical faculty elected Charles Hooker (figure 10) as the first dean of the medical school—the first dean of any graduate school at Yale. Hooker was listed as dean in the medical-school catalogue of 1845, although the Yale Corporation did not appoint him officially until 1853. His demeanor was unusual. "Dr. Hooker's mental alertness found expression in a somewhat tumultuous speech, a mixture of hesitation and precipitancy. . . . There was an odd jerky, flitting unexpectedness to his movements, which used to remind by-standers of some of his more agile rodents."[3] Despite these mannerisms, Charles Hooker remained as dean until his death in 1863.

In 1839, prior to his decanal appointment, Hooker had attended the Africans awaiting trial in the Amistad incident; he found four of them suffering from chronic diarrhea and one from pleuritis. The Africans were "the most accommodating of patients" and liked medicines so much that they devoured any brought into the cell.[4] The schooner Amistad was a slave ship carrying fifty-three West African captives who had been sold as slaves to a Spanish planter in Havana.[5] During the voyage, the captives rebelled and took control of the ship, killing the captain and the cook. They then demanded that the crew sail them back to Africa. Instead, the crew sailed the ship in the opposite direction and landed at Montauk Point, Long Island, where the Africans were arrested. The forty-three survivors were placed on trial for murder in New Haven.

Josiah Willard Gibbs, professor of sacred literature at Yale and a noted philologist, located an interpreter who understood the prisoners' language. A New Haven judge eventually ruled that the prisoners had not been legally enslaved and were not guilty. The judge's ruling was upheld by the U.S.

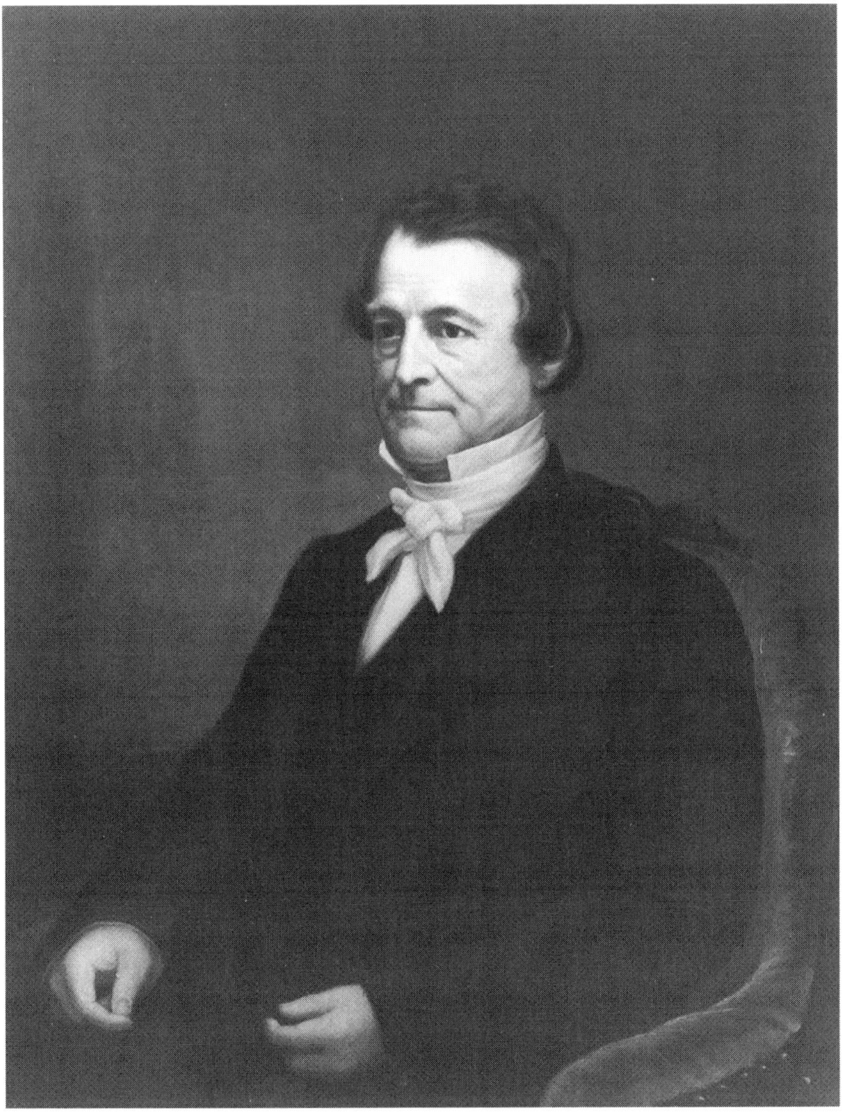

Figure 10. Charles Hooker

Supreme Court, which decreed on March 9, 1841, that the Africans could not be considered property as they had not been purchased prior to their arrival in Cuba.

During this period the opening of other medical schools in New England and the disappearance of luminaries like Nathan Smith had led to the Medical Institution of Yale College becoming primarily a school for Connecticut residents. It is surprising that more medical schools were not incorporated in Connecticut, given the trend in the rest of the country. An act incorporating the Connecticut Homeopathic Medical Society was passed by the legislature in 1864. It allowed the society to confer the degree of doctor of medicine "on the same term of study and attendance of lectures required by the Medical Institution of Yale College, but it was never implemented."[6] Whether the close relationship between Yale and the Connecticut Medical Society blocked the establishment of other medical schools in Connecticut is unclear.

Few medical students at the Medical Institution of Yale College had entered with a college education. Yale catalogues show that in the mid-1800s only 26 percent of medical students had a college degree; the overall number of Yale medical graduates with a baccalaureate degree in the nineteenth century as a whole reflects similar proportions.[7] More highly educated students chose to study divinity or law. Prior to 1846, 34 percent of Yale graduates chose to read law, 31 percent the ministry, and 12 percent medicine.[8] At the end of the nineteenth century, 30 percent of living Yale graduates were lawyers, 7 percent ministers, and 8 percent physicians. Of these, about 25 percent of Yale Law School and Yale Divinity School graduates subsequently engaged in other forms of professional activity, as compared to 10 percent of medical-school graduates.

The stringent entrance requirements and course work for the medical school proposed in 1827, which included more preparation and a three-year course for college graduates, had been abandoned in 1832. Because the other northeastern medical schools had not followed suit in imposing the higher standards that they had agreed on, medical-student enrollment at Yale began decreasing. Unhappily, Yale students decreased in quality as well as in number. In an uninspiring address to Yale medical students in 1856, Dr. Benjamin H. Catlin, a representative of the Connecticut Medical Society, declared that students were entering medical school "because they had failed in every other branch of business, or had nothing else to choose."[9]

Convinced that four months was too short a period in which to teach medicine well, the faculty announced a private supplemental course of instruction that would continue through the four months of the regular course and also run for twenty-six weeks in the spring and summer. There would be one recitation in each course each week during the regular course and two recitations daily in the spring course. Instead of purely didactic lectures, there would be daily textbook recitations, demonstrations, and experiments. Yale College libraries and museums would be open to the "private" school students.[10] The private course was announced in the annual circulars of the

Medical Institution, which by 1866 was referred to in the Yale College catalogue as "The Yale Medical School."[11] The course went beyond the authority of the charter granted by the Connecticut Legislature, and not all members of the Connecticut Medical Society, which had joint responsibility for the Medical Institution with Yale College, were in favor of the added instruction. Nevertheless, the supplemental curriculum continued—with about one-third of the Yale medical students enrolled in it—until the Medical Institution formally adopted a year-long integrated medical course in 1875.

Despite the faculty's concerns about the quality of the medical students, the *Boston Medical and Surgical Journal* had this to say of the school in 1839: "We feel a respect for the medical department at Yale because no effort seems ever to have been made to force it into undue notoriety. A plain dignified course has characterized all its operations: the faculty, distinguished for their scientific attainments, have never been obtrusive nor manifested a disposition to increase their importance by defaming or undervaluing the neighbors."[12] Jerome Van Cortland Smith, editor of the journal, continued to laud the Medical Institution at Yale in editorials. Whether out of respect for Yale or pique at Harvard is not clear.

General concern among the nation's medical-school faculties about the quality of medical students persisted. Demands for higher academic standards, a medical code of ethics, and a national organization to enforce the standards led to the formation of a national committee and the development of a constitution to found the American Medical Association. We recall that Jonathan Knight chaired the organizing committee and in 1846 and 1847 was president of the convention that formed the AMA. In 1853 he was elected as the second president of the association.

At a time when the quality of the medical students was declining, the quality of science at Yale College was increasing.[13] Silliman's laboratory attracted a number of stellar individuals. Charles Goodyear was working on a process to vulcanize rubber in a building on what was called Sodom Hill, now Congress Avenue, and tested his preparations in Silliman's laboratory.[14] Dr. William Beaumont sent Silliman samples of gastric juice for analysis and acknowledged Silliman, Knight, Ives, and Hubbard in his classic work on experiments in digestion.[15] In 1846 Silliman, with the support of the Yale College faculty, convinced the corporation to create two new professorships, one in "agricultural chemistry and animal and vegetable physiology" and one in "chemistry and kindred sciences as applied to the arts."

His son, Benjamin Silliman Jr., Yale 1837, was appointed to the professorship in applied chemistry. Silliman and John Pitkin Norton, the professor of agricultural chemistry, received no salary and were dependent on fees from students. Yale College lacked funds to support them, and if funds had been available, they probably would not have gone to professorships in science. The importance of natural science as part of a Yale College education was not appreciated. "Chemistry, like virtue, must be its own reward."[16]

The elder Benjamin Silliman retired in 1853 after forty years of service to Yale and the medical school. Like the death of Nathan Smith in 1829, his departure marked the passing of an era for the Medical Institution of Yale College. Eli Ives, who had also been on the medical faculty for forty years, retired at the same time. Worthington Hooker (figure 11), Yale 1825 and Harvard M.D. 1829, who had been a practitioner in Norwich, Connecticut, for twenty-five years and was a second cousin of Charles Hooker, was appointed professor of the theory and practice of medicine in 1852 to succeed Ives. Worthington Hooker's 1849 book *Physician and Patient* has been described as "the only comprehensive view of professional ethics published in book form by a North American practitioner before 1900."[17] Hooker was also interested in introducing natural science into the curriculum as early as elementary school.[18] Timothy Beers stepped down as chair of obstetrics and was succeeded by Pliny Adams Jewett, Yale M.D. 1840, in 1856. Charles Augustus Lindsley, Yale M.D. 1852, from Orange, New Jersey, was appointed professor of materia medica and therapeutics in 1860, succeeding Henry Bronson. Lindsley, the first non-New Englander and a popular general practitioner in New Haven, was elected dean in 1863 upon the death of Charles Hooker.

The younger Silliman was appointed to the chair of chemistry in both Yale College and the Medical Institution in 1846, while James Dwight Dana was appointed to the chair in geology in 1850. The Department of Natural Science was reorganized in 1854 as the Yale Scientific School. Four years later Joseph Sheffield bought the Medical Institution building at College and Grove streets for $165,000 and presented it to the Yale Scientific School as the future home for the Sheffield Scientific School. Biomedical science had begun to flourish. In 1855, the German pathologist Rudolph Virchow demonstrated that the cell was the locus of the disease process, displacing the humoral theory. Four years later, Louis Pasteur formed the basis for the germ theory of disease. But although science was now ensconced at Yale, total acceptance by the college was not forthcoming. Sheffield students were awarded a degree of bachelor of philosophy rather than a B.A. after a three-year course and were not permitted to sit with the regular Yale College students in chapel.

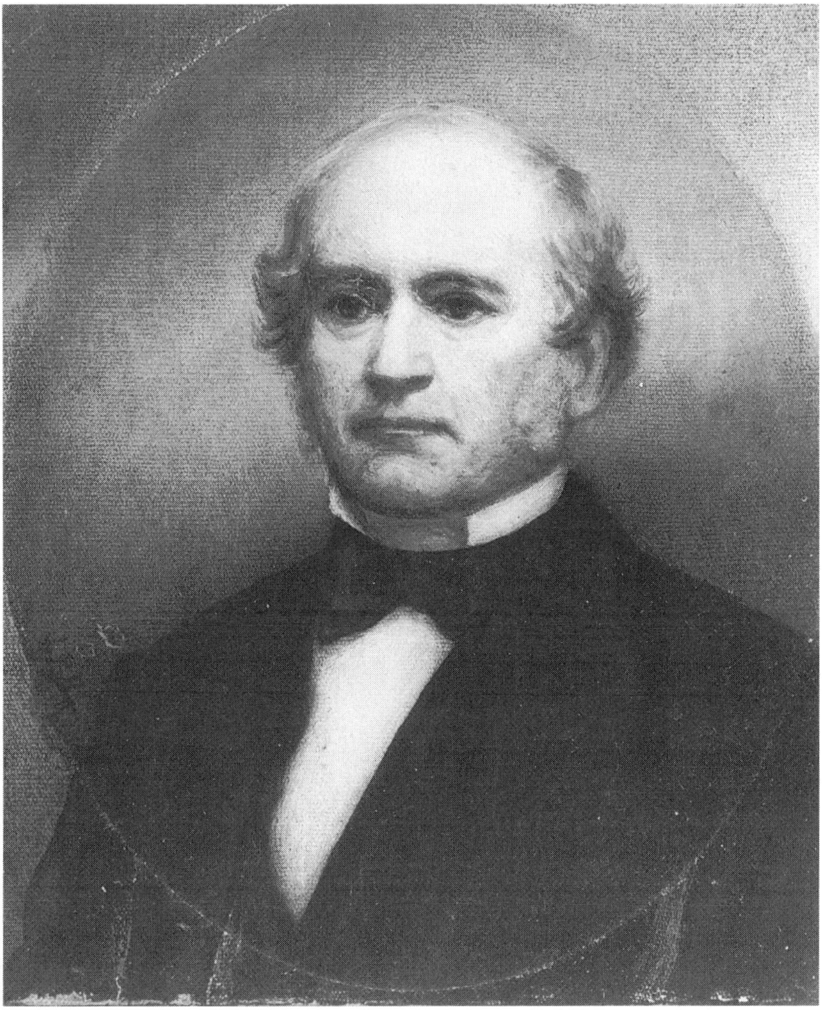

Figure 11. Worthington Hooker

With the proceeds from the sale of its building, the medical school built a three-story structure at 150 York Street (figure 12), which it occupied from 1860 to 1925. The first laboratory at the medical school came into existence shortly after the move with the introduction of the microscope by Moses Clarke White. White taught botany at the Sheffield Scientific School in 1862 and 1863 and also became an instructor at the medical school. He was promoted to professor of microscopy and pathology in 1867.

The medical school had a new building but was hanging by a financial thread, with virtually no support from the Yale Corporation. Faculty salaries,

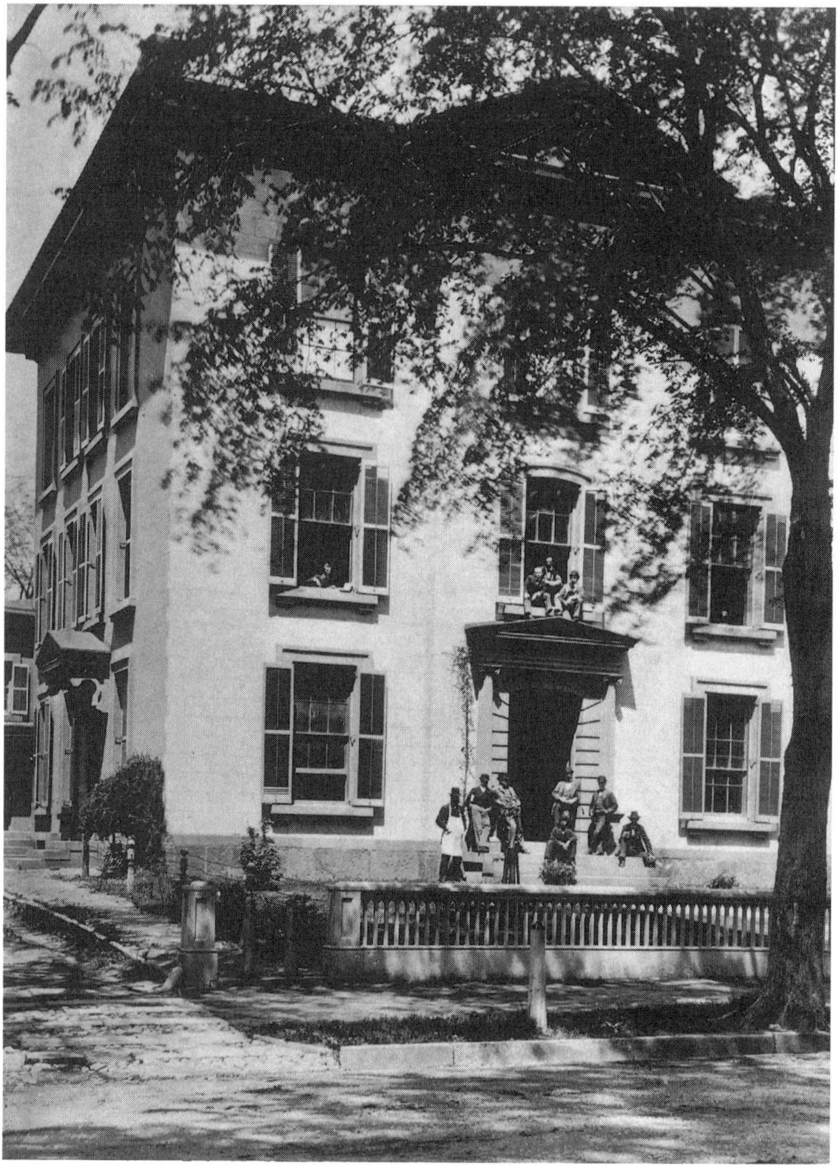

Figure 12. The Medical School at 150 York Street

which depended on student fees, were woefully inadequate because of the depressed student enrollment. Students who did attend had difficulty paying their fees. The Civil War was raging. When President Lincoln instituted a draft for military service, some medical students chose to buy their way out of conscription. In 1863 Edwin Gardner, a recent graduate, wrote to Dean

Lindsley explaining that he could not meet his debts to the school because he had had to pay $500 to avoid conscription in the war. Gardner commented, "Perhaps money is not so hard with Professors as it is with young practitioners of medicine."[19] Although the Civil War had little impact on the medical school as a whole, the hospital was taken over by the military and renamed the Knight Hospital (figure 13).

Finances were so tight that there was not enough money for alcohol to maintain the specimens in the medical museum. The precarious condition of the medical school at this time was later described by Francis Bacon in a historical essay: "There have been some critical moments when this institution has seemed ready to add one to the long list of defunct American medical colleges, but its possession of a small fund and something of the necessary plant, in the way of apparatus and building, has served not so much to make continuance in life satisfactory as to make dying inconvenient."[20]

At this financially inopportune time, the president of the Connecticut State Dental Association, Asa Hill, wrote a compelling nine-page letter urging the Yale president and medical-school faculty to start a dental school within the medical school. "The specialty [of dentistry]," he wrote, "is no longer a simple Mechanical Art, or calling, supplying an additional fee to the Barber-Blacksmith or Tinker, but a necessary, and indispensible [sic] auxilliary to the general practice of Medicine and Surgery [that] must needs be provided for. It has been . . . treated as a Bantling for too long. . . . It needs the foster care of its own mother [being] as much a legitimate Child of Medicine as general Surgery. . . . If a knowledge of Anatomy Phisiology [sic], Hygiene and Chemistry are essential to its successful practice, where can these be so well taught as in the Medical Schools of our country."[21] Hill's timing could not have been worse. The Yale Corporation was withholding financial support from the medical school on the one hand and was perceived as encroaching on the role of the faculty on the other.

In 1868 Dean Lindsley complained to President Theodore Dwight Woolsey that the corporation had assumed the power of appointing faculty in the medical school by having designated a demonstrator of anatomy and curator of the museum without faculty consent.[22] Although not opposed to the designated individual, the medical faculty was opposed to the process and wanted the corporation to reverse the appointment. Woolsey acknowledged that, because it lacked the approval of the medical faculty, the appointment was an administrative error. But he did not want to involve the corporation, and such an error would not occur again.

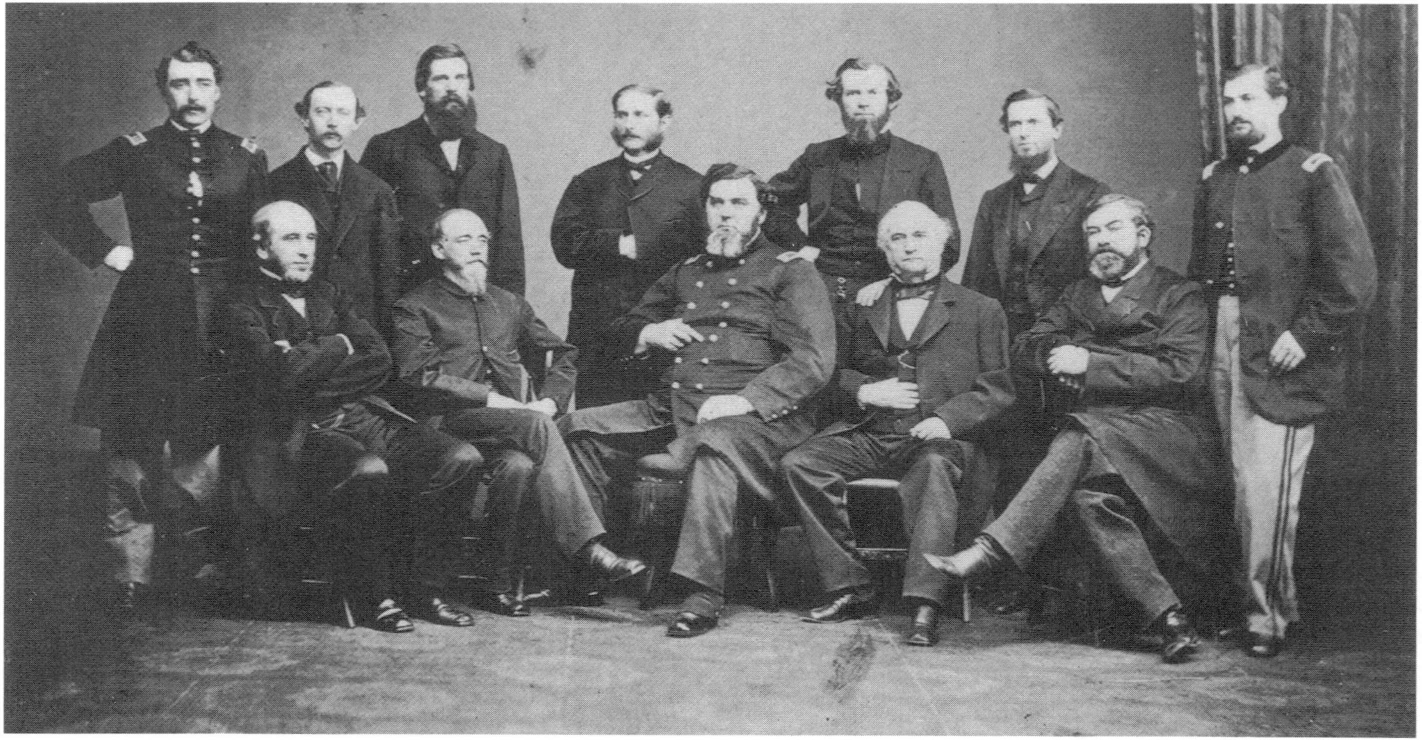

Figure 13. Physicians at Knight Hospital

In 1871, the medical faculty submitted to the corporation a document entitled "Needs of the University," which outlined curriculum revisions. Financial support from the university was needed to implement the revised curriculum, but the necessary funds were not forthcoming. Support for the Medical Department did come from certain quarters of Yale College, however. That same year Professor Timothy Dwight commented that there should be faculty in the Medical Department "who shall be wholly given to science while others mingle with the scientific the practical element, in their daily work so that the students can derive the full benefit of both."[23]

What was called the "critical condition" of the school was addressed in a forthright manner two years later, on March 25, 1873, in a signed "Memorial" to the corporation on behalf of the medical faculty. Its authors, Dr. Bacon, Dr. Hubbard, and Professor Silliman, alluded to the fact that the plan for revising the curriculum had been formulated as early as 1865. "While our remuneration has been nothing worth mentioning . . . income from the fund is not equal to the expenses of the Department. . . . The deficiencies are paid by ourselves." The members of the medical faculty considered themselves part of Yale College and complained that, although "countenance, encouragement and sympathy were given to the other Departments" by the corporation, the medical school had suffered "neglect." The memorial ended with a strong statement about the future of the medical school: "We would feel mortified if the question of its abandonment should be forced upon us. How long in the present plan can the medical department be continued?"[24] The members of the medical faculty were committed to high-quality medical education. Rather than lower standards, they even supported the school from their own salaries, accepting IOUs so that the medical-school building could be maintained.

The memorial went on to mention that Harvard Medical School had implemented virtually the same plan the medical faculty at Yale had proposed to the corporation in 1871. In 1869 the Massachusetts Medical College of Harvard University had been described as "a money-making institution, not much better than a diploma mill."[25] That year, however, Charles W. Eliot became president of Harvard University. A chemist, he understood the need to teach medicine in a more rigorous fashion and made reform of the medical school his immediate objective.

Money was not an issue at Harvard, but there was strong opposition from senior faculty, including Oliver Wendell Holmes and Henry Bigelow. According to Bigelow, "no successful school has thought it proper to risk large existing classes and large receipts in attempting a more thorough education."[26] Despite these formidable foes, Eliot succeeded in introducing a number of reforms at the medical school. Whether Yale's medical school was "successful" during this period is open to question, but its faculty took a major financial risk by raising standards at the expense of enrollment. Money rather than courage prevented the Medical Institution from implementing curriculum change. At Harvard, under President Eliot's strong hand, the medical school was integrated into the university. A graded three-year program with nine-month terms was instituted, and laboratory sciences were emphasized.

On June 24, 1873, having received no answer from the corporation to their March plea, the members of the faculty wrote yet another memorial, calling attention to their previous communication and requesting funds to buy property for the medical school.[27] The corporation had attempted to obtain $100,000 from the Connecticut Medical Society in an effort to provide funding to the medical school while sparing college funds. The attempt was "unproductive of practical results." At the same time as it requested desperately needed funds to keep the medical school viable, the June memorial repeated the necessity of lengthening the educational process so that graded courses could be given throughout the school year, as outlined already in 1871. A graded curriculum meant specific courses assigned in logical order to each year of study.[28] In its March memorial the medical faculty had urged the corporation to ratify a change in the curriculum that would entail entrance requirements for admission and would extend the course over the entire year, with recitations as well as lectures.[29] For the first time, instead of merely listening to lectures and taking notes, medical students would be expected to discuss the lesson in class. Examinations would be required for advancement.

Despite the financial state of the medical school, the faculty continued to pursue increased educational standards. At a time when the professors were being paid less than $1,000 a year, by 1874 they had advanced $1,556 from their own funds to keep the school afloat, with the expectation of reimbursement from the university.[30] Undaunted by corporation indifference, the medical faculty made another plea for funds in 1874 on behalf of the medical museum, to which, once again, there was no response. Finally, the corporation voted the grand sum of $500 for the medical school. When in 1875 the faculty sent a bill to the corporation for various medical-school expenses, it added a note stating that "the creditors are clamorous."[31]

When Charles Ives stepped down as professor of the theory and practice of medicine in 1873 because of ill health, David Paige Smith (figure 14), grandson of Nathan Smith, was appointed to the position. Smith had written to President Noah Porter about the position, indicating that although he had been earning $15,000 a year, he was interested in "study and improvement in his profession" rather than "interminable fee-taking."[32] Smith relinquished the chair in medicine for the chair in surgery in 1877 but he died two years later; he was succeeded by William Henry Carmalt. Carmalt graduated from the College of Physicians and Surgeons in New York City in 1861 and, following an internship at St. Luke's Hospital, engaged in general practice in New York until 1869. During this period he specialized in ophthalmic surgery, becoming a charter member of the American Ophthalmological Society. From 1870 to 1874 he studied in Europe; after his return he started a practice in New Haven and joined the Yale medical faculty as professor of ophthalmology and otology, prior to his appointment to the chair of surgery.[33]

In June 1878, the Yale College treasurer, Franklin Bowditch Dexter, sent a letter to the medical faculty on behalf of the corporation: "They regret that they have no funds at their disposal for any further aid to the Medical Department."[34] (The corporation had designated the Yale treasurer to manage the financial affairs of the Medical Institution in 1880. By making the treasurer responsible for the medical school's finances, the corporation had de facto accepted the Medical Institution as an integral part of Yale College!) The continuing economic drought resulted in a statement in the 1884 report of the president that the Medical Department was in financial distress. This was clearly a cry for help.

The Yale Corporation had accepted bylaws for the governance of the medical school in 1875 that "vested [the government of the department] in the President and Medical Professors." Previous bylaws, set forth in "An Act in relation to the Medical Institution of Yale College" and approved in 1834, with subsequent amendments enacted in 1866, were expanded.[35] The new bylaws provided that "the Medical Professors shall constitute a Board [that] shall direct the details of the courses of Instruction . . . and at their pleasure may elect a dean."[36] There was now a structure in place to allow decisions to be made on behalf of the medical school.

The Connecticut Medical Society, originally chartered as a degree-granting body by the legislature in 1792, had shared this authority with Yale College in an amiable but awkward arrangement. By the second half of the nineteenth century, however, the Medical Institution was essentially operating independently of the state society, and the charter under which the school had been founded was no longer applicable. In 1879 a new charter

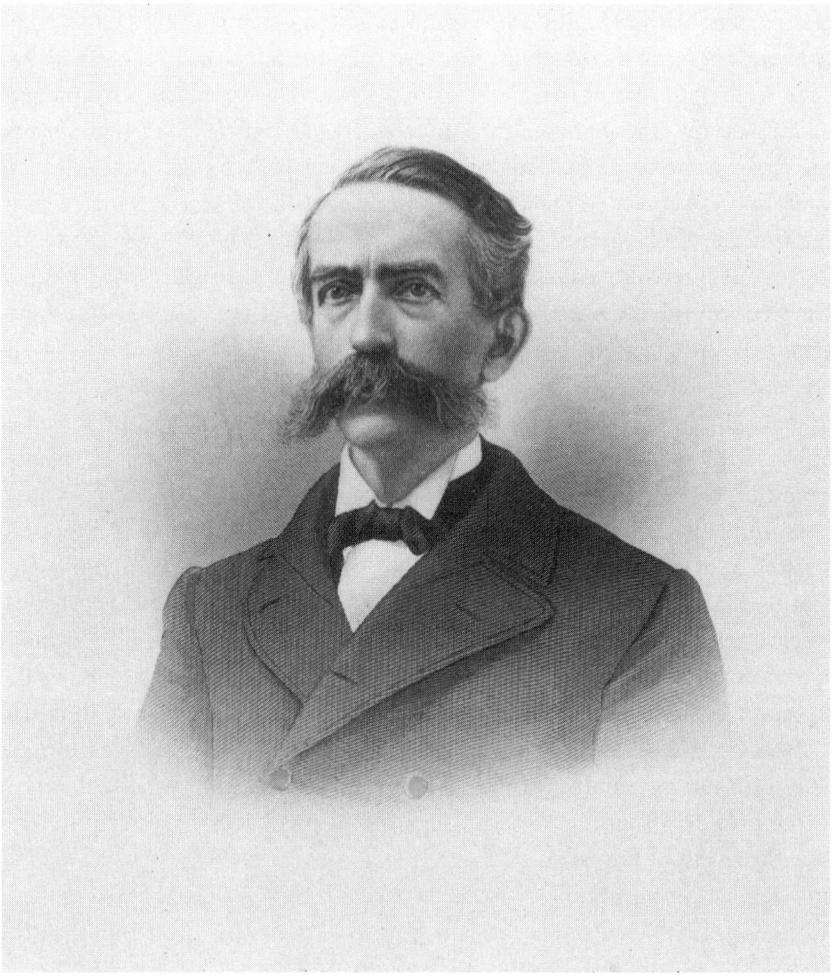

Figure 14. David P. Smith

was enacted by the Connecticut Legislature that allowed the two institutions to break their tie by mutual agreement rather than by legislative fiat, which would have raised hackles: "Such an act of dissolution may be consummated by mutual agreement without further legislative action."[37]

Relations between the Medical Institution and the society were good, and passage of the bill in this manner allowed the two parties to remain friendly. With the passage of the act in 1879, the name of the school was changed from the Medical Institution of Yale College to the Medical Department of Yale College, thus reaffirming the medical school as an integral part of Yale College. Five years later the partnership between the state medical society and the college dissolved, ending an interesting and mutually beneficial relationship. The alliance had allowed high standards of practice to be maintained within Connecticut and had probably prevented the proliferation of proprietary medical schools in the state.

The new charter afforded the Medical Department of Yale College a wider degree of latitude in which to develop, with no limits on the size of the medical-school faculty or on the faculty's right to determine the curriculum. Timothy Dwight had stated in his 1886 report that "the rapid rationalization of medicine is throwing more and more weight upon the earlier, more fundamental and scientific parts of medical education." This view fitted well with the new subject of biology at the college, which had been developed by James Kingsley Thacher. Thacher, a graduate of Yale College, had received a medical degree from Yale in 1879 and was appointed professor of physiology, a position he held from 1879 to 1891. An "eminent comparative anatomist, abreast of modern physiology and clinical medicine," he was responsible for a number of changes in the medical curriculum.[38]

A graded course of study over three full academic years was instituted in 1879.[39] More radically, a matriculation examination became a requirement for students lacking a college degree. This was truly a bold step. Yale and Harvard were the only medical schools in the Northeast to set such high standards. The medical faculty at the University of Michigan had considered raising educational standards but expressed concern that setting the bar too high would encourage prospective students to apply elsewhere.[40] Interestingly, Yale abolished the thesis requirement at the same time, for reasons that are not clear, and did not list it as a stipulation for graduation until 1888. Most medical schools' admission requirements at the time consisted simply of the applicant's signature and a fee of five dollars.

Setting higher standards required fiscal courage, and Yale's curricular innovations were very nearly fatal, resulting in a drop in medical-student enrollment from fifty-eight in 1878 to a nadir of twenty-one in 1881. The average matriculation rate at the medical school did not exceed thirty students until 1889. Funds available to operate the school as well as pay the salaries of the professors amounted to only $25,000, of which $9,000 went to capital improvements. As had happened so often in the past, the medical faculty hunkered down and pared the school budget down to the bone.[41]

The school had benefited from the opening in 1872 of the New Haven Dispensary, which delivered outpatient medical care to the underprivileged of New Haven. Because Yale medical students were barely tolerated in the hospital, the dispensary was important for clinical teaching. Oversight was provided by an independent board made up of prominent members of the community. Under the existing arrangement, however, members of the medical faculty were basically guests in the dispensary, lacking administrative as well as clinical authority. Within five years of opening its doors the dispensary was treating more than five thousand patients, and the demand for care had outgrown the available space.[42]

In 1877 the medical faculty proposed that Yale purchase property on York Street next to the school for renting to the dispensary, and the Yale Corporation agreed. The rental agreement stipulated that "the Medical Faculty shall have the right to nominate the medical attendants, and the medical students of the Institution shall have the privilege of viewing medical and surgical practice."[43] In 1879 the medical faculty thanked the corporation for its help in relocating the dispensary adjacent to the medical school, which had made it possible for medical students to have access to an additional six thousand or seven thousand patients.[44]

In tandem with improved clinical teaching came greater emphasis on the basic sciences. William Carmalt pointed out that the "rapid rationalization of medicine" was making the sciences more important, and that a medical school connected with a university offered better opportunities than one that stood alone. "It is possible to make here, in the near future, a medical department, good in its clinical and preeminent in its scientific structure."[45] Medical science was developing rapidly in the late nineteenth century. In Europe, the study of disease had evolved from the earlier clinical observations of Pierre Louis through improved methods of observation, examination, and diagnosis of patients. The introduction of the stethoscope, the ophthalmoscope, and the laryngoscope improved the technological aspects of medicine. By the late 1800s, laboratory medicine was thriving in Germany, where decentralized universities and adequate funding fostered laboratory research and modern medical investigation.

In the United States, physiologic observation had been performed as early as 1833 with Beaumont's famous *in vivo* studies of digestion. But American medicine was slow to integrate the scientific method. At the end of the Civil War there were still no academic research laboratories or provision for training in experimental science. The establishment of a professorship in physiological chemistry at the Sheffield Scientific School and the appointment of Russell H. Chittenden to that position in 1882 were of the utmost significance to the medical school. Chittenden maintained his interest in the school well into the 1930s. He would arrive for meetings at the Sterling Hall of Medicine on his bicycle, a dignified elderly gentleman with a well-trimmed goatee. In 1934 the Connecticut State Medical Society invoked its ancient prerogative and bestowed an honorary degree of doctor of medicine on him.

The medical faculty at Yale had recognized early on the importance of training in basic science. A first step in that direction had been taken with the introduction of preparatory studies in 1879. Now, in the 1880s, despite financial problems, the medical-school faculty wanted to increase the size of the faculty, in order to teach the disciplines of histology and pathology separately. The time was propitious. After the groundbreaking work of Louis Pasteur and the German bacteriologist Robert Koch, the link between germs and disease had been definitively established, forging a bridge between basic and clinical science.

A proposal was made at the medical school to appoint a professor of histology. One of the candidates under strong consideration was T. Mitchell Prudden (Yale Ph.B. 1872, M.D. 1875), who at the time was studying in Germany.[46]

Despite his "true blue" lineage and his affection for Carmalt, Prudden decided to remain with Francis Delafield, professor of anatomy at the College of Physicians and Surgeons in New York, who had given him a full-time research job. According to Prudden, both the research facilities and the remuneration were better in New York than in New Haven.[47] At the urging of Carmalt, the medical faculty at Yale was so convinced of Prudden's importance to the future of the medical school that it offered him a salary of $1,200 to come up from New York once a week to teach.

This arrangement, however, was not greeted with universal enthusiasm by the faculty, who had agreed in 1880 that the stipend for all professors would be $300. Any additional revenues that might have come to the faculty in the past would be used for laboratory apparatus and capital maintenance. Moses White, the venerable and respected professor who held the chair that was being divided into pathology and histology, received only one-quarter of the amount paid to Prudden for part-time histology lectures. Resenting the inequity, and seeing it as a threat to the future of the financially shaky institution, White wrote to President Noah Porter in June 1882: "I enter my formal protest against the whole plan proposed, as a wild and ill considered scheme."[48] At the same time, White sent a ten-page letter to the Prudential Committee of the Yale Corporation in which he expressed his fear that the course his colleagues were taking would be the ruin of the medical school.[49]

Trying to hold onto the past, Moses White lamented the drift away from the Connecticut Medical Society and the strained relations between the hospital and the medical school. He was disturbed enough to contact the secretary of the medical society, who in turn advised President Porter in March 1883 that the medical faculty had not known about or consented to section 6 in the new charter.[50] The act of 1879 allowed the articles of agreement between the Connecticut Medical Society and Yale College to be dissolved without legislative approval. Section 6, which was purported to be in different handwriting, actually repealed all previous acts, in effect dissolving the partnership. It appears that nothing further was done to determine how section 6 had been inserted. Like so many others before him in a time of change, White longed for the good old days. But change was inevitable.

A June 1882 faculty memorandum to the president and fellows, which White had refused to sign, raised the serious question whether the medical school should continue operating in its current, underfunded circumstances: "It is possible to establish and maintain here a school of medicine, which shall depend solely on the fees of its students for its support, which will be a reputably strong and efficient member of the University." The memorandum went on to explain that the development of a scientific basis for medicine demanded more courses and increased expenses: "There is need for extended and well adapted courses in anatomy, pathology, chemistry and physiology. These things are real needs for very practical ends. They are not luxurious embellishments. They are not even the anticipated needs of the future. They are the needs of the present time."[51] The faculty proposed new appointments of lecturers in chemistry, histology, and physiology, each with an annual stipend of $1,200, which would need an immediate endowment. Aware of the discomfort of White and his colleagues, the authors of the memorandum recommended that appointments should be made without causing ill feeling in any member of the faculty. The Yale Corporation received the memorandum but, true to form, did not increase support or commit to future increases in funding for the medical school. Nevertheless, responsibility for the medical school now rested entirely with the corporation.

President Noah Porter addressed a letter to the medical faculty in December 1885 in which he stated that "as the entire control of the medical department has now been assumed by the corporation, it seems a favorable time for the reorganization of the school." He went on to ask for a plan "best calculated to establish and maintain a school of superior merit."[52] The faculty submitted a proposal emphasizing the scientific advances and development of medical education in Europe. The recurrent theme that New Haven was not large enough to support a clinical program was addressed. According to the faculty, New Haven had an advantage in that it was small enough for both scientists and clinicians to interact and thus accomplish "the object of a medical school [which] should be to make science tell upon art in the future professional life of its students."[53] The faculty evidently shared the view Sir William Osler, the great Canadian physician, expressed in his aphorism that "the practice of Medicine is an art based on science."[54]

Because Yale College received all fees and income generated by the medical school and paid the salaries and expenses of the medical faculty, the corporation had total control of the direction of the medical school. This was unlike most other medical schools, where the direction belonged to the professors. The arrangement at Yale was intended to offer "greater security to benefactors."

Not surprisingly, the plan the medical faculty suggested was similar to the one submitted to the president three years earlier, only with greater emphasis on the need for an endowment, now amounting to $500,000. Endowment funds were requested to support professorships in chemistry, physiology, anatomy, and pathology, including assistants and expenses, in addition to general expenses of $40,000 a year. Part of the plan was to increase the number of instructors in the "practical branches": "These subjects should evidently be taught by men in active practice, and no provision by endowment is recommended for these departments as it is believed that the interested services of the best of our practitioners could be obtained with such funds as you have from the fees of the students."[55] Endowments were helping Yale's competitors to expand. Harvard had erected a building that cost more than a quarter of a million dollars. Columbia had received half a million dollars for land and building from William H. Vanderbilt. Andrew Carnegie had built a laboratory for Bellevue Hospital in New York, and Johns Hopkins had endowed the new university and hospital in Baltimore with $7 million.

Charles Lindsley, who had served as dean since 1863, stepped aside in 1885 to devote his full time to the chair of medicine. The corporation appointed Herbert E. Smith to the deanship as well as to the chair of chemistry, which had been vacant since the death of Benjamin Silliman Jr. Smith was a graduate of the Sheffield Scientific School. In 1882, immediately after receiving his M.D. degree from the University of Pennsylvania, he had joined the Yale faculty as an instructor in chemistry, assisting Silliman. Smith had also studied at the University of Heidelberg and been exposed to the scientific approach taught in German universities.

The deanship of Yale's medical school was not regarded as a plum: "In 1885 Professor H. E. Smith was persuaded to undertake the thankless task as Dean. Doing so involved the sacrifice of the career in chemistry, in which he had addressed initial success in exchange for the cares and responsibilities of a business man at the head of a complex industry, but without the possibility of the material rewards of a successful business."[56] During the ensuing ten years, from 1885 to 1895, the policy of the school seems to have been based on the principle that when trouble comes from doing well, do well the more. Dean Smith followed this maxim, and by 1894 the entire endowment had been "borrowed"—and there was additional debt of $6,301.

President Porter, who had little interest in the medical school, stepped aside in 1886, and Professor Timothy Dwight, son of former president Timothy Dwight, became president of Yale. Dwight had a decided interest in medicine, which augured well for the plans set forth in 1871.[57] The new president's first move was to change the name of the institution from Yale College to Yale University, and his first report to the Yale Corporation made no mention of the plan for the medical school that his predecessor, Noah Porter, had solicited.[58]

Following the medical schools at Michigan, Harvard, and Pennsylvania, the medical faculty at Yale had added a third year to the medical curriculum in 1879, resulting in a significant decrease in the number of medical students. Dwight mentioned the drop in medical-school enrollment but at the same time commended the increase in educational standards responsible for the decrease. He also reinforced the need for an endowment to support a full-time medical faculty: "The establishment of a strong Medical School here for all coming time will be of the highest advantage and importance to the life of the University."[59] An additional required year was added in 1896, bringing the total curriculum to four years.

At the tenth anniversary of the medical alumni association President Dwight spoke about the desirability of increasing funds as well as student numbers, which was tantamount to increasing revenues.[60] He urged the alumni to make an effort to direct students to Yale, because it would be a misfortune for Connecticut and the university if the medical school were to die. His speech was followed by a keynote address in Battell Chapel by William Henry Welch on "Some Advantages of the Union of the Medical School and University." Clearly, a concerted effort was being made to save the medical school.

In 1894 students founded the *Yale Medical Journal*, with the stated desire to bring students into closer contact with one another and with the medical profession. Members of the medical faculty, including Dean Herbert Smith and William Carmalt, chairman of surgery, acted as an advisory board.[61] Articles were solicited from faculty as well as from the medical profession in general. In 1895 the editors commented on the rise in medical-student enrollment at Yale during the previous five years from 65 to 130, which was attributed in part to the emphasis on "personal instruction." The editors did, however, view the lack of ready access to medical journals as a problem, because the university library was not close by. But they were excited about the "case method" of teaching medicine put forth by Walter B. Cannon, the Harvard physiologist, at the turn of the century. The intent of the case system was to provide actual patient histories so that "the student may be thoroughly trained to do just the kind of thought and work which he will be obliged to do when he gets into practice."[62] By 1906 the journal was in favor of a combined course that would allow students to obtain both a bachelor's and a medical degree in six years.[63] They would have the advantage of spending four years in college residence, taking the science courses of the medical curriculum as well as undergraduate courses. The editors did not believe that medical schools should require four years of college as a minimum entrance requirement.

The editorial page of the *Yale Medical Journal* reflected the rising discontent with the quality of medical education in the United States. Two years before the Flexner Report, an editorial in 1908 suggested that there should be expert scrutiny of medical schools without absolute uniformity. The journal also thought that the lack of control of hospitals by medical schools was a bar to the progress of medical education in the United States as compared to Europe.[64] Whether these opinions reflected the views of the medical students or those of their faculty advisors is not clear. The journal had come out strongly in 1897 against "contract physicians," supporting the resolution "that the Connecticut State Medical Society declares it to be derogatory to the dignity of its members to render professional services at a stipulated fee per capita per annum."[65]

During the 1890s, despite the continuing financial crisis, the medical faculty was bolstered by the appointment of men who understood the importance of scientific research and the need for improving clinical care. From 1893 the teaching of physiology and physiological chemistry was supervised by Russell H. Chittenden, who expressed the firm belief that "medicine in the end would profit most from a broad development in physiological chemistry."[66] Research of this kind required laboratory space, which was in short supply at Yale. President Dwight recognized the importance of laboratory work in the development of the medical school, and with his help a three-story laboratory building was built in 1893, mainly for chemistry and physiology. Dwight's presidential report for 1893 stressed the importance of science, stating that "indeed, the proper development of this feature appears to be essential to the future success and highest usefulness of a medical school which is located as ours is, and which like ours, forms a department of a university."[67] Dwight backed up his rhetoric with financial support. In 1897, he allocated a budget of $50,000 to the medical school. The Spanish-American War in the following year had little impact on the school, although the hospital cared for an influx of 202 military patients. Of those, one hundred had typhoid fever and fourteen reportedly died of the disease.[68]

In 1899, Arthur Twining Hadley, the first nonclerical president of Yale, accepted the "diadem of the Presidency," which Ezra Stiles had called a "crown of thorns." Even though the college had prospered under Dwight, the "university" had been realized in name only. As George Pierson, the eminent Yale historian, commented, "The 'outside' schools had been strengthened but not admitted to equality." Sheffield Scientific School "had grown into a rival rather than a partner. . . . The sciences had not prospered." Pierson wondered whether Dwight fully understood how much the world was changing and how profound the changes were for all colleges: "The inevitable question, accordingly, was whether colleges could keep pace with the advances in science and technology and the widening vocational ambitions. And for Yale the special, additional problem was whether its gradualism was any longer adequate or its traditionalism safe."[69]

Hadley, grandson of a medical-school lecturer and son of a Yale faculty member, grew up on Elm Street in New Haven where Calhoun College now stands.[70] A brilliant scholar, he was valedictorian of Yale College Class of 1876. He was well liked and was class secretary, despite suffering from poor vision and being deaf in one ear. Hadley was a strong proponent of Yale as a university extending beyond the confines of Yale College. In 1899 he appointed Russell Chittenden, then director of the Sheffield Scientific School and professor of physiological chemistry, to the post of professor of physiology in the medical school. The appointment not only strengthened the teaching of physiology but, more important, also built a bridge between Sheffield and the medical school.

When Yale University celebrated its bicentennial in 1901, William H. Welch delivered a keynote address in Battell Chapel on "The Relation of Yale to Medicine."[71] Dean Herbert Smith was asked to comment and lamented to Welch that, as the medical faculty heightened the matriculation requirements, registration fell off, reaching a nadir of twenty-one students in 1881.[72] Smith considered the minimum admission requirement of a high-school education a weakness but was concerned about raising standards further.

Smith subsequently told Welch that the university officers were interested, sympathetic, and ready to listen. He also, however, wondered "if the President fully appreciates from what we say the opportunities which exist in medicine." In spite of Smith's comments, Welch was not impressed with the support that Yale had provided to medicine. He had written to his sister, Emma, that "the subject 'Relation of Yale to Medicine' is about the most barren theme I ever tackled. The relation is so slight that I shall have to beat around the bush and talk on side issues. If they had only asked me to talk on the relation of Yale to Calvinism or football there would be something to say."[73]

In his address, Welch concentrated on the history of Yale College and its relation to medicine since its founding in 1701, emphasizing the contributions the college had made to medicine in the United States. He ended with a plea for support of the medical school: "Medical teaching and research can no longer be successfully carried on with the meager appliances of the past. They require large endowments, many well-equipped and properly supported laboratories, and a body of well paid teachers thoroughly trained in their special departments. With an ampler supply of such opportunities as these there is every reason to believe that the Yale Medical Department would take that important position in the great forward movement of modern medicine to which its origin, its honorable history, and the fame of this ancient University entitle it. May the next Jubilee find medicine holding this high position in Yale University!"[74] These were the same themes that the corporation had heard for years without significant response.

Welch's concern for the medical school and its students (figure 15) continued unabated. When John Slade Ely, who was professor of medicine, died in 1906 after being thrown from his horse, Welch was consulted about Ely's successor. He recommended George Blumer, a Californian, who had been a graduate-student assistant at Johns Hopkins from 1893 to 1896 and had worked under Welch, Halsted, and Osler as an assistant in medicine and pathology.[75] After working in New York, Blumer had returned to California in 1903 to practice medicine and serve as associate professor of pathology at Cooper Medical College (the forerunner of Stanford University School of Medicine). Blumer was promised a salary of $3,000, the highest yet paid to a full-time appointee, which was raised to $4,000 a year later, when this salary was offered to the chair of surgery.

Another faculty member who came from Johns Hopkins at this time was Ross G. Harrison, Bronson Professor of Comparative Anatomy. Shortly after

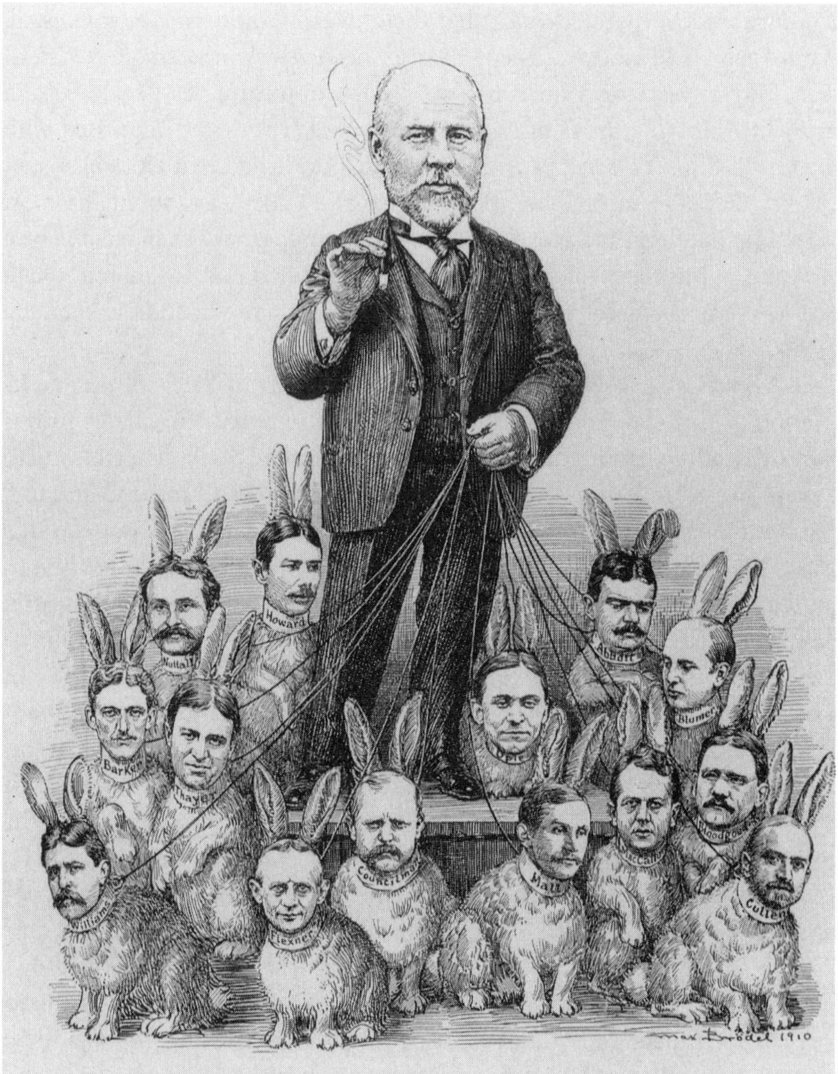

Figure 15. Welch's students

arriving in New Haven, he produced his work on the explanation of neurons, for which he was voted a Nobel Prize, although his prize was never awarded because of World War I.[76]

In 1906 William Carmalt announced that he would retire from the chair of surgery. The appointment of his successor was a crucial one. Medicine

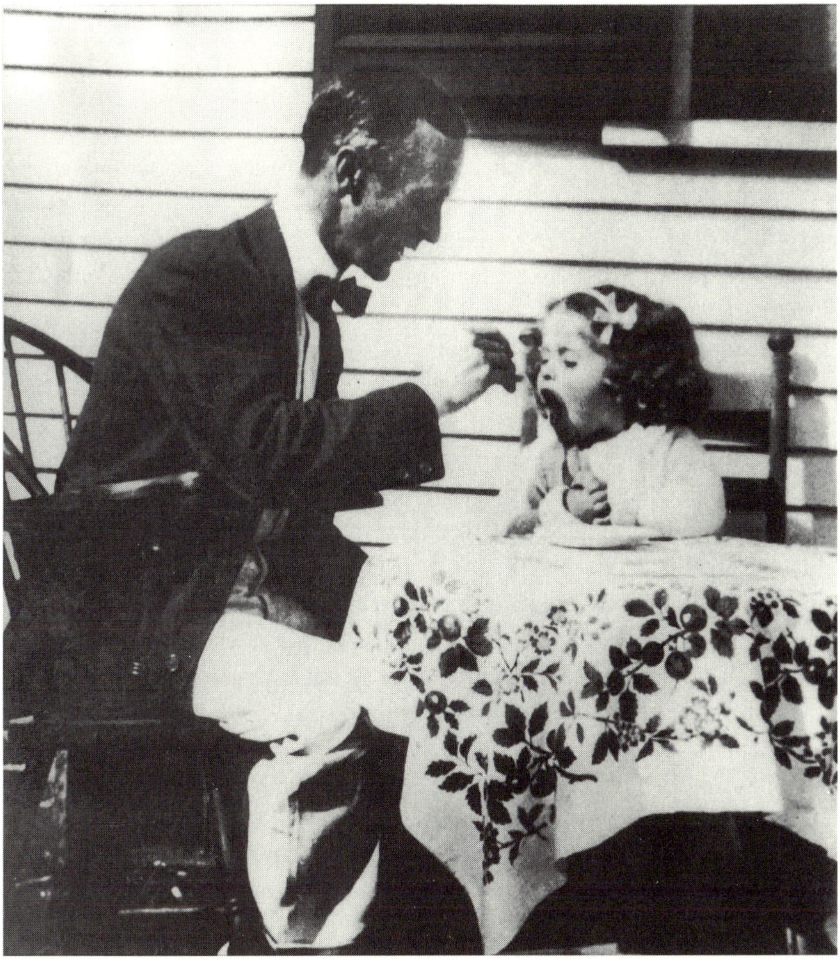

Figure 16. Harvey Cushing and his daughter Betsey

and surgery were—and still are—the dominant departments in a medical school. If Yale's medical school was to thrive, it needed an individual who could work with Blumer to raise the standard of the school. Harvey Cushing (figure 16), Yale B.A. 1891, had gone to Harvard Medical School and was a pioneer in neurosurgery at Johns Hopkins.

Carmalt was soliciting funds to gain academic control of the hospital in order to recruit Cushing, "for he is satisfied with all other conditions and wants to come to Yale to teach." Carmalt described "the want of a close hospital connection" as one of the major problems for the medical school: "The hospital is to us a foreign corporation." In his letter soliciting funds, he admitted that the school had "more or less deteriorated" from 1865 to 1885: "Until 1880 it was carried on in the usual commercial basis of medical schools in the country. The professors were paid from the fees of the students and they attempted to underbid the metropolitan schools in the price of their 'tickets,' and with this cheapening of the fees the effect was inevitable, the neglect of instruction."[77] Carmalt had been appointed professor of surgery in 1881, two years after the adoption of the graded curriculum, and along with James Thacher and Herbert Smith had promoted excellence irrespective of medical-student enrollment.

President Hadley took an uncharacteristically active role in Cushing's recruitment. The inability of New Haven to support a medical school because of its small size had been a persistent issue, fanned by prominent Yale alumni in New York. Hadley, influenced by this advice and by differences of opinion with the dean, Herbert Smith, was dubious about creating a first-class medical school in a city the size of New Haven.[78] Cushing, however, dismissed this as a significant factor. In a 1906 letter to Hadley, he expressed the view that "as . . . in Germany, the small select schools in relatively small cities will become those whose degrees are most sought after by the best class of students. . . . It is not an *abundance* of patients that makes for the most successful clinical teaching, but the way in which the *small number* is utilized as a means of instruction."[79]

According to Cushing, the major issue was the need to control the New Haven Hospital on a year-round basis; the medical faculty had charge of the wards for only three months a year. Cushing also strongly supported the addition of a fourth year to the medical-school curriculum, which Yale had instituted in 1895. At Harvard he had been in the first class to take a fourth year and had benefited from the experience. He stressed the need for tougher admission requirements, even if they meant that fewer students would enroll. More stringent admission requirements in addition to a fourth year would ensure that there would be "more mature students with whom to work . . . who in their fourth year could safely have the freedom of hospital wards."[80] In 1902 the student editors of the *Yale Medical Journal* had pushed to devote the fourth year of medical school to hospital work, followed by one year of internship, rather than have two years of internship. "Most of our hospitals have too few internes, work them too hard, and keep them too long. . . . Hospital internes have no time for reading, much less for original research."[81]

Cushing's final point in his 1906 letter to Hadley was that "the one pressing need of the school was a hospital with a continuous service for those occupying the clinical chairs. Without a hospital in which they have clinical and teaching privileges the year round, clinical professors are as destitute of opportunities for instruction and investigation as a chemist or a physicist would be without a laboratory."[82] The ability to see private patients was important to him, as it was to William Osler. In contrast, full-time clinical practice without private practice was a theme that would be promoted fervently by Abraham Flexner in coming years.

After strenuous efforts by Carmalt, President Hadley, and the Reverend Anson Phelps Stokes, secretary of the university, an agreement was reached with the New Haven Hospital. The professor of surgery was given control over one-quarter of the surgical service and the professor of medicine control over one-sixth of the medical service for the entire year.[83] Despite these efforts, Cushing declined the position. A lot of time would have to be given to the reorganization of teaching, and he would have to devote "much of his energies" to building a private practice. He felt that his professorial duties were almost certain to become subordinate to his outside professional ones. He thought that Yale could become one of the choice medical schools, but "to accomplish this a strictly university hospital is needed and a large endowment is necessary, for a small school is relatively more expensive than a large one."[84]

In 1907, a group of New Haven physicians led by William F. Verdi, a Yale medical graduate, founded the Hospital of Saint Raphael with the help of the Sisters of Charity.[85] At the laying of the cornerstone for the new hospital, Father Edward Stone stated that "Catholic doctors" had been excluded from "the avenues of hospital staff and hospital practice in New Haven."[86] A February 1907 newspaper article about Saint Raphael's stated that prior to 1906 the hospitals of New Haven (that is, the New Haven Hospital) bordered on a "closed corporation." Hospitals did not in fact exclude Catholic physicians, but they did prevent visits by a patient's family and family physician. The Hospital of Saint Raphael, on the other hand, would allow patients to be cared for by their own physicians: "The Catholic hospital will bar no patients who apply for treatment, either on account of creed or color, . . . and one feature which is unique in this city so far as hospitals are concerned, will be that the hospital will be open for all physicians to treat their own patients."[87] This was soon emulated by the New Haven Hospital. By 1910 New Haven had about forty-three thousand foreign-born residents, of whom almost a third were Italian, so there was a ready-made patient base for the Hospital of Saint Raphael. Besides being the driving force of St. Raphael's, Verdi admitted 262 patients to the New Haven Hospital in 1909, compared to 227 admitted by the professor of surgery, Joseph Marshall Flint.[88]

In addition to dissatisfaction with opportunities for clinical teaching, the medical faculty had long been uncomfortable with its minimum requirement of a high-school education for matriculation. In 1905 it proposed a curriculum plan combining the preclinical sciences with undergraduate education, leading to both a B.A. and an M.D. degree in six years.[89] In 1906 the corporation announced that as from 1909 candidates to the medical school would need to have completed two years of college.[90] Also, students at Yale College might elect a six-year program that would lead to B.A. and M.D. degrees at completion. These were steps toward the "ideal" requirements of accepting more college graduates, which had been established at Johns Hopkins and other schools, and which were the harbinger of unsuccessful attempts in the 1970s to shorten the length of physician training. Yandell Henderson, chairman of physiology, was concerned that these standards would cause even greater problems for the medical school because there would be "a very considerable, even if temporary diminution in students," with a concomitant diminution in tuition revenue. A potential decrease in revenue had real significance, as by dint of hard work the school had managed to pay off its debt in 1907.

Although there were several individuals at the medical school who championed laboratory sciences and scientific medicine, clinical teaching was woefully inadequate. As William Carmalt put it on the occasion of the hospital's centenary in 1926, "The directors of the hospital and a portion of its medical staff were indifferent, even at times, antagonistic, to the function of the hospital as a factor in medical education."[91] The new professor of surgery, Joseph Flint, agreed with Carmalt: "The medical students were there on sufferance, and then only during the winter months when the professors were on service. At most they were onlookers, not participants."[92] President Hadley had turned to Flint, also a Hopkins man, to succeed Carmalt. Part of the gap that had developed between the hospital and the medical school reflected town-gown tensions, and university officials were not helpful in lessening these strains. "There was a certain aloofness if not an assumption of superiority on the part of the conservative college circle."[93]

In spite of the tensions, there was a feeling among the faculty in the first decade of the twentieth century that the medical school and the hospital would ultimately become closely affiliated. To that end the university purchased almost the whole front of Cedar Street facing the hospital, confident that the medical school would ultimately be located there.

This vision of the future had sustained the medical faculty, particularly Ferris in anatomy (figure 17), Henderson in physiology, Carmalt in surgery,

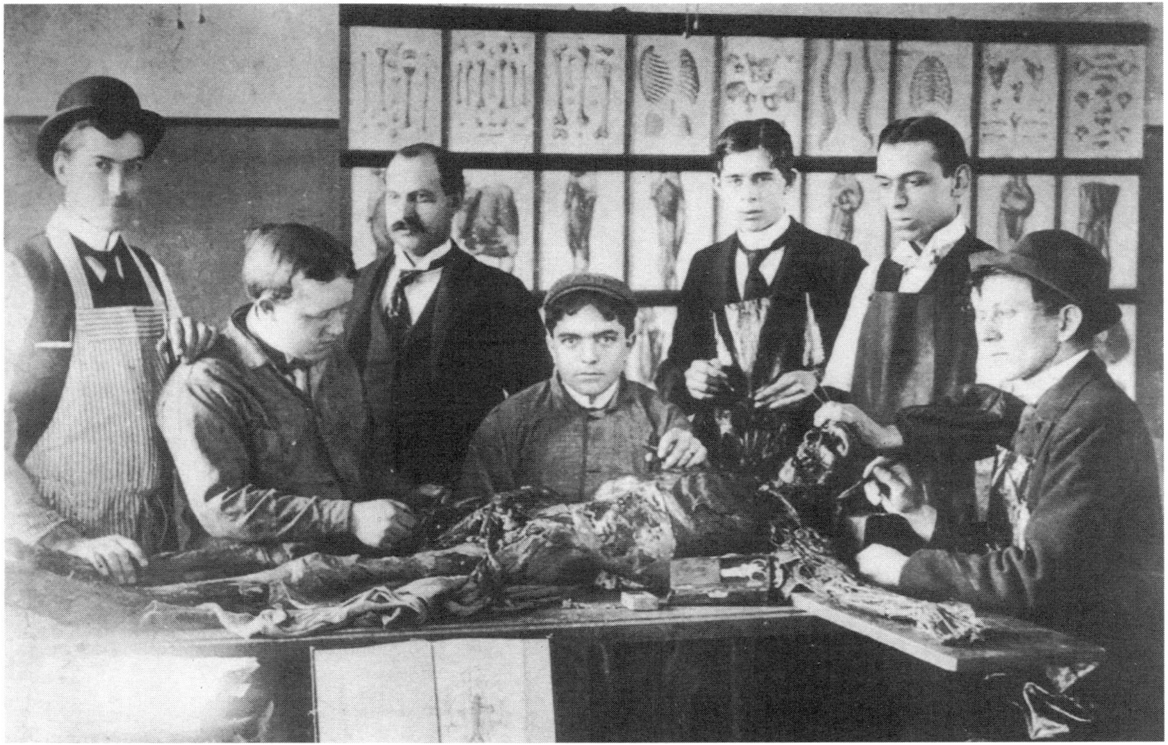

Figure 17. Anatomy class with Dr. Ferris

and more recently Blumer in medicine. Their vision persisted despite almost insurmountable obstacles, above all the apathy and indifference of the central administration and the Yale Corporation. The administration viewed the Sheffield Scientific School as a rival of the medical school with its increasing emphasis on laboratory science. Clearly, the medical school would not thrive in this sea of institutional ambivalence. Something would have to happen if the school were to flower rather than vanish, and 1910 was to become the pivotal year.

4

FLEXNER'S REPORT AND BLUMER'S DEANSHIP

The Defining Years

During an otherwise uneventful Yale Corporation meeting on March 21, 1910, two items of business shaped the future success of the medical school. "The Secretary read the confidential report prepared by Dr. Abraham Flexner on the condition of Yale Medical School,"[1] and later in the meeting "the President spoke of possible changes in the scope of Professor Smith's work in the medical school, but no formal action was taken."[2]

Flexner's report had been prompted by growing discontent with medical education amid a proliferation of proprietary schools across the country. The Council on Medical Education of the American Medical Association approached Henry Pritchett of the Carnegie Foundation for the Advancement of Teaching about conducting a study of medical education in the United States and Canada. Pritchett had been impressed by Flexner's critical review of the American college system and asked him to undertake the study.[3] Flexner, a graduate of Johns Hopkins University, used Johns Hopkins as the benchmark for his survey of American medical schools. Although he was not a physician, his brother, Simon, had trained at Johns Hopkins with Welch and later became director of the Rockefeller Institute for Medical Research.

During 1909 and 1910, Flexner visited every medical school in the United States and Canada. His report, entitled *Medical Education in the United States and Canada*, was published in 1910 as the fourth Bulletin prepared under the auspices of the Carnegie Foundation.[4] It was broad and comprehensive, although questions have been raised about its thoroughness, and it became the impetus for fundamental change in medical education in the United States. Of the 155 medical schools Flexner visited, he deemed only thirty-one worthy of survival. Within a few years following publication of his report, the number of North American medical schools had decreased from 155, about half the total worldwide, to one hundred.

Flexner visited Yale in January 1910. His report read as follows: "General Considerations. . . . As the school now stands, it would, in point of facilities, still have to be classed with the better type of those on the high school basis; for, though it has advanced to a two-year college basis, there has been as yet no corresponding improvement of facilities. In order to deserve the higher-grade student body, which it invites, a more liberal policy ought to be pursued. The laboratory branches ought to be better manned, so that the instructors may create within them a more active spirit. A university department of medicine cannot largely confine itself to routine instruction, certainly, not after requiring two years of college work for admission to its opportunities. For the same reason the clinical facilities should be extended, probably through a more intimate connection with the present hospital. . . . To make these improvements, larger permanent endowment is required. As the school is one of a very few in New England so circumstanced as to have a clear duty and opportunity, it behooves the university to make a vigorous campaign in behalf of its medical department."[5]

Herbert Eugene Smith was dean and professor of chemistry at the medical school during Flexner's visit, having served as dean since 1885. The "changes in the scope of Professor Smith's work" mentioned in the March 1910 corporation minutes referred to his stepping down as dean, paving the way for the appointment of George Blumer. Recruited to Yale from San Francisco in 1906 on the recommendation of William Welch and Harvey Cushing, who was a passionately loyal Yale College alumnus and a Johns Hopkins faculty member, Blumer had received the invitation from Dean Smith to succeed John Slade Ely as professor of medicine the evening before the San

Francisco earthquake, which may have made his decision easier. Blumer had graduated in 1891 from Cooper Medical College in San Francisco and had worked in pathology with Welch at Johns Hopkins and then in Albany before returning to San Francisco. Minutes of the Yale Corporation and correspondence between Harvey Cushing and Yale President Arthur Hadley make it clear that Smith was pushed aside, and that the appointment of Blumer as dean and Smith's retirement were carefully orchestrated.[6] In a January 30, 1910, letter to President Hadley, Blumer wrote, "While we freely admit that it may not be in the best interest of the school to retain Dr. Smith as the Dean, we do believe that he should still hold a professorship."[7] Retiring with an annuity on June 30, 1910, Smith commented that he had "made the choice that seemed to be expected of [him]."[8]

President Hadley had essentially delegated the affairs of the medical school to the highly competent secretary of the university, Anson Phelps Stokes, an independently wealthy Episcopalian minister. Stokes in turn relied heavily on advice from William Welch, who was a loyal Yale College graduate in addition to being founding dean of the Johns Hopkins medical school and a major architect of the modern era in American medicine. On June 20, 1910, the Yale Corporation acted on the following items from its March 21 meeting: "Resolved that the corporation concurs in the opinion of important experts such as Dr. Flexner in his report to the Carnegie Foundation, that there is an unusual opportunity for developing in New Haven a small university medical school of the highest standard and that special conditions make the present a most opportune time for placing the school on a satisfactory and permanent foundation.

"Resolved, that it is important not only in the interest of medical education in the state of Connecticut but of general university reputation and service that the medical school should be adequately endowed and equipped."

"Resolved, that the Corporation approves the purpose of the medical faculty to raise a fund of at least $2 million to commemorate the one hundredth anniversary of the school which was chartered in 1810 and opened in 1813 and pledges hearty support to this movement."[9]

Flexner's identification of Yale and Harvard as the only two medical schools in New England that merited survival clearly had a salutary effect on the Yale administration's view of the medical school's importance. The unsuccessful attempt to recruit Harvey Cushing four years earlier had also helped. President Hadley had previously been influenced by the perception fostered by New York alumni that New Haven was too small to support a medical school. Clinical facilities were considered inadequate given the city's proximity to Boston and New York. Cushing had disagreed: "I see no reason why a school of the first rank, in all of its departments, should not exist in New Haven."[10]

According to the corporation, the most pressing needs for the medical school were an increased endowment, extension of the hospital facilities, and new laboratories. To Blumer, the chief deficiencies of the school were lack of an adequate endowment (the university was contributing only $30,000 a year to the school), lack of clinical material, inadequate house staff, and inadequate laboratory facilities for clinical investigation.[11]

Blumer assumed the deanship on July 1, 1910, with a pledge of "hearty support" from the corporation for the medical school to raise $2 million. The original wording of the resolution had pledged support "in trying to accomplish this," which was strengthened in the final version to "support to this movement." The "hearty support" had limits, however. The corporation was nervous about decreasing enrollment, and it voted not to support the medical faculty's request to increase entrance requirements for the medical school beyond two years of college preparation "until a large increase in endowment [was] assured."[12]

Thus a major capital campaign had to be launched. The campaign opened with an article in the *Yale Alumni Weekly* by Blumer explaining why the medical school needed $2 million. Publication coincided with the hundredth anniversary of the opening of the medical school in 1913, and the university strengthened its case by publishing the results of Abraham Flexner's visit to Yale in the same issue.[13]

But progress in bolstering the school was slow. Within a year of assuming the deanship, Blumer advised Secretary Stokes that "we must either put the school into a satisfactory condition or abandon it. Progress in the development of the medical departments is very rapid in other places, and unless we can do something within a comparatively small number of years, we will be entirely unable to compete with other schools."[14] Blumer softened his complaint five days later, sending Stokes a letter conceding that the university had been generous to the medical school in recent times. Nevertheless, the need for additional faculty was pressing. Blumer submitted an academic budget of $58,828, with a projected deficit of $37,542 for the year, which provided little comfort to the financially wary central administration.

Blumer certainly tried using his good connections for the benefit of the school. A widower, he had remarried into a prominent New Haven family, had joined local and state medical societies, and had been appointed to the

Prudential Committee of the New Haven Hospital Board. At a board meeting of the General Hospital Society of Connecticut in 1911, Blumer proposed that the board "consider the future relation of the Hospital and Medical School."[15] A committee was appointed to work on this proposal and to examine Flexner's report. In his committee report entitled "The Relation of the Medical School to the Hospital," Blumer provided a model for the way the two institutions should interact. In place of lectures or observation, "the student must learn his work by actually doing it himself, under supervision . . . under the ordinary type of American hospital organization, instruction of this kind is impossible." In the most advanced medical schools, Blumer pointed out, fourth-year students actually formed part of the hospital system, working on the medical wards as "clinical clerks."[16] This meant that medical students in the third and fourth years would learn clinical medicine by the same methods used in their preclinical years of laboratory training. Blumer envisioned the kind of medical school–hospital relationship in place today, with a series of hospital divisions, each of which would have a chief responsible for overall care of the patients and for divisional policy. Under the divisional chief would be members of a hierarchical staff, responsible to him and to one another. Blumer admitted that using the wards for teaching purposes would cost more, but "it is in teaching hospitals thus organized that the patient receives the best possible treatment."[17]

Relations with the hospital were the major obstacle that had deterred Harvey Cushing from accepting a position at Yale. He particularly objected to the fact that the university had charge of the wards for only three months, "a condition almost unheard of in other civilized countries."[18] In the hope of luring Cushing from Johns Hopkins to Yale, the system had been changed in 1907 so that the professor of surgery had control of one-quarter of the hospital beds throughout the year. In exchange, the university had provided funds to recruit a hospital pathologist. Medical-school control over interns and medical staff appointments was still lacking, however. A separate university hospital had been discussed within the Yale administration but had been ruled out because of lack of available funds and because New Haven already had a number of hospitals.

In January 1912, Blumer's committee to examine relations between the hospital and the medical school recommended to the directors of the General Hospital Society "that closer relations be established between the Yale Medical School and the New Haven Hospital, and that an increase in continuous service be made, provided a satisfactory financial arrangement can be made between the two institutions."[19] Although both parties would benefit, Blumer had earlier pointed out that the university and the medical school would have to raise the funds needed to build and maintain a laboratory for pathological and clinical work, an estimated $720,000 in all.[20] In return, the medical school would be able to nominate the attending physicians and surgeons and to use the wards for teaching.[21]

The plan was not without its detractors. Francis Bacon, a professor of surgery at the medical school from 1864 to 1877 and an attending surgeon at the hospital until the time of his death in 1911, vehemently opposed it.[22] In 1877 he had resigned from the faculty, though not from the hospital, because of irreconcilable personality differences with the professor of obstetrics and diseases of women and children, Stephen Hubbard, a very difficult individual who was ultimately forced to resign.[23]

Prominent and wealthy, Bacon left an estate of $713,000, which he initially intended to be divided between the hospital and the university.[24] In 1907 he added a codicil that use of the hospital for medical-school teaching should be secondary to patient care. If using the hospital as a means of education were not helpful to the sick, his money would go instead to the Yale College library. Just before he died, he revoked his bequest to the hospital and left the remainder of his estate to Yale College for scholarships. Although Bacon was clearly unhappy with the plan for medical education in the hospital, his distress did not affect his loyalty to Yale College, which received his largesse of $195,000 in 1912. One of the major reasons that an agreement was reached between the hospital and Yale despite Bacon's powerful opposition was that, by 1911, most of the hospital directors were associated in some manner with Yale University.

The ambivalence that had characterized the relationship between the university and the medical school persisted, however. Despite—or perhaps because of—the hospital agreement, the Yale Corporation remained uneasy that the medical school might become a permanent burden on the university's income. The school's deficit in 1912 was about $25,000, and it was predicted to increase the next year. To lessen this drain on university resources, the corporation again voted support to raise $2 million, of which $1.2 million would be used for the medical-school endowment.[25]

The agreement between the hospital and the corporation would lapse if the funds were not raised by July 1, 1914. President Hadley and Eli Whitney, chairman of the hospital board, signed the agreement only a little more than a year before the July 1 deadline. Flexner was sent a copy of the contract and commented that "it is an admirable one, one of the very best that have yet been made in this country to procure for universities the advantages offered by existing hospitals."[26] After a visit to Yale in 1913, Sir William Osler (figure 18) wrote to Secretary Stokes, "That seems a very satisfactory arrangement that you have made with the New Haven Hospital."[27]

Dean Blumer prepared a memorandum, "The Yale Medical School, Its Present Condition and Needs," which was published in 1913 and 1914 for fund-raising purposes.[28] The Rockefeller Foundation through its General Education Board was considered the prime source for the funds needed to amalgamate the medical school with the hospital. Stokes, having asked Flexner to support Yale's approach to the foundation, sent a letter to the General Education Board on April 22, 1914, less than three months before the agreement with the hospital would expire.[29] The letter outlined the reasons for his urgency. If the funds could not be raised by July 1, it was not at all clear that the hospital's board would extend the agreement. Stokes indicated that the university had expected support from the Carnegie Foundation but had been turned down by Andrew Carnegie, despite the recommendation of his foundation directors. In addition, Stokes reported, "a friend forgot her definite assurance" to President Hadley to be part of a small group that would provide $2 million for the medical school. The formal proposal to Rockefeller asked its General Education Board to pledge "at least" $250,000 toward the medical-school endowment, contingent on the university's securing $1 million by July 1, 1914, to fulfill the agreement with the hospital. Further, the foundation should pledge an additional $250,000 toward a second million dollars, to be raised by January 1, 1916.

The General Education Board, however, had resolved to consider aiding medical education only "in so far as it concerns the installation of full-time clinical teaching" and turned down Yale's application.[30] Rockefeller said that if it were to be a source of funds, the medical school would have to institute a full-time clinical program. Convinced by the Johns Hopkins experience, Flexner had persuaded the General Education Board that full-time clinical positions were necessary for medicine to flourish in the United States.[31]

July 1, 1914, was fast approaching, and George Parmly Day, the university treasurer, urgently solicited the support of wealthy donors in the months before the deadline. Despite Herculean efforts hardly any funds had been raised. Harvey Cushing remarked to Day that "the continuance of the school on the old basis is impossible, and its status has been a humiliation to all loyal Yale men who have been aware of the progress in medical education made and in the making elsewhere."[32]

In March 1914, just four months before the deadline, the university began a formal fund drive led by a corporation Committee on Medical School

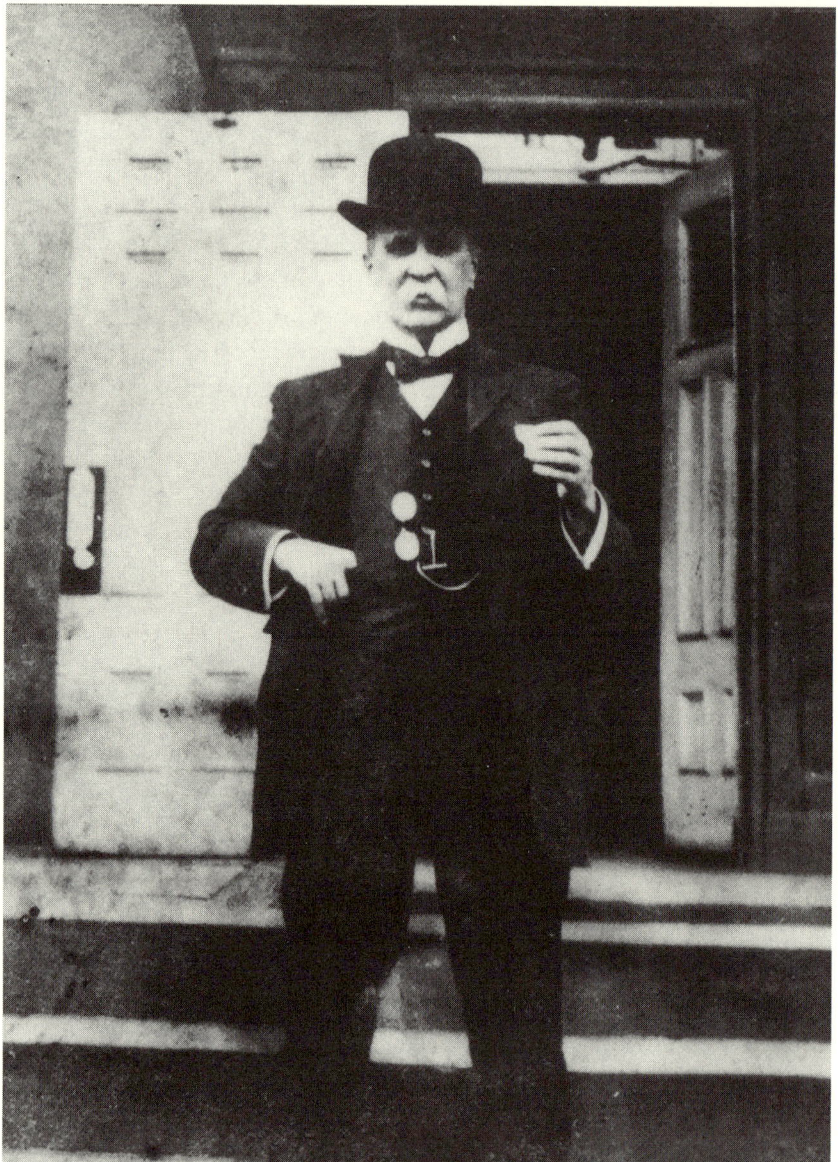

Figure 18. Sir William Osler

Development, composed of physicians who were Yale College graduates. The committee distributed a confidential letter of appeal endorsing the proposed agreement with the hospital and urging "prompt action that the opportunity now open to Yale may not be lost. . . . Not only the future of Yale Medical School, but also to a large extent the future of Yale as a University is now to be decided."[33] There was a long fund-raising road to travel and very little time left. Blumer was becoming anxious: "I do not believe that it will be possible to hold the school together, even in its present state of development, if there are no possibilities of progress . . . the position of dean . . . can hardly be regarded as an attractive one if a condition of stagnation in development takes place."[34] The possibility of asking for an extension of the deadline was discussed but dismissed.

Day wrote a number of masterful letters in an attempt to solicit funds. Two of his friends succeeded in interesting the wealthy philanthropic Brady family in donating $600,000 for the pathology laboratory.[35] The Bradys set aside an endowment of $500,000 in the form of a foundation, the income from which would support the laboratory. If the university successfully raised an additional $2 million, the endowment would go to the university outright. The Harkness brothers, Charles and Edward, each pledged $100,000. The Yale Corporation still wanted to be assured of an endowment large enough to prevent the medical school from being a drain on university funds. Rockefeller's General Education Board, anxious to expand the experiment of a full-time clinical program beyond Johns Hopkins, pledged $500,000 to the medical school if the university agreed to organize the clinical departments on a full-time basis and raised $1.5 million by January 1, 1916.

The notion of full-time academic clinicians was not popular among the medical profession. As the Council on Medical Education of the AMA reported in 1914, "The grotesque plan is proposed that these men may do private practice but that fees from the practice are to be turned into the university treasury. . . . This plan has not been well-received by the clinical teachers and finds its supporters almost entirely among laboratory men."[36]

If academic control of the hospital were achieved, Blumer as professor of medicine and Joseph Marshall Flint, the professor of surgery, were willing to accept the conditions of the full-time clinical system set by Rockefeller's General Education Board, and the other heads of the clinical departments would support them.[37] With a commitment from the General Education Board, the Yale Corporation signed the contract with the hospital, which marked the beginning of the medical school's rise to international prominence. William Welch wrote to President Hadley, "The advantages of the union of the medical school and the university can now be exemplified as never before."[38]

The success in obtaining funding coincided with the medical school's centennial, which was celebrated during the week of June 15, 1914. To commemorate the occasion, honorary degrees were awarded to an exceptional roster of honorees.[39] Doctor of science degrees were conferred on Harvard physiologist Walter B. Cannon, French surgeon and father of transplantation Alexis Carrell, and George Crile, the distinguished endocrine surgeon from Cleveland. Surgeon General William Gorgas, who had made construction of the Panama Canal possible by eliminating yellow fever and malaria from the area, received an honorary doctorate of laws, and Mary Emma Woolley, president of Mount Holyoke College, was awarded an honorary master's degree. Other master's degree recipients were Elliot Joslin, an 1890 Yale College graduate, recognized for his work in diabetes mellitus, and William F. Verdi, who had been instrumental in founding the Hospital of Saint Raphael and was an 1894 graduate of the medical school. Fred Towsley Murphy, a graduate of Yale College and Harvard Medical School and a Yale Corporation member who was to play a key role in the future of the medical school, also received an honorary degree.

A centennial volume carried President Hadley's announcement that "towards the $2,000,000 sought for endowment needed to develop the Yale Medical School, independent of the sum required for the alliance with the Hospital (the $625,000 given by the Brady family), the University has received, as heretofore announced by the General Education Board, an offer from the board of $500,000 conditioned on the remaining $1,500,000 being secured by January 1, 1916, and upon the departments of Medicine, Surgery, and Pediatrics being placed on a full-time university basis."[40] The president went on to say that other pledges had raised all but $900,000 of the $2 million required.

Having voted in June 1914 to thank Rockefeller's General Education Board with the "earnest hope" that the university would be able to meet the conditions of the full-time clinical system, the Yale Corporation appointed a Committee to Consider Full-time Professorships in Clinical Subjects. While this committee was deliberating, Blumer wrote to a number of distinguished individuals at other institutions that had, or were considering, a full-time clinical section.[41] George Dock at Washington University in Saint Louis favored the idea but cautioned that clinical facilities should be excellent and the staff large, expert, and paid sufficiently. Dock was concerned about consultation fees and departmental pooling of funds. Theodore Janeway at Johns

Hopkins ended his letter of response by commenting, "If the university hospital, with its full time staff, cannot teach the art and practice as well as the science of medicine, then the full time plan is going to ruin clinical teaching in this country." David Edsall of Harvard wrote that although uncertain at first, he came to believe that it was the "most satisfactory solution that has been proposed by the situation in clinical medicine and its teaching." Edsall felt that "men with both scientific and clinical training have and will always have . . . a higher market value . . . than the men trained solely in laboratory branches."[42]

The "Report of the Committee on the Full-time Professorship in Clinical Subjects" was positive, finding that "the conditions, therefore, under which the clinical departments of most medical schools are now organized are, from the academic standpoint, decidedly unsatisfactory."[43] To the committee, the full-time plan simply meant that the clinical professor would teach and do research under the same conditions as the academic professor. Various full-time plans were in fact already in existence elsewhere.[44] The Peter Bent Brigham Hospital had put forth a full-time plan that allowed Harvard faculty to see private patients in the hospital, a provision that had been attractive to Harvey Cushing.[45] The plan at Johns Hopkins, where all consultation fees were turned over to the Clinical Fund, was considered the most satisfactory from an academic point of view. The committee felt that if a physician elected an academic career, he should be willing to receive a salary comparable to salaries paid elsewhere in the university. But, reflecting the enduring medical-school commitment to excellence, the committee realized that securing "men of the first rank" was the primary concern and that economy should not interfere with quality. It was also aware that a high salary might lead the hospital or university to exert pressure for more clinical work, decreasing teaching and research time.[46]

Stokes, anxious about cost, proposed to Blumer that $6,000 was a reasonable salary for a full-time clinical professor.[47] Blumer replied that the remuneration of heads of departments had to be sufficient to allow them and their families "to live at a level to which they had been accustomed." In response to the question of whether some full-time professors might receive compensation for consultation work in the hospital, Blumer pointed out that this was the case at Harvard, where Harvey Cushing received $5,000 each from both Harvard and the Peter Bent Brigham Hospital. Large salaries in the medical department might cause dissatisfaction in other schools of the university. Apparently, discontent already existed in the law school. Blumer told Stokes that if the demands set forth by the committee were not met, "the full time scheme must be given up, or it must be modified along the lines of the Harvard plan, or the University must ask for the resignation of the heads of departments who feel they cannot meet its wishes and appoint younger men in their places."[48] Flexner, too, was concerned about salaries, and in reply to him Stokes raised the possibility of the "Cushing solution," which would allow full-time professors to have private consultations within the hospital. Stokes cited the example of professors of engineering, who were allowed outside consultation fees, and professors of theology, who were permitted to take fees for outside preaching.[49]

After discussing the full-time issue with both Flexner and President Hadley, Blumer told Stokes that he had revised his ideas about the full-time concept "materially": "When I stated professional salaries were too low, I did not mean that Yale University was the worst sinner in that respect, nor did I desire to attach any blame to the authorities of the University for this unfortunate state of affairs."[50] During the course of his deanship Blumer periodically vented his frustrations to Stokes. When Stokes chided him, Blumer became contrite and reaffirmed how much the university was doing for the medical school.

The cost of the full-time plan was estimated to be $50,000 a year, which was twice the endowment income that would be provided by the General Education Board's conditional pledge of $500,000. As the difference would have to be made up from general university funds, the committee did not believe that it would be possible "to carry the plan into effect."[51] Once again the Yale Corporation was reluctant to support the medical school financially. Blumer advised Flexner of the shortfall, commenting that "this fact has, I think, alarmed some members of the corporation, and even the President himself, occasionally shows signs of doubt."[52]

Newman Smythe, a fellow of the corporation and a Congregational minister in New Haven, questioned whether Yale should accept the offer of the General Education Board at all, given the conditions attached. He worried that such financial power might be used in the future to secure an educational policy not welcomed by the university. "Stronger Universities like Yale and Harvard should be watchful to resist the beginning of such deflections of education by powerful outside attraction."[53]

Although there were many critics of the General Education Board's rigid insistence on full-time medicine both within and outside the medical school, Blumer commented that "irrespective of any subsidy from the General Education Board, the faculty of the medical school is for the most part strongly in favor of the full-time plan."[54] An editorial in the *Commercial and Financial*

Chronicle stated that the full-time concept would deprive medical faculty of living in the "real world."[55] Welch was asked by Flexner to write a rebuttal but apparently never got round to it. Despite opposition within the corporation, efforts to institute the full-time plan persisted. The General Education Board agreed to give the university until July 1, 1917, to raise the $1.5 million needed to meet the conditions of the grant.

Medical-faculty support for the full-time clinical program formed part of its goal to improve the academic quality of the school. Three months after the hospital agreement had been ratified in 1914, the Executive Committee of the school's Board of Permanent Officers had appointed a committee to consider whether a college degree should be required for entrance to medical school, as had been the case at Johns Hopkins since its inception in 1893. After prolonged deliberation the committee reached the conclusion that two years of college and a four-year medical course would in general suffice for medical practice. A few medical schools should admit students interested in more prolonged training in "the methods of science as applied to clinical medicine." In order for such a plan to be successful, a highly qualified faculty and a high faculty-to-student ratio with adequate resources would be essential. Because fees would be insufficient, a large endowment would be needed to support the program. The committee also discussed what proportion of active clinical work would produce the best results within eight years of combined premedical and medical education. It felt that students with college degrees would be more "mature" and have broader interests. These students, however, would receive an M.D. degree at an age that some committee members thought was too late. Too much time in college was spent in "frivolous pursuits like fraternity politics," and a fourth year of undergraduate education would be wasted. The committee eventually proposed that three years of preparation for medical school was an adequate compromise.[56]

The medical-school curriculum was in "a condition of extreme congestion." If scientific practitioners and teachers were to be developed, there needed to be adequate elective time. Although attempts to introduce electives had been made at Johns Hopkins and Harvard, they had not been entirely successful. The Yale committee's solution, which was never implemented, was to recommend five years of medical school, not including internship, of which 30 percent would be elective or research time. "In a word it combines the best of the American system of developing the average man with the ideal of the German system of concentrating on the exceptional man."

Medical education for women in the United States had begun in 1847, when Elizabeth Blackwell gained admission to Geneva Medical College, although none of the prestigious medical schools immediately followed suit.[57] The first major traditional medical school in the East to admit women was Johns Hopkins in 1893. This landmark event was less due to an enlightened view of women's role in medicine than to financial exigencies. The university and hospital had been founded with the legacy left by Johns Hopkins, but decreases in the endowment and the cost of recruiting faculty like William Halsted and William Osler had left insufficient funds to open the medical school. Elizabeth Garrett offered to donate $500,000 if women were admitted and if four years of undergraduate preparation were required for admission.[58] Osler commented that the experiment of admitting women to medical school was a failure but that the "die was cast."[59]

The question of admitting women medical students to Yale had lain dormant since 1872, when the Prudential Committee of the medical school voted to admit women provided that other schools at Yale were willing to do so. In 1915 the Board of Permanent Officers again discussed the matter and voted to admit women to the medical school if $1,000 could be found for necessary alterations to the physical plant. Bathroom facilities for women would have to be provided. Henry Farnam, professor of economics and a member of the Executive Committee of the hospital board, wrote to President Hadley offering to provide funds for the women's bathroom.[60] His daughter, Louise, a graduate of Vassar and the recipient of a Ph.D. in physiological chemistry from Yale in 1916, wanted to apply to the medical school.

The *Bulletin of the Yale University School of Medicine* for 1916 and 1917 stated that "a limited number of graduates of recognized colleges for women who can meet the special requirements in sciences and languages will be admitted to the school of medicine." Men did not have to be college graduates to apply to the medical school until 1924, and their number was unlimited.

Louise Farnam went on to graduate at the top of her class.[61] She and her classmate, Helen May Scoville, were among only seven students who graduated cum laude.[62] Following graduation, Louise Farnam went to Johns Hopkins for further training and then to China as a faculty member at Yali, a Yale-sponsored medical school in Changsha. She remained there for nine years until driven out by Mao's army in 1930. Other Eastern medical schools began to admit women at about the same time Yale did. The medical school of the University of Pennsylvania had admitted women in 1914, and the medical school at Columbia University began enrolling women in 1917. The Harvard Medical School, however, did not admit women until 1945. The Yale Law School did not officially admit women until 1918.[63] The Yale Divinity School records do not include female matriculants until 1920, at which time there were five women students out of a total enrollment of 111; the divinity-school faculty, however, did not vote until 1932 to admit women to its bachelor's program.[64] The Yale Graduate School of Arts and Sciences, which originated from the Department of Philosophy organized in 1846, was officially established in 1892 and admitted women doctoral students in the same year.

Student educational issues were important, but one of George Blumer's great academic achievements as dean of the medical school was the creation of the Department of Public Health in 1915 with a gift of $500,000 that established the Anna R. Lauder Chair of Public Health. The chair was filled by Charles-Edward Amory Winslow (figure 19), one of the leaders in public health in the United States. Shortly after coming to Yale, Blumer had chaired a committee to consider the establishment of a department or school that would educate individuals to work with public-health bureaus and philanthropic or charitable organizations. Irving Fisher, a professor of political economy at Yale, pointed out that Yale was particularly well equipped to take advantage of the public-health movement because of the combined interests of the medical school, the Sheffield Scientific School, and the Department of Economics. But the Committee on Graduate Education and President Hadley thought the committee's proposed plan for public health was too diffuse, and the recommendations were not implemented.

The newly formed Department of Public Health also offered courses in public health to students in Yale College. The medical school and the Sheffield Scientific School had developed a curriculum leading to a certificate in public health for individuals who had completed a bachelor's degree or two years of medical study.[65] As chairman of the Department of Public Health, Winslow also chaired the new Board of Health of Yale University, which was responsible for the students' health care. The board began its work by examining all students engaged in organized athletics as well as "competitors for the editorial staff of the *Yale Daily News*."[66]

In June 1915, amid all these educational initiatives, financial pressures, and the gathering clouds of World War I, Blumer sent Treasurer Day three sets of plans about the future space needs of the medical school and the hospital.[67] Almost two years later, he informed Hadley that the hospital's requirements still included a new private-room pavilion, a "psychopathic" pavilion, a pavilion for specialties of eye, ear, nose, throat, and skin, as well as an institute for physical therapy, remodeling of the wards, and a nurses' home.[68]

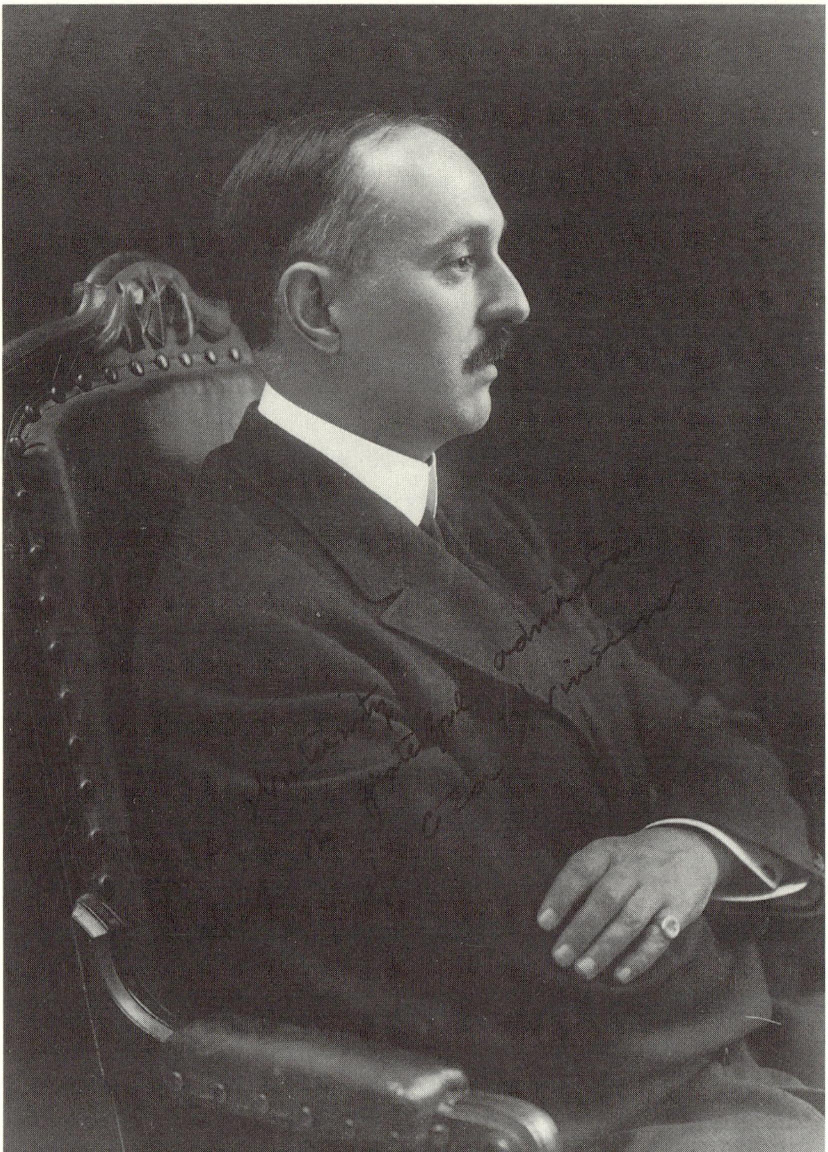

Figure 19. C.-E. A. Winslow

Blumer was convinced that the medical school should remain in the neighborhood of the hospital, because difficulties would arise with the New Haven Hospital Board if the school moved elsewhere. Blumer's plans called for great sums of money for buildings and especially endowment, "for without endowment we cannot have men and without the right kind of men we cannot build up a great institution." The needs of the medical school in 1915 were estimated at $4.75 million for endowments and $3.25 million for buildings and land, a total of $8 million.[69]

Although Blumer's plans presented a majestic vision of what Yale's medical school could become, there was an immediate pressing need to raise $1 million in order to make the school eligible for the Brady endowment and the money promised by the Rockefeller Foundation's General Education Board. The university, after securing funds to solidify the hospital relationship, had once again withdrawn from active support of the medical school. Day raised the specter of dissolution: "In the present state of University finances, it may well prove impossible to continue to make large appropriations from university income to cover the annual deficits in the medical school . . . with the heavy demands from other sources it will no longer be possible for the university to do this without impairing its funds."[70] The very future of the medical school was at stake. With the passage of time, the cost of living had increased as well as the cost of buildings and salaries. Blumer informed Stokes in 1916 that it would require $1 million rather than $500,000 to put the school on a full-time basis. He mentioned that "the appropriation they offered was in any event never large enough."[71]

Blumer pointed out that the nursing situation in the hospital and dispensary was also critical. The Connecticut Training School for Nurses was urgently in need of funds to upgrade its educational program. For the university to provide a suitable nurses' training school, $750,000 would be required. "I present these figures for your consideration, because I think it would be better to fail than to half-way succeed, and I believe large plans often appeal to donors more than small ones." He ended his letter to Stokes by saying, "It is very trying for the Medical School to have to go on year after year hanging on, so to speak, by the skin of its teeth and it is equally trying for the University to have to go on year after year providing for the Medical School out of the income of its General Funds."[72]

Stokes replied that although the fund-raising campaign had been temporarily held up, he was sure the necessary money would be raised. He went on to say that it was discouraging to find the cost of medical education increasing by leaps and bounds. Blumer pointed out that the medical faculty had never been consulted about the funds needed for full-time clinical professorships and that he was not in favor of adopting the full-time plan unless it could be done properly.[73] Stokes indicated that if the endowment were not raised, there would have to be serious discussion of limiting the work of the medical school. Blumer found the possibility unacceptable: "The effect on the faculty would be most deplorable."[74] Yale could have either a two-year medical school or a first-class school in the preclinical years and a second-class school in the clinical years as currently constituted. The latter was not tenable. Yale would have a two-year medical school unless the necessary endowment were raised.

This scenario never came to pass. The opposition of the Yale Corporation to the full-time concept dissipated, and on April 16, 1917, it passed the following resolution: "Voted, that the Corporation commits itself to the continuance of the full four-year medical course; and to the option of the full-time basis in all departments of the medical school as soon as the necessary endowment is secured, and urges that every possible effort should be made by the administrative officers of the University to secure . . . the additional endowment fund."[75] Stokes wrote to Flexner of his delight at the resolution, which committed the corporation to medical education. "I have been very much troubled by the attitude of two permanent members of the Corporation who have been more or less hostile to the full-time plan, and one of them even in favor of our confining ourselves to pre-clinical instruction."[76]

By June 1917 the university could announce unconditional gifts and pledges of $1,067,100 toward the $1.5 million needed to secure the contingent pledges of $500,000 each from the Brady family and the General Education Board. America had entered World War I by this time, and by including pledges for the Yale Mobile Military Hospital and bequests, the university could meet the conditions. Because these latter gifts were not within the provisions of the General Education Board award, however, the amount still required to reach the goal was $322,000. This shortfall was occurring at a time when Yale faced a war deficit of more than $250,000. Fortunately, once again the angels appeared. The Carnegie Foundation for the Advancement of Teaching promised $250,000, and the General Education Board increased its original pledge by $82,900 to make up the total Yale needed to qualify for the award.[77]

In addition to feeling discouraged at the lack of university support, Dean Blumer, who was also chairman of the Prudential Committee of the hospital board, was glum about the hospital. He had become chairman when Harry G. Day, a Yale graduate and member of the Yale Corporation, developed tuberculosis and went to the Trudeau Sanatorium at Saranac Lake. During the influenza pandemic of 1918, the hospital had treated one thousand patients. An entire ward in the isolation pavilion was filled with nurses who had contracted the illness. Despite this great influx of patients, the hospital still ran a deficit of $16,000. Blumer told George Day that sitting as chairman of the hospital's Prudential Committee while he was dean was a conflict of interest, but Day replied, "I do not know what either the Hospital or the University would do if you were not willing to continue to act as you have done in caring for the interests of both institutions."[78]

Before Yale could sign the contract with the General Education Board, the agreement between the university and the hospital had to be amended to permit reorganization of the wards for full-time teaching. The hospital directors were sympathetic and voted unanimously in favor of the full-time concept on May 1, 1918, declaring that "the control required by the General Education Board's offer is desirable in the interest of the hospital." Blumer prepared the ground for the full-time clinical program in an article about the success of the fund drive. "The necessity for teachers of the medical sciences giving their whole time to their work has been conceded for the past 20 years. The necessity for teachers in the clinical branches occupying a similar position is a principle which is now being fought for." The full-time plan could not be implemented formally, however, until the faculty members returned from the war.[79]

Blumer outlined the changes that had occurred during his tenure as dean, including the reorganization of the Department of Pathology and Bacteriology and the Department of Obstetrics and Gynecology as well as the development of the Department of Public Health. Pathology had been a particular problem. In February 1917 Blumer and the Executive Board of the medical school informed President Hadley that a complete reorganization of the Department of Pathology was imperative. The chairman had to be replaced; Charles J. Bartlett was incapable of first-class research and was an uninspiring teacher. There was a need to develop departments of pediatrics, psychiatry, and orthopedics. Blumer also emphasized the importance of nursing and social work to the medical school, and he pointed out as well the need for a new medical-school building with modern laboratories close to the hospital.[80]

Blumer was convinced that the full-time proposal would meet with opposition from physicians trained under the traditional rotating system. The disappearance of rotating control of the wards would put the community physicians at a distinct disadvantage. To smooth the path, Stokes suggested in December 1917 that a confidential report on hospital organization and administration would be of great value. He recommended Winford Smith, superintendent of the Johns Hopkins Hospital, which was operating on a full-time clinical model.[81] Smith's opinion was devastating: "The New Haven Hospital at the present time judged by modern standards is a poor hospital, due to faulty organization, faulty administration, lack of endowment, and old, poorly equipped, and poorly planned hospital buildings." He made a number of recommendations and stressed that "an alternating service composed of men who are not teachers is bad and absolutely impossible in a teaching hospital."[82]

All the issues facing the medical school were compounded by the entry of the United States into World War I in April 1917. The Yale medical faculty answered the call to arms and mobilized for war. Joseph Flint, who had served as a surgeon for a summer in an Athens hospital during the Greco-Bulgarian War and for six months in a French military hospital at Passy, conceived of a mobile hospital unit manned by Yale personnel.[83] Flint was largely responsible for its formation and organization, with the help of the Yale Corporation, which voted $50,000 for the preliminary equipping of a mobile military hospital to be organized by the medical faculty. In June 1917 the corporation announced a gift of $200,000 to equip the hospital under the command of Flint, with the proviso that the unit be sent to France as soon as possible, for use by the French military authorities until they transferred it to the Americans.

Besides being the commanding officer of the Yale Mobile Hospital (figure 20), Flint was responsible for obtaining the finances to support it during the year and a half it was in France.[84] The mobile unit consisted of surgical tents, X-ray equipment, sterilizing apparatus, and stretchers, arranged for easy transportation in fourteen trucks. The purpose of the unit was to treat the wounded sooner than they would be if they were first transported to ordinary stationary base hospitals. The unit was composed of forty physicians and nurses, as well as civilian personnel, including fifty Yale College graduates, among them Archibald MacLeish, Class of '15. President Hadley mentioned in his 1917 report that the mobile hospital gave students an opportunity both to render service in the field and to obtain instruction from Yale faculty. He went on to say, "The activity of the Yale Medical School on many lines of war service has already justified the faith of the Corporation in its future and the very considerable expenditures of money which that body has made without prospect of immediate return."[85]

To aid the war effort, a Yale Committee on Research was formed in 1917 to cooperate with the National Research Council; Russell Chittenden of the Sheffield Scientific School served as chairman, and Charles-Edward Amory Winslow was the medical-school representative. The National Academy of

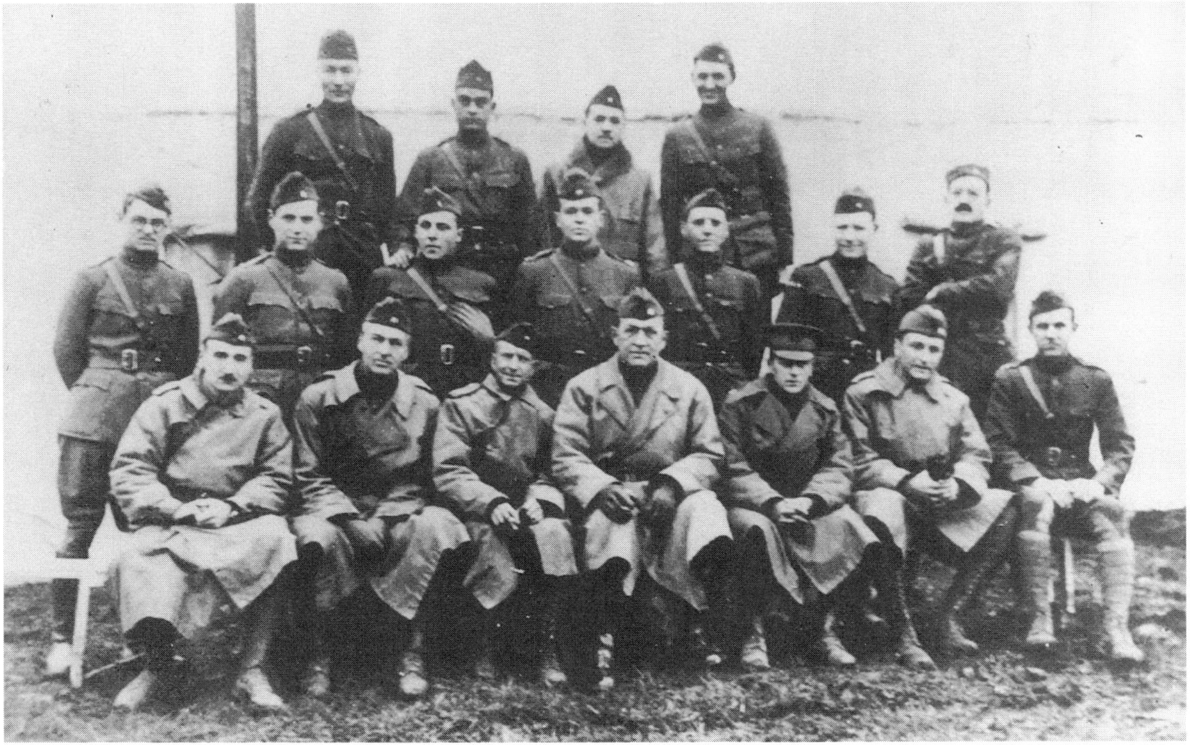

Figure 20. World War I: the 39th Mobile Hospital

Sciences had organized all the scientific resources of the country for war, and the National Research Council had been formed to deal with the issues. Yale's medical faculty duly responded to the need for scientists for military purposes.

The introduction of poison gas in warfare by the Germans led to the development of the Chemical Warfare Service within the War Department. The Bureau of Mines had had a great deal of experience dealing with poison gases and was in a good position to investigate the gases used in war. Yandell Henderson, who had been a consultant to the bureau, was placed in charge of the United States Board of Gases in Warfare and in turn recruited Milton Winternitz, Henry Barbour, and Frank Underhill from the medical school.[86] Winternitz had come to Yale from Johns Hopkins in 1917 shortly before the United States entered the war, but was fully involved with Henderson's poison-gas program and was chief instructor in pathological laboratory histology for the laboratory school.

The laboratory training school was housed in a temporary building—the "Barracks"—near Brady Laboratory. The university purchased the former private Elm City Hospital, which eventually became a Yale School of Nursing dormitory, for the use of the government and transformed it into a gas laboratory. Winternitz was in charge of a similar war gas laboratory in Washington and traveled to Washington each Sunday, then to a gas plant in Lakewood, New Jersey, on Tuesday, and back to New Haven for Thursday, Friday, and Saturday, where he taught and directed research.

By the 1918–1919 school year, all medical students not in the fourth year were required to enlist in the Students' Army Training Corps. According to Blumer, "The Students' Army Training Corps furnished an experience in medical education which neither the students nor faculty would care to repeat." It demonstrated that "medicine and militarism do not only not mix but will not even make a decent emulsion."[87] The experience did, however, highlight the medical students' lack of training in public health. So many of the medical faculties across the country had joined the war effort that the suggestion had seriously been made to put all the medical schools under the control of the Surgeon General's Office. World War I was seen as "the war to end all wars," and Yale's medical school had been fully committed to it, although there was some concern about a militaristic approach to medical education, which was to recur in World War II. After the war, on August 24, 1919, the medical school submitted the first federal grant application ever made by the university. It was to the United States Inter-departmental Social Hygiene Board and contained four proposals on various aspects of venereal disease, requiring a grant totaling $8,000. Three of the four proposals were successful, with grants going to the surgery, pathology, and bacteriology departments. President Hadley had definite reservations about the propriety of receiving a grant of this kind from the government. Hadley believed that such money was not well used and that, as a rule, money for local needs should be raised locally. He expressed this sentiment to Josephus Daniels, chairman of the Social Hygiene Board, who was in the process of requesting $2.5 million from Congress.[88] The adverse consequences of opposition from a man of Hadley's stature was pointed out to Blumer.[89] Hadley finally allowed the grant, but only because he considered venereal disease a major problem.

By the beginning of the 1919–1920 academic year, the Department of Surgery and the Department of Obstetrics and Gynecology had full-time staffs, with a single chief who was also a full-time professor at the medical school and salaried accordingly. The Department of Pediatrics would not be organized for another year. Blumer, the school's first full-time professor of medicine as well as dean, indicated that all the clinical branches had adequate house staffs. For the first time, the full-time medical-school faculty had complete control of the hospital's public wards.[90] As community physicians no longer had control, they were to cause difficulties in the future by not admitting patients to New Haven Hospital.

The hospital had been founded by physicians in 1826 in part to serve as an "auxiliary" to the Medical Institution of Yale College in order to foster the teaching of clinical medicine. This commitment of the hospital to medical education was renewed with the development of the full-time clinical system. As a result of the 1918 report by Winford Smith, superintendent of the Johns Hopkins Hospital, the hospital's Prudential Committee expanded and became known as the Executive Committee, which excluded both community and faculty physicians. Subsequently, three members of the Yale Corporation were appointed members of the Executive Committee. Physicians were represented by the Medical Board, which was created to advise the Executive Committee on professional policy and consisted of the full-time heads of the hospital departments of medicine, pathology, surgery, and obstetrics and gynecology.

The disruption the war had caused within the hospital and the medical school hampered the effort to raise endowment and implement the full-time plan. The magnitude of the influenza epidemic further aggravated the situation, and the hospital was finding itself in ever-greater financial difficulty. A Committee on finance for the hospital, which had been formed in response to the critical review of the hospital by Winford Smith, delivered a report in January 1919.[91] Henry L. Galpin, representing the Union and New Haven Trust Company, stated in November 1918 that the hospital was virtually bankrupt.[92]

Blumer considered finances to be the hospital's major problem. The medical school's ability to nominate the superintendent of the hospital would help, but no one would take the job given the hospital's current financial status. In January 1919 Blumer wrote to Secretary Stokes, "If the plan ultimately succeeds, we shall have sacrificed the best years of our lives for the benefit of the succeeding generation. . . . I am very pessimistic . . . as regards adequate support being obtained from New Haven."[93] Several weeks later, Blumer told Stokes, "I am also decidedly in doubt as to the advisability of the University actually taking control over the New Haven Hospital."[94] Blumer went on to reiterate that taking over the hospital would not be necessary if the university had "complete control of nominations," including that of the superintendent, and if the Executive Committee of the hospital were controlled by individuals sympathetic to the university.

The difficulties were heightened by the perception on the part of the hospital administration that the decreased bed census was partially due to the new arrangement with the university. Colonel Isaac M. Ullman, chairman of the hospital Executive Committee, asked Stokes what "improvements" had been made in the services of New Haven Hospital since the contract with the university had been signed in 1913. In a three-page reply, Stokes cited better care of patients, better records, a better X-ray department, and improvements in pathology, surgery, and obstetrics and gynecology. "The use of the hospital for teaching purposes . . . can only justify itself, in the last analysis, by improvement of the resulting service to the Hospital."[95] To assuage any concern the hospital might have about a university takeover, Stokes assured Ullman that during his twenty years as secretary the only matters to come before the Yale Corporation regarding the New Haven Hospital had been appointments and terms of agreements.

There were no doubt discussions within the Yale administration as to whether the university should try to assume control of the hospital or terminate the agreement after ten years, but the topic was never brought to the corporation for a vote. In April 1919 Stokes informed Ullman that the corporation had endorsed the full-time clinical concept and had established a committee to see what the university might do to help the hospital. "The University is increasingly concerned that the welfare of the New Haven Hospital and of the Medical School are intimately related and has determined to do all in its power to cooperate with the citizens of New Haven in building up a group of institutions for the treatment of disease that will be superior to anything in New England outside of Boston."[96]

There was concern in the medical school not only about the hospital but also about the university. As part of what was termed "Reorganization of the University" in 1919, a new scheme of university-wide departments was inaugurated, and the Board of Permanent Officers was apprehensive about its effect on the medical school. The board recommended that deliberations of the medical faculty, including discussions about the budget, should be carried out under the dean of the medical school. To counteract a drift toward the college, the board thought that the various preclinical sections should be grouped together and be located near the hospital. Facilities for investigation were necessary because students must learn at least the methods of research, for every patient they, as clinicians, see presents problems that require investigation. Clinical sections of the medical school obviously required close affiliation with the hospital, which would have added benefits because donors would be assured that their contributions would serve a triple purpose—the care of the sick, the instruction of students, and the advancement of medical knowledge.

In response to an announcement that the General Education Board would distribute $20 million for medical education, Blumer prepared a "Memorandum to the Yale Corporation on the Development of the Yale Medical School." Although he also noted favorable factors, Blumer emphasized the problems. Among the unfavorable points he mentioned was the opposition to the full-time plan for clinical instructors. "The progress of the Hospital and consequently of the Medical School is now delayed by the open antagonism of the medical profession and its friends." He went on to make the point that physicians trained under the traditional system "bitterly resent the loss of their vested interests. . . . Success of the full-time system will depend on full financial support of the educational foundations which are convinced of the wisdom of the principles involved."[97]

Blumer indicated that the multiplicity of organizations participating in clinical work—hospital, nurses, dispensary, and so forth—was a drawback; "with all these incoordinate agencies inclined to give rather than receive direction, progress is greatly retarded." The new arrangement whereby the hospital's Medical Board reported to the Executive Committee of the hospital was also a problem. "The assumption of arbitrary powers by the laymen with lack of consideration for the opinion of the Medical Board and want of sympathy with the teacher can only result in loss of efficiency and impaired morale. The methods of the political caucus are not applicable to successful hospital management."

Blumer expressed concern that the hospital appointments were annual, with no assurances of renewal to the faculty. "The Directors of the Hospital may terminate the services of a useful teacher without considering the fact that they are sacrificing University Privileges and Principles." Despite these problems, the Medical Board did not feel that a new hospital was needed. "Such a step we believe was uncalled for."[98] There was a strong sense, however, that the Yale Corporation and the directors of the New Haven Hospital had to operate in unison to promote the interests of the medical school.

Blumer also considered the development of the nurses' training school an essential factor in the requirements of the medical school. "Efficient nursing not only promotes the comfort of the patient but is fundamental to the efficacy of the treatment the physician prescribes." The Medical Board thought that the nursing profession had grown beyond the hospital and required a position as dignified as other professional schools. The Yale Corporation had approved a school of nursing as a department of the university in May 1918, on certain conditions.

Blumer included a strong statement to the effect that the university should resolve its ambivalence toward the medical school: "The moral support of the University will be assured only when there is no longer an expressed or implied doubt on the part of the University Authorities regarding the wisdom of supporting the Medical School." Blumer ended the memorandum with a challenge. "The University should be given a free hand in the selection of men to administer the school: and your Board favors the resignation of all members of the present faculty as the ideal method of attaining this result."

The memorandum recommended that:

1. the hospital, dispensary, and Nurses' Training School be unified in a way to ensure university control;
2. the preclinical sections, including physiological chemistry, which was located in Sheffield Scientific School, be located on Cedar Street;
3. sections of pediatrics and neuro-psychiatry and a nursing school be developed;
4. "the best personnel available be chosen to effect the full-time plan and bring it success";
5. the corporation express its intent to support and finance the medical school;
6. the university should ask the General Education Board for almost $5 million.

This was a truly remarkable document. The Board of Permanent Officers was asking the Yale Corporation to take over the hospital's board and bring the hospital, the dispensary, and the Connecticut Nurses' Training School under university control, as well as asking for the resignation of the entire medical faculty and hiring back only the best. Having struggled for years in a hand-to-mouth existence, donating their own earnings to keep the medical school solvent, the faculty members had been encouraged by the Flexner report. Academic control of the hospital, construction of the Brady Laboratory, and the full-time clinical plan were a reality. But the faculty found "Camelot" ruled by a lay hospital board that did not understand academic medicine, a clinical enterprise with different organizations working against each other to deliver health care, and a university persistently ambivalent about supporting a medical school.

With the faculty morale low and student enrollment falling off, a meeting was held in June 1919 at Secretary Stokes's office. Blumer, unable to attend, wrote a memorandum venting his frustration: "American Universities are obsessed with the importance of organizations . . . the important things in any branch of a university are not organizations but teaching and research. Let this idea simmer in your brainpans for a while. . . . No attempts to improve the quality of the students will be necessary if the quality of the school improves. . . . One of the dangers of the full-time clinical plan is that it will result in a breed of clinicians who will not be in touch with the profession in the surrounding country. The description of scientific work done by the school has been featured from time to time in the annual report of the President. Unfortunately, very few people read the annual report of the President."[99]

In a recurring drama, the hospital edged toward bankruptcy once more. The full-time clinical issue was a significant contributing factor, as the community physicians boycotted the hospital in protest. In May 1920 the hospital's board voted to hold a special meeting "to consider what action shall be taken if it appears impossible because of financial conditions to continue operation of the hospital under the existing contract with Yale University."[100] The meeting was never held, but matters were grave. The university again turned to the General Education Board, with George Day stressing that "the future of the New Haven Hospital seems in jeopardy. The adequate maintenance of this hospital is essential to clinical instruction in Yale Medical School. Unless relief can be found from some source in the near future, a serious curtailment, possibly an entire breakdown may occur in the clinical opportunities of the school."[101]

Blumer and George Towsley Murphy, a supportive member of the Yale Corporation, met with Flexner to obtain his support for funding from the General Education Board.[102] Blumer reported that the university would have to continue supporting the medical school financially. Flexner responded aggressively that if the university did not intend to back up its medical school, he did not see how they could ask the General Education Board to do so. Blumer had the impression that Flexner thought the proposed budget for the school was "financially impracticable," rather than extravagant. Previously, Flexner had mentioned to Stokes that Yale's proposed medical-school budget was larger than that of Johns Hopkins, which had a student body four times the size and twice the number of hospital beds.[103]

The General Education Board had little choice. Collapse of the full-time clinical plan in New Haven would have greatly strengthened opponents of such plans throughout the country. The board's appropriation of $1 million contingent on Yale raising $2 million helped the New Haven Hospital over the immediate crisis and provided the time needed to increase the hospital's endowment.[104] The board allowed $50,000 a year of the interest on the gift to be paid to the hospital to support the educational process.[105] The money was earmarked for extra house officers and nurses, ten to fifteen free beds for special cases, and utilities and animal care at Brady Laboratory.

After dealing with continual crises for ten years, George Blumer decided to step aside as dean in 1920. He also submitted his resignation as chairman of the Department of Medicine, transferring from the John Slade Ely Professorship to the David Paige Smith Professorship. In his letter to President Hadley, Blumer mentioned that the question of his "fitness" to hold the full-time professorship in medicine had been raised at an open meeting of the Board of Permanent Officers in 1918, and that he had accepted the professorship only after he had received the board's formal approval. Blumer went on to say that if he had been choosing a full-time professor in 1918, he would not have chosen himself, but he had accepted the position in order to implement the full-time plan and because "the school was only just seeing daylight after passing through a critical period under my administration." Blumer felt that he did not have the training necessary to combine research with medical practice on a full-time basis, as the chairman was committed to do under the new plan.[106]

In a letter to Flexner, Blumer explained that "I had no college education, that the instruction which I received in the pre-clinical sciences, was a farce, and that I have never been able to fill the gaps in my training. I feel that a full-time chair so important should be filled by a very much younger man who has been thoroughly trained both in the pre-medical and pre-clinical sciences."[107] Flexner sent the letter to his brother Simon, director of the Rockefeller Institute for Medical Research, who replied, "I think he is right, not so much perhaps because of imperfect early training as because of a certain slowness of mental movement, which was characteristic of him in Baltimore, fully twenty-five years ago. He was the substantial kind with a narrow range. Hence he did not really keep up with the forward strides of medicine along the more exact sciences."[108]

In his final report to the president, Blumer gave credit to the administrative officers of the university for their "unremitting efforts" on behalf of the medical school. Certainly Secretary Stokes and Treasurer Day had been the driving forces in raising money for the school. Investments between 1910 and 1923 grew tenfold to $2.8 million. The annual contribution from the university during this period increased from $15,000 to $75,000 and the medical-school budget from $43,000 to $225,000. Blumer considered the reorganization of the Department of Pathology and the Department of Obstetrics and Gynecology as the most important accomplishments during his tenure as dean, along with the creation of the Department of Public Health and the Department of Experimental Medicine. "Pathology is the great link between the pre-clinical and clinical departments and is one of the most important subjects in the curriculum. The School was fortunate in obtaining Professor Milton C. Winternitz to head this department."[109]

The success that came later to the medical school was based on the solid accomplishments of George Blumer in his ten years as dean, during which time he was also chairman of the Department of Medicine. Reaching agreement with the hospital was the defining event that led to the full-time clinical plan, the Brady Laboratory, and an increased endowment. These achievements were the cornerstone on which the spectacular advances of subsequent years were constructed. Although he felt frustrated when he left the deanship, Blumer deserves far greater credit than he has so far received. Stokes and Day had been convinced by Blumer's vision of the medical school and had sought the funds necessary for its implementation. President Hadley played little part in Blumer's accomplishments and was not generally supportive of the medical school. Although the financial support from the university that the medical school so desperately needed came sporadically and often at the last moment, the support was absolutely crucial for the school's survival.

A news release from the office of Anson Phelps Stokes on March 1, 1920, perhaps best summed up the contributions of George Blumer as dean: "Dr. Blumer was chosen Dean in 1910 and his administration covers by far the most important period in the whole history of the School."[110]

5

"A STEAM ENGINE IN PANTS"

The Boom Years

At a meeting of the Faculty of the Yale Medical School held on May 7, 1920, the following action was taken for transmission to the Corporation. Voted to nominate Professor Milton Charles Winternitz to the Corporation as Dean of the medical school for a period of five years."[1] The new dean was a man who evoked strong emotions. He was described by his friends and colleagues as a "vital and vivid man, an intense fountainhead of energy, an inexhaustible generator of ideas and constant stimulator of the imagination." Others, while acknowledging his accomplishments, portrayed him as a "martinet," "a terrible little guy who dissipated the financial resources of the school on impractical schemes."[2]

During his fifteen years as dean, Winternitz firmly brought the medical school into the fold of the university by assuring that the medical faculty met the university's academic standards and by reorganizing medical-school departments as university departments. Under his firm hand, the full-time system for clinical teachers was hammered into place. He tirelessly raised funds for buildings and facilities. Winternitz believed strongly in all he did, but he was particularly adamant that medical students should be treated as graduate students—a view that led to the creation of the "Yale system" of medical education.

Accomplishments of this magnitude cannot occur without cost, especially when achieved in so short a time. Diplomacy in human relations was not always one of Winternitz's strengths. Levin Waters, a pathologist trained by and devoted to Winternitz, took the view that "though his methods may continue to evoke controversy, there will always be agreement that Winternitz was the right man in the right place at the right time for the Yale School of Medicine."[3] John Fulton, physiologist, medical historian, and friend of Winternitz, described him as "of Napoleonic temperament and stature and a thoroughgoing autocrat but honest as the day is long and possessed of a broad and sympathetic nature."[4]

Milton Charles Winternitz was born in 1885 in East Baltimore, the son of an immigrant doctor from Czechoslovakia. The Winternitz family was part of the Jewish community in Baltimore but was not particularly religious and did not attend synagogue. Winternitz repeatedly recounted growing up in "moderately straitened circumstances." But they could not have been too "straitened," as his father sent his shirt collars to Paris to be properly laundered![5] Winternitz's granddaughter, Susan Cheever, recounted that as he became more successful, his childhood was made out to be increasingly sordid and difficult.[6]

Winternitz was four when the Johns Hopkins University School of Medicine opened its doors in East Baltimore in 1893, four years after the founding of the Johns Hopkins Hospital. Growing up near the medical school must have been a powerful influence on a neighborhood boy whose father was a doctor. Hopkins's founding dean, pathologist William Henry Welch, had brought the excitement of German scientific medicine to the young school, which was to become the model for modern medical education in the United States. Despite his claims of poverty, Winternitz was financially secure enough during his medical-school years to visit the University of Chicago, where an effort had been undertaken to make medicine a part of the School of Biological Sciences. Perhaps this influenced his future thinking. He published his first paper, on the enzyme adenase, while in his second year of medical studies. An outstanding student, he applied for a house-staff position in surgery under William Halsted, but he was turned down and went to work with Welch in pathology (figure 21).[7] Welch, a Connecticut native

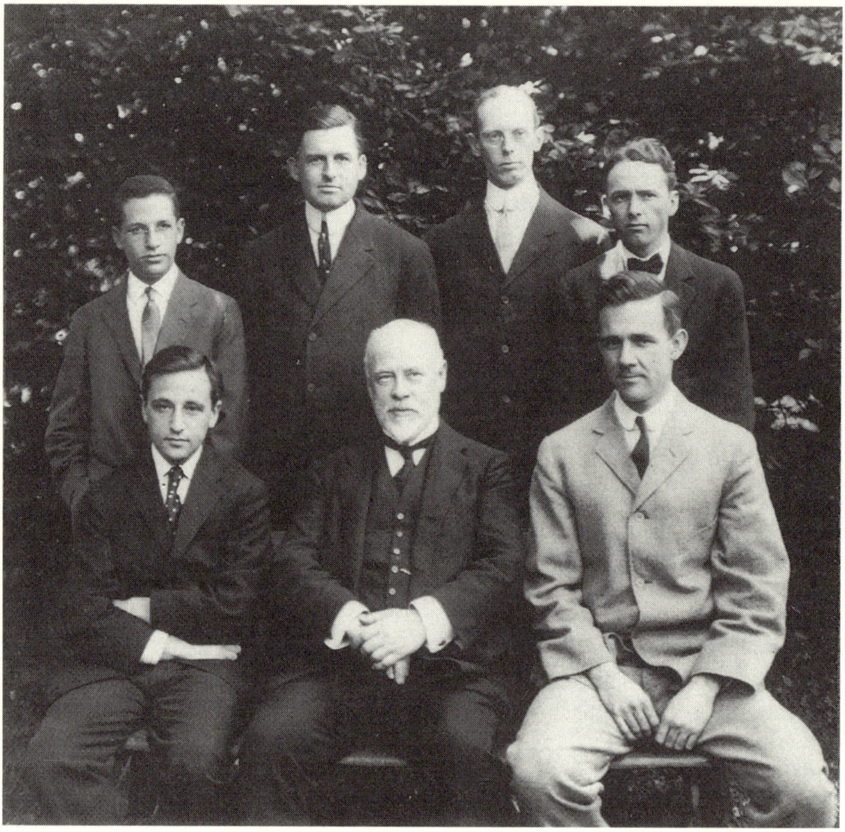

Figure 21. Welch and Winternitz (front row: center and right)

and a staunch Yale alumnus, was a dynamic and stimulating teacher. Winternitz was enthralled with Welch as a role model, followed him into pathology, and was awarded a teaching position at Hopkins.

As Welch was in constant demand and traveled frequently, junior members of the faculty were often asked to fill in as lecturers at the last minute, and Winternitz developed a capacity for "extemporaneous elegance." Like his mentor, he also made a number of trips, including several short visits to Leipzig, Berlin, Freiburg, and Vienna. Despite his idolization of Welch, Winternitz developed a very different teaching style. Whereas students described Welch as "a kindly and infinitely wise old gentleman" who went out of his way to be helpful, they saw Winternitz as a martinet who taught by terrorism. John Paul, who had been a second-year medical student at Johns Hopkins, could not understand how "Welch tolerated him as a member of his Department, for even as long as a decade."[8]

Winternitz was a man of many facets. Susan Cheever described her grandfather as a "a short man with a tyrannical manner, an intense charm that could make you feel that you were the only person in the world—and a raging temper that could make you wish you weren't." He utilized his great charm to attract and marry Helen Watson, whom he pursued with "the sweetness of a kitten and the ferocity of a lion."[9] A Wellesley graduate and a medical student at Johns Hopkins, she was beautiful, smart, Protestant, and the daughter of Thomas Watson, who with his friend Alexander Graham Bell had invented and developed the telephone. Overcoming formidable obstacles, Helen Watson and Milton Winternitz were married in 1913.

Winternitz had hoped to remain at Johns Hopkins and eventually succeed Welch as chairman of pathology. But this was not to be. Several authors have attributed Winternitz's ultimate lack of success at Hopkins to anti-Semitism.[10] Welch told Thomas Watson at a chance meeting that Winternitz was entirely capable of succeeding him but that his scientific contributions, although of high quality, were not yet voluminous enough. Watson relayed Welch's comments: "Age he intimated was the only objection against your election."[11] Being Jewish would not have helped his chances, but there were clearly other reasons why Winternitz was not chosen to succeed Welch.

It was almost certainly on Welch's recommendation that Winternitz was appointed professor of pathology at Yale in 1917.[12] He was the first Jewish professor at the medical school, and Dan Oren recounts that to the disappointment of many, "Winternitz rejected Jews, Judaism, and Jewish associations in his drive for achievement." Oren has described him as "almost a caricature of the American Jew striving to become part of the gentile society." He had married a non-Jew and, when she died, took a second wife who was gentile. Some Jewish colleagues saw him as the "most anti-Semitic person on the faculty. He hated them."[13] Others could find no evidence of anti-Semitism in their relations with him.[14] Winternitz's "anti-Semitism" was certainly in evidence during the course of his deanship with regard to medical-school admissions.

Winternitz himself encountered prejudice when he moved to New Haven and wanted to buy a house on Prospect Street. The local residents sought unsuccessfully to block the sale because of his Jewish background. When Winternitz was appointed dean in 1920, he was proposed for membership of the Graduate Club, the semiofficial faculty club, but was rejected. Twenty-five letters were sent in his behalf, including one from William Howard Taft, former president and soon to be chief justice. George Dudley Seymour, a Yale alumnus and later fellow of Berkeley College, wrote to Taft thanking him: "I am rather amused to find myself in the position of carrying the 'banner of the Jew,' but it did seem a shame to betray the original purpose of founding the Club and to embarrass the University, also to throw any more stumbling blocks in the way of the solution to the very difficult problem of the Hospital and the Medical School."[15] Yale President Hadley, too, provided a letter of support and proposed that Winternitz be invited to become a member of the club as dean of the medical school, unless there were stronger objections than "the fear that the Hebrew element in the Club may become too large."[16]

Winternitz was scheduled to start at Yale just as America entered the Great War. Welch attempted unsuccessfully to delay Winternitz's departure in order to have him work with the Hopkins medical unit. Winternitz arrived at Yale as chair of a pathology department in a medical school that was deeply involved in the war effort. Yandell Henderson, the professor of physiology, who had been a consultant on gases for the Bureau of Mines, enlisted Winternitz's aid in the war gas project. With a flair for organization that was to serve him well, Winternitz established a center for the biological study of war gases as well as an army training school for laboratory medicine. In 1920 he published a monograph on the results of these studies, *Collected Studies on the Pathology of War Gas Poisoning*.[17] That same year he published *The Pathology of Influenza*, which he had cowritten in the wake of the postwar pandemic.[18] Although he had been at Yale for only three years and had been heavily involved in the war effort, the faculty elected him fourth dean of the medical school in 1920.

When Milton Winternitz succeeded George Blumer as dean of the Yale University School of Medicine, academic control of the beds in the hospital had been achieved and a full-time clinical program had been organized, although not yet fully implemented. The General Education Board's criteria had been fulfilled, ensuring solvency of the hospital, at least in the short term. But academic control of the hospital was complicated by the profusion of health-care organizations involved in patient care. There was ongoing opposition to the full-time clinical system from both the community and long-term members of the faculty, and the hospital board was making decisions that were not in the interest of medical academia.

President James Rowland Angell commented that Winternitz became dean at a time when the medical school faced its most disheartening prospects.[19] There was a perception that the "outlook was as unpromising and depressing as could be imagined."[20] Yet the saga of the School of Medicine had contained many equally bleak periods before. All the goals for which the faculty had fought to achieve in the school and the hospital had been reached, but Camelot remained elusive. After having worked so hard for so long, the clinical faculty still did not have academic control.

When Winternitz took over the deanship, his first priority was to fill the ranks of the senior faculty. Blumer had resigned as chair of medicine, exchanging the John Slade Ely Professorship for the David Paige Smith Professorship, and had immediately taken sabbatical leave. Morris L. Slemons, founder of the first full-time clinical Department of Obstetrics and Gynecology in the United States, had left to return to California. Joseph Marshall Flint, the professor of surgery, who had experienced persistent pulmonary problems since the war, had retired.

Yandell Henderson, who had been professor of physiology for ten years, had long been dissatisfied with conditions in the department and had actually announced his resignation in 1917. He did not resign, however, but continued through the years to complain to the president. Finally, President Angell sent him a letter saying that he was impossible—in effect firing him.[21] Henderson tried to explain that it was all a misunderstanding, but he was ultimately transferred to the Graduate School and given an appointment in applied physiology. These departures left only seven members of professorial rank to constitute the entire medical-school faculty.

In contrast to the somewhat muted George Blumer, Winternitz—whether liked or disliked—was a "steam engine in pants" and incapable of floating in a sea of uncertainty.[22] A number of events occurred within the university that helped Winternitz navigate that sea. In 1921, President Arthur Twining Hadley, a Yale man and a traditionalist, was succeeded by James Rowland Angell, a psychologist and the first Yale president from "elsewhere" since Abraham Pierson. It was the era of the postwar boom, and funds to build facilities were becoming increasingly available. In addition, the Yale Corporation had yet again examined the future of the medical school and had issued a ringing statement of affirmation. A wealthy Detroit physician and corporation Fellow, Fred T. Murphy, had been asked to review the school. On the basis of his investigation, the Committee on Educational Policy unanimously recommended the following policy:

1. That there is a clear and definite obligation of the University to Medical Education;
2. That the Yale School of Medicine is a valuable nucleus of men and material and sound traditions, which richly justify the development of an institution for medical education of the highest type;

3. That the Corporation accept as policy the development of a Medical School of the highest type to include the pre-clinical and clinical years of instruction upon such principles of medical education as may be approved by the Corporation, after conference with the Medical Faculty; and
4. That every effort should be made to obtain at the earliest date the necessary funds with which to expand and develop the buildings, the equipment and the research and the service, in accordance with the best ideals of modern medical education—as an essential unit of our University plan of development.[23]

Meanwhile, the central university administration had been thrown into a state of turmoil in 1919, fomented by alumni. In the immediate postwar period the secretary, Anson Phelps Stokes, and the treasurer, George Parmly Day, had conceptualized the need for long-range planning and had persuaded the corporation to create an alumni Committee on a Plan for University Development. Stokes and Day were primarily interested in further growth of the university and an increase in the endowment, leading to higher faculty salaries.[24] Discontent among alumni, particularly from the West, had been growing, however, and the committee became a device to press for reform. Thus the Stokes-Day plan for a bigger and better university was turned into a demand for reform.

For unknown reasons, the faculty of Yale College had never been convened to consider possible reforms or been systematically consulted about them. Imagine the faculty's response when the alumni committee visited New Haven on November 23, 1918, and voted a number of extraordinary recommendations, which included a common course for all undergraduate instruction, consolidation of the college and Sheffield Scientific School, and emphasis on teaching rather than research in the undergraduate college.

President Hadley, who had been timid in these matters, appeared to have his resolve stiffened by the impetus of the alumni committee. The faculty members, on the other hand, were angry that they had never been given a hearing, but they were not well organized.[25] The corporation appeared to be deliberately forcing reorganization by a strategy of divide and rule. When Hadley wavered, the corporation replaced him on the Reorganization Committee, a move that amounted to a vote of no confidence in the president of Yale University. The faculty, too, had lost confidence in his leadership and had held a meeting to which Hadley was not invited. By any definition, when both corporation and faculty have lost confidence in the president of a university, a major crisis exists.

The denouement came when the alumni committee proposed the abolition of the Board of Permanent Officers and of permanent tenure. "Fortunately, the President was not so weak, nor the Corporation so reactionary, as to countenance anything so drastic."[26] Hadley had considered the educational and organizational implications of the reorganization, but had paid little heed to the administrative or management implications. If the head of an organization loses the confidence of his board or faculty over fundamental issues, he has effectively lost control of the organization.

Although the members of the faculty may have been "resolutely conservative," they had devoted their lives to academic matters. To have educational decisions made by businessmen who had spent four years in higher education was to set a very dangerous precedent. As Charles Seymour, a future Yale president, wrote to one of the corporation members, "The Faculty is responsible for the active application of the education given at Yale. The welfare of Yale demands that that they should feel the responsibility as theirs."[27]

Most of the alumni committee's recommendations were accepted. Despite the cataclysmic nature of the reorganization, it did solve the problem of the college and the Sheffield Scientific School as two separate schools. In addition, professors with similar interests were brought together. The professional schools were given new status, and the graduate school increased in stature. As a result of the reorganization, Yale had been converted into a better-balanced institution with a strengthened administration and a broader university focus.

It is unclear whether Hadley himself felt that his presidential powers had been weakened after the reorganization. In the winter following the March vote of the corporation on reorganization, however, he let it be known that upon reaching the age of sixty-five, after twenty-two years as president of Yale, he would retire. Samuel H. Fisher, the driving force on the Reorganization Committee, was named chairman of the corporation committee that would seek alumni opinion and identify presidential candidates. The obvious successor—and Hadley's choice—was Stokes. But because Stokes had long served as scapegoat for Hadley, some alumni and faculty members were so hostile to him that his appointment to the university presidency would have been difficult or even impossible. Law, divinity, and business were represented on the five-member search committee for the presidency, but not scientists (although Fred T. Murphy, a corporation member, was a surgeon).

From the medical school's point of view, Stokes was the perfect candidate. George Pierson recalled that "when the President was staggered by the costs of the medical school and considered abolishing it, it was Stokes who had backed the school and secured the support which guaranteed its continuance."[28] When Stokes realized that he was not going to be offered the appointment, he resigned to leave the way clear for the new president. In September 1920, Angell's name surfaced, perhaps through a recommendation by Abraham Flexner. William Welch also wrote a letter recommending him. Angell was president of the Carnegie Foundation at the time, and no one knew whether he was interested in the job. Otto Bannard, a blustery businessman from Ohio who was a member of the corporation committee but a stranger to Angell, reportedly walked into his office and said: "Look here. Would you consider going to Yale?"[29] In conversations with Hadley, Angell wanted to know about the mood of the alumni and the issue of nominating professors. He must have been aware of the reorganization and Hadley's loss of administrative control but according to Pierson, was reassured after his discussions.[30] Although deeply hurt, Stokes graciously urged Angell to assume the presidency.

Angell's educational credentials were impeccable. His father, like Hadley's, was a college professor and became president of the University of Michigan. The young Angell had graduated from the University of Michigan, did graduate work there and at Harvard, and after holding academic positions at several universities, became dean of the faculty at the University of Chicago. Angell was interested in the presidency of the University of Chicago, and when that did not happen, he accepted the chairmanship of the National Research Council, followed by the presidency of the Carnegie Foundation. His desire to be a university president remained, however, and when approached by the Yale Corporation on February 19, 1921, he accepted. Thus, six months after becoming dean, Winternitz was faced with not only an unfamiliar president but also the loss of Stokes, who had been a strong supporter of the medical school.

Winternitz's major priority was the recruitment of faculty, and he used the university reorganization plan to place all the available resources in the "fundamental" sections of the medical school while eliminating sections that were not crucial. The plan was supposed to unite the various schools with the university, thereby furthering the development of an increasingly unified university with a coordinated scheme of instruction that would eliminate duplication of courses. The members of the faculty were to be Yale University faculty, designated to teach where their talents were most needed, rather than individuals owing primary allegiance to distinct schools within the university. One of the chief duties of the newly created office of provost was to partake in discussions concerned with the educational development of the university, in an attempt to foster this integration.

Using the university plan as a shield, Winternitz avoided the major confrontations that occur when medical-school departments are reorganized. He committed the school's support to anatomy, physiology (including chemical, physical, and biological physiology), pharmacology and toxicology, pathology and bacteriology, public health, medicine, surgery, pediatrics, and diseases of women (including obstetrics and gynecology). He planned to establish a section of psychiatry and to develop some of the medical and surgical subspecialties, but he felt it unlikely that any of them would develop to the importance of major sections. The issue of what constitutes an academic department continues to be debated. Often the determining factor is not academic principle but a powerful section chief who threatens to leave unless his or her section is made into a department, with no assurance that a replacement can be recruited.

Winternitz immediately began to strengthen his faculty, recruiting Francis G. Blake as chairman of medicine, who brought with him John Punnett Peters, a Yale '08 and Columbia medical graduate. Peters and William T. Stadie constituted the chemical, or metabolic, division of the Department of Medicine (figure 22). James D. Trask, a pediatrician, and Arthur B. Dayton were appointed to the biological division of the department. Harold M. Marvin was recruited to direct the work in electrocardiography, which resulted in less emphasis on the stethoscope and "heart murmurs," a trend that has continued to this day. These recruitments marked the beginning of specialization in the medical school.[31]

Joseph Marshall Flint, the professor of surgery, retired in 1921 due to ill health incurred during his military service. Samuel Clark Harvey, who had received both his undergraduate and medical degrees from Yale, succeeded him as chairman.[32] Graduating from the medical school in 1911, he spent two years in pathology in New York, followed by four years as a resident with Harvey Cushing in Boston. In 1917 he returned to Yale as an instructor. Harvey was appointed an assistant professor of surgery at Yale in 1920 and was promoted to associate professor and acting chairman a year later, a meteoric rise. His rapid promotion to the chair of surgery must have raised some eyebrows, but Winternitz emphasized that he was a good candidate: "For the past two years, Dr. Harvey has been associated as first assistant with Dr. Flint and has been carefully trained to assume responsibility as

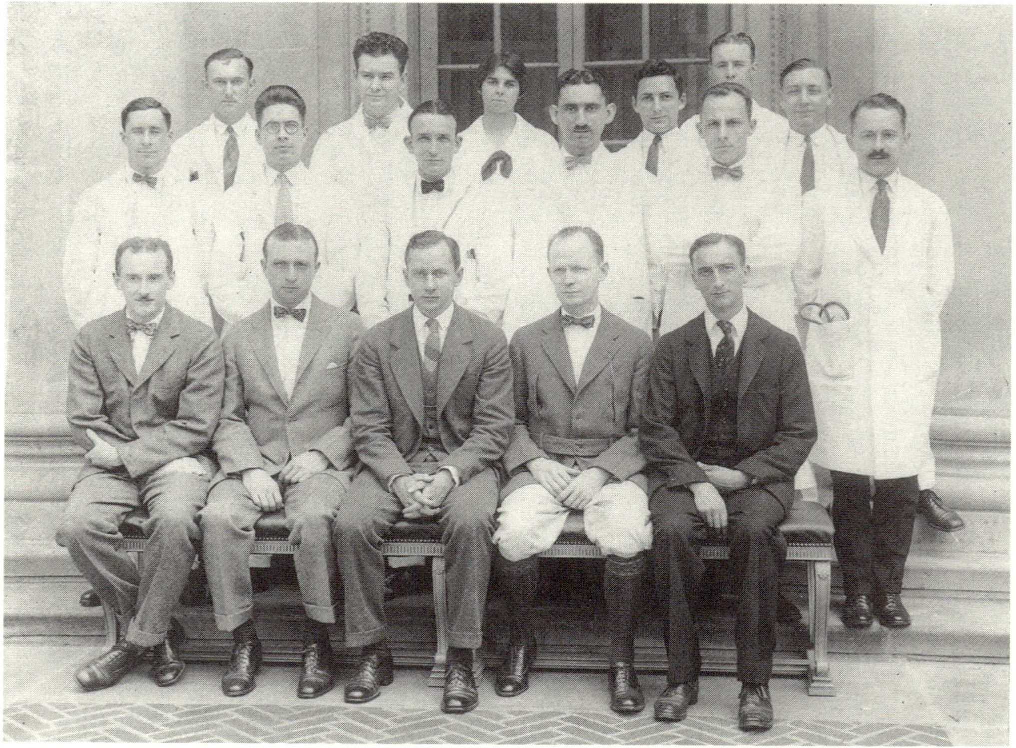

Figure 22. The Department of Medicine. *Front row, from left:* Stadie, Marvin, Blake, Peters, Trask

chief of the clinic."[33] Winternitz himself retained his position as chairman of pathology.

When Morris L. Slemons resigned as chairman of obstetrics and gynecology in 1920, Arthur Morse, who had been a Yale faculty member since 1915, was appointed to the post. Morse was said to be one of the very few men in the country capable of conducting a women's clinic. Indeed, George Blumer had mentioned the Women's Clinic as one of the high points of his deanship.

A full-time pediatrics section had been one of the conditions for the grant from the General Education Board. Edwards Park, Yale College '00, was recruited from Johns Hopkins as professor of pediatrics. Park and his assistant, Grover Powers, had done outstanding work on dietary deficiencies in children. After six years at Yale, Park confided to Angell that he was not pleased with some of the appointments and was not confident about the future of the school.[34] James Gamble from Harvard urged Park to return to Johns Hopkins, where he would "find much better students to teach and proper men to lead into research presenting much more frequently."[35]

Park did indeed return to Johns Hopkins but during his stay in New Haven had recruited Martha Eliot, a former Johns Hopkins student, to be his chief resident and an instructor in pediatrics.[36] Ethel Dunham, who had arrived a year before Eliot in 1919, was the first woman house officer at the New Haven Hospital. When Eliot subsequently left Yale for a full-time post at the Children's Bureau, Dunham became head of the bureau's research division in child development. During Yale's search for a chairman of pediatrics, the ever-intrusive Flexner pushed his family physician very hard for the position, disparaging Powers's abilities in the process.[37] Angell commented to Fred Murphy that although Powers was good clinically, "nobody has any illusions about Dr. Powers' qualifications, least of all Powers himself."[38] As it turned out, both Flexner and Angell were wrong. Powers went on to have a brilliant career as professor of pediatrics at Yale (figure 23). He was an autocratic, controlling individual who was determined that every child should be well cared for and that all his staff, including the medical students, should consider this a top priority.

In the midst of making appointments to strengthen the school, Winternitz had, as always, to consider ways to attract funds. He sent Flexner a cartoon in 1920 showing submarines from the university, faculty, hospital, and community firing torpedoes at one another (figure 24).[39] The medical school was portrayed as a small boat containing two rowers going in opposite directions, with a life preserver marked "$5,000,000" and "G.E.B.," a clear message that

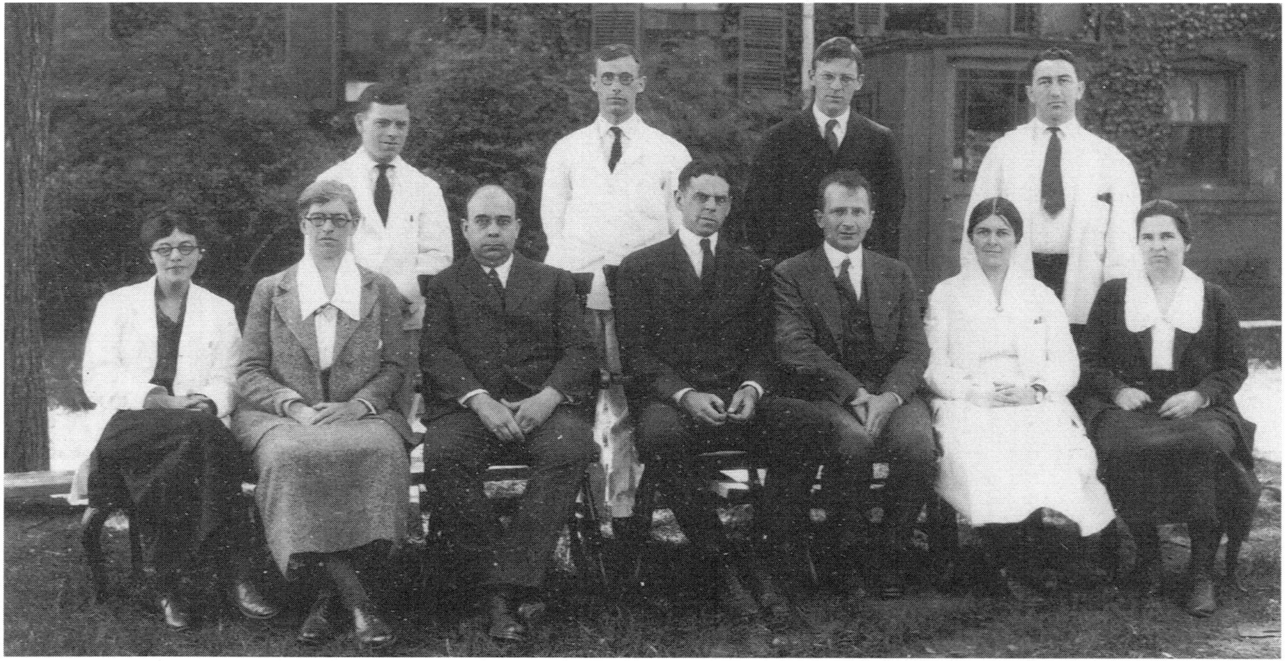

Figure 23. Grover Powers (first row: third from left) and the Pediatric House Staff

Flexner and the General Education Board were capable of bringing Winternitz's dreams to fruition. The cartoon was effective. Flexner replied: "You have certainly devised the most poignant and appealing form of application that was ever presented to our Board."[40]

In 1922 the cartoon was published in a pamphlet Winternitz entitled "The Past, Present, and Future of the Yale University School of Medicine and Affiliated Clinical Institutions including The New Haven Hospital, The New Haven Dispensary, and The Connecticut Training School for Nurses." The title itself linked the diverse institutions together, thus addressing one of the frustrations that the faculty had discussed in a letter to the corporation. Winternitz wrote that his pamphlet was to be "a summary of the past, lest we forget what has been done," and even more important, an outline of future plans, so far as they had been developed.[41] The pamphlet described the organization of the school, instruction in the various departments, proposed changes in the curriculum, nursing, and plans for the future.

By 1920 the number of medical students was gratifyingly higher than it had been a few years earlier. When George Blumer became dean in 1910, there were eighty-three students enrolled in the medical school. The tougher admission requirements instituted the year before had scared off many applicants, and enrollment dropped to a low of forty-two students in the 1912–13 school year. Enrollment then gradually increased, reaching a total of 118 in the last class selected by Blumer, in 1919. With the improved enrollment, Winternitz was able to raise admission requirements to three years of college work for all entering students, as well as increase tuition to the same level as Yale College. Although tuition fees at the medical school and the college were similar, costs were very different. In 1922 the average university expenditure for a student in Yale College was about $700 a year, while the expenditure for a medical student was close to $2,500, by far the highest in the university.[42] Space limitations, particularly in the clinical years, made it necessary to limit the size of the class to fifty, which meant that, because of the success in expanding the pool of qualified applicants, not all qualified applicants could be accepted. A member of the admissions committee, Harry Zimmerman, said that Winternitz's instructions to the committee were explicit: "Never admit more than five Jews, take only two Italian Catholics, and take no blacks at all."[43]

In 1934 the president of Wesleyan University had advised Jewish premedical students that it would be difficult for them to enter medical school in view of the fact that half of all applicants were Jewish. Medical-school deans were asked to comment on Wesleyan's approach, and Winternitz drafted a

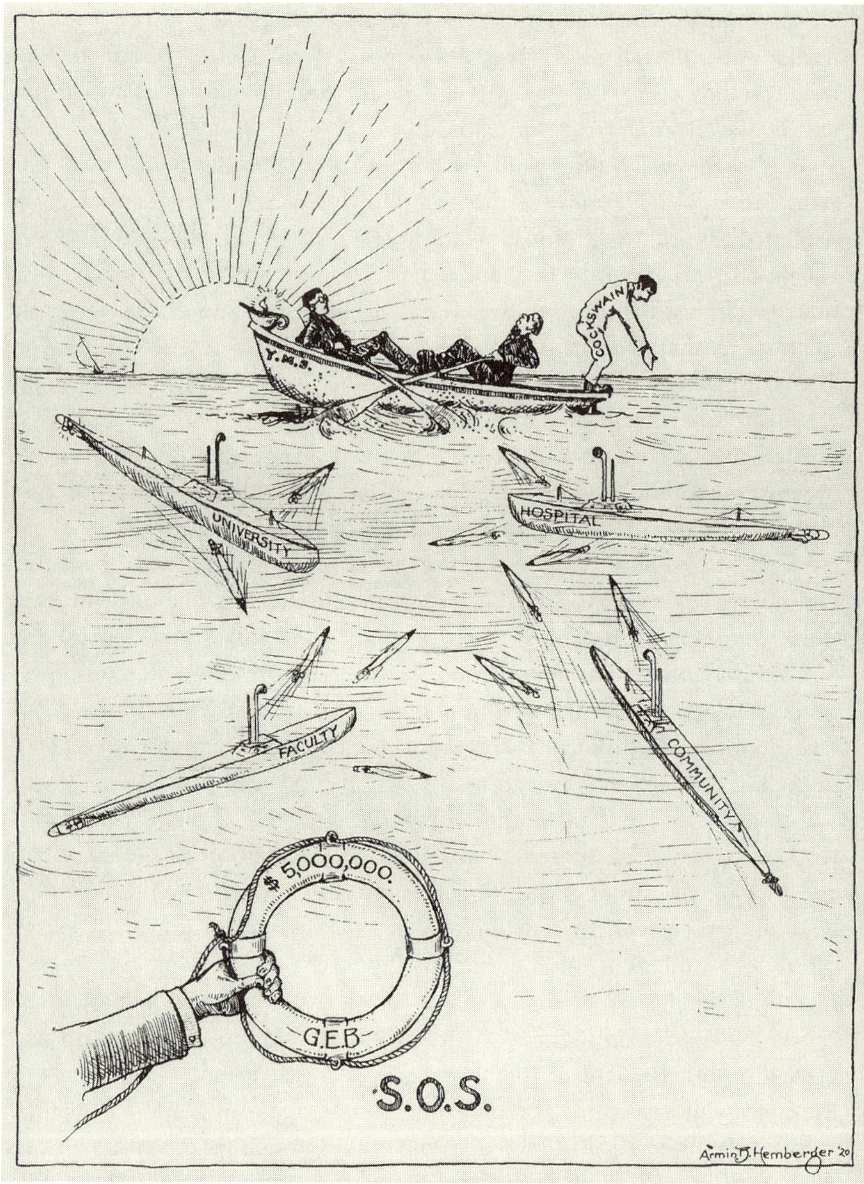

Figure 24. The Situation of the Medical School in 1920

letter of response that was never sent. In it he stated that Yale applied the same standards to all applicants, but that the "proportion of applicants who can qualify for admission, nevertheless, seems smaller among the Jewish than non-Jewish."[44]

When Winternitz was asked in 1934 whether the proportion of Jewish prospective physicians was too large, he responded affirmatively, indicating that so long as the population was mixed, there was a need for diversity. Whether Winternitz truly believed in the need for diversity or was providing a cover for his own anti-Semitism is a key question. He was a man of violent likes and dislikes, and his detractors' perceptions of discrimination may have been linked to personality clashes.

Miriam K. Dasey, the registrar, prepared two memos, in October 1934 and February 1935, that presumably reflect Winternitz's views of the admission procedure: "The composition of a class should be balanced, and on the basis of the general population, racial, institutional and geographic ratios are preserved. The number of women is restricted; students trained in some religious institutions where the viewpoint has proven to be too narrow, are limited, as are some racial groups. In a final analysis, many of the students in these groups are not fitted for medicine, and their reasons for selecting this profession are fallacious. The group from which the largest number of applications are received is the Hebrew: 55 percent of all applications. The result is that with a limitation of acceptances in this class, the result seems like discrimination, when as a matter of fact, this is not the case. All students are subjected to the same standards and the rating is the same; an unprejudiced evaluation of the man." The final paragraph contains advice for the successful Hebrew applicant: "Particularly important is a friendly approach and friendships with many different types."[45]

These comments certainly go beyond merely ensuring diversity in a class. When Stanhope Bayne-Jones succeeded Winternitz, applicants were further categorized as Americans, Hebrews, and women; no notations of this sort were found in the admission folders of the Winternitz era.

In his report to the president of 1921–1922, Winternitz stated that medical education in the United States was in a "state of flux." Several systems of clinical teaching had evolved, and controversy raged over the relative merits of the various systems, particularly the full-time clinical system, which Yale had adopted in 1915. At Yale, "now more of the major clinical divisions are on a solid and comprehensive full-time basis than in any other school of the world. . . . Indeed, a small medical school as a part of a great university like Yale is particularly well adapted to pedagogical experiment, and it is to be hoped that such experiments, judiciously carried out, will be one of the means by which this school will aid medical education and give character to itself."[46]

Winternitz also indicated in his report that "radical changes" in the curriculum had to be made, because of the overloaded course schedules. He wanted to give students more free time, to allow individuals to develop at their own pace, faster or slower. As someone on the Curriculum Committee said, the hope was to "teach the student less but learn him more." By "judicious pruning" the medical course could be cut by a quarter, and the candidate for the degree of doctor of medicine would still receive a broad, well-grounded training in the fundamentals of medicine. The extra time would give the challenged student more of a chance to review, while the gifted student could elect to do research or special work. With less teaching time available, the instructor would in theory concentrate on basics rather than simply talk faster. With more free time, medical students would develop a particular interest and expertise in a particular area of medicine. Winternitz concluded that the equivalent of one year's work had been salvaged from the required courses—a major accomplishment, as anyone who has been involved in curriculum reform can attest. The student was expected to use a third of this time for electives, and he could pursue research or other interests during the rest of the time.

In his annual report on the pathology section, Winternitz commented that group teaching along interdepartmental lines would be advantageous. He cited as an example that the physiology, anatomy, and histology of the heart and lungs, as well as their pathology and bacteriology, could all be studied together. In his role as chairman of pathology, Winternitz was particularly interested in improving the curriculum in Pathology by emphasizing gross pathology and eliminating the "busy work" for students of routine staining and preparation of histological specimens. Emphasis would be placed also on clinical-pathological correlations throughout the clinical years.

Curriculum revision reversed the sequence of the clinical years, so in the third year students concentrated on ward medicine, which entailed acute illness and intensive therapy. On the other hand, fourth-year students, who had more clinical maturity, concentrated their efforts in the dispensary, which allowed the more mature students to acquire knowledge of disease in an outpatient setting, gain an appreciation of epidemiology, and develop an interest in preventive medicine. Dispensary patients were to be encouraged to come for consultations even when they did not have a problem, so that the dispensary would be a "health clinic" as well as a "disease clinic."

It was hoped that the time made available by curriculum revision would also result in research theses of higher quality. The research thesis had been a requirement for the doctorate of medicine at Yale almost continuously since the inception of the school. The first thesis found in the school's historical library was written by Charles Hooker, later dean of the School of Medicine, in 1823. In spite of this long history, no time had ever been allotted in the curriculum to do the necessary research. Now more advanced research could be undertaken.

Winternitz indicated in his report for 1924–1925 that by allowing time for the student to pursue his particular interests, the opportunity for study in selected fields would be expanded, compatible with a true graduate education.[47] Winternitz's vision was imaginative and exciting, and although it was not completely realized, it formed the basis of the Yale system of medical education. Winternitz stated that the annual grading system would be abolished and that the student would be allowed to select the sequence of studies from the courses offered in the school. The number of courses and the time taken to complete them would depend on the student, who would require the instructor's permission. Group examinations and the research thesis would be used to monitor the student's accomplishments. Closer cooperation with the graduate programs in the biomedical sciences would occur. During the preliminary part of the medical curriculum, students could be enrolled in both the graduate school and the medical school. Winternitz's plan would have allowed graduate students to switch to the medical school if their interests became more clinical.

The medical faculty adopted many of these components as educational policy at the beginning of the 1926–1927 academic year, including elimination of the traditional annual "class" system, elimination of "final" examinations, and greater educational freedom for students, which would place greater responsibility on them. Instead of final examinations, there would be a comprehensive, week-long examination twice a year, qualifying students to pursue clinical medicine. The third and fourth years of medical school would remain unchanged, with emphasis in the fourth year on the natural treatment and study of disease.[48] Although the "university" aspects of a joint medical school–graduate school venture were not included in his 1924–1925 report, Winternitz had outlined the Yale system of medical education as we know it today.

With the increasing size of the faculty, issues requiring the dean's attention burgeoned exponentially. At the same time, Winternitz was involved in a number of major initiatives that added to his workload. He conceived of a Department of Medical Education, centered in the Office of the Dean, to relieve some of these pressures. Although this concept did not solve Winternitz's problems, Arthur B. Dayton was appointed as assistant dean, to shoulder some of the administrative burden. Winternitz also made increasing use of committees and hired two administrative assistants, who became fixtures at the Yale Medical School. Miriam K. Dasey, the long-time registrar, knew each student, and Lottie G. Bishop, the dean's executive secretary, lived for the institution and ran her part of it with an iron hand.

Both Winternitz and Blumer before him considered a high-quality nursing program essential to the success of the hospital and championed the cause of a school of nursing within the university.[49] A solution to the shortage of nurses appeared unlikely unless the nursing profession were made more attractive. The Board of Permanent Officers submitted a report during the 1921–1922 school year to the Visiting Nurses Association, the New Haven Hospital and Dispensary, and the Connecticut Training School for Nurses. Both the Visiting Nurses Association and the hospital had associated nursing schools. The activities of the schools were divided into practical nursing and classroom education, with the latter supplied in a haphazard fashion by the faculty of the medical school. The solution was to create a Yale School of Nursing, with a dean and a board that would include the superintendent of the Connecticut Training School for Nurses and a representative of the Visiting Nurses Association. The educational requirements would be like those of other university schools and would stipulate a high-school education for matriculation. On completion of a two-year course the graduate would receive a certificate; after an additional two-year period of specialized training, the student would be a candidate for the degree of bachelor of nursing.

The thought of men entering this profession apparently did not cross the Board of Permanent Officers' collective mind. It concluded that the manual and domestic labor that was part of nursing training would not be appropriate in the Yale School of Nursing: "The work would have to be relegated to paid employees such as used to do this same work in office, factory or home. The choice between these or other possibilities is difficult."[50] The Yale Corporation voted approval of the plan, provided that the school could be coordinated with the university's work and that the university would be relieved of all financial obligations.

In his 1922 document "The Past, Present, and Future of the Yale University School of Medicine and Affiliated Institutions," Winternitz discussed the physical unification of the School of Medicine. "Sweeping changes are contemplated and indeed steps have been taken to assure much more." On November 13, 1920, the corporation had voted "That the permanent University laboratories of Physiology, Pharmacology and Anatomy be located in connection with the group of Medical buildings near Cedar Street as soon as funds can be provided." This vote was important for several reasons. On the one hand, it provided for the foundation of the Sterling Hall of Medicine, and on the other, it stated that the preclinical departments would be located in proximity to the medical school and not to the college. The corporation requested the Sterling Trustees to set aside $1,320,000 for a medical-school building.[51] By the time Winternitz's pamphlet was published, plans had already been completed for what was to be the Sterling Hall of Medicine. At the same time, a number of changes and additions were being made to bring the hospital into the twentieth century.

The construction of Sterling Hall combined the disparate departments formerly scattered in antiquated buildings into a "real Medical school." At the time, anatomy was taught in two old and inconvenient buildings at 150 York Street, while training in physiological chemistry was provided by the Sheffield Scientific School. Physiology and public health were located in Nathan Smith Hall. The Anthony P. Brady Memorial Laboratory, the only adequate modern building, was crowded with several departments—pathology and bacteriology, obstetrics and gynecology, medicine, and pediatrics. In addition to departmental space, the Sterling Hall of Medicine (figure 25) would provide a library for approximately twelve thousand volumes, an amphitheater for 250 people, administrative offices for the dean, faculty rooms, and students' commons, as well as toilets and locker rooms for men and for women. Physical physiology and pharmacology would be located in the Broad Street wing (B wing). Physiological chemistry (biochemistry) and anatomy would be in the Cedar Street wing (C wing).[52] These departmental locations have persisted to the present day.

Subject to assured funds for building the Sterling Hall of Medicine, a conditional gift of $370,000 was requested in 1921 from the General Education Board to build additional laboratory space near the medical wards of the hospital, to be the Laboratory for Medicine and Pediatrics. President Hadley contacted Flexner about the possibility. Hadley did not want to jeopardize the grant from the General Education Board, but neither did he wish to hurry the Sterling Trustees, "because Mr. Church like many other good businessmen hates the idea of being rushed and reacts somewhat against

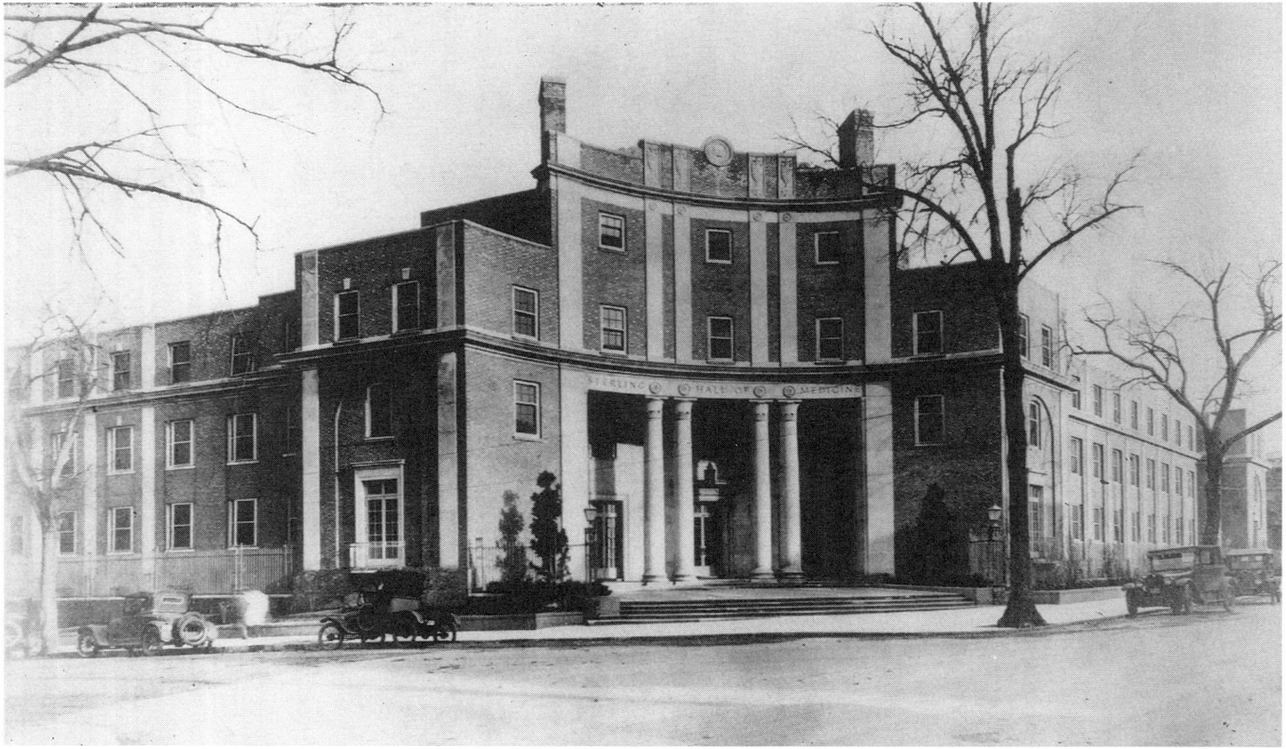

Figure 25. Sterling Hall of Medicine in 1925

it."[53] The fact that Hadley wrote to Flexner rather than the Sterling trustees is an indication of how sensitive he was about "rushing" their Mr. Church. Hadley soon received word from Flexner that the General Education Board had awarded an appropriation of $185,000, provided the university secured assurance of funds for the Sterling Hall of Medicine. Flexner followed with a letter to Hadley the same day, stating that to his "very great regret and discomfort" Stokes and Winternitz might have formed the impression that the board was going to give the entire $370,000, which was not what Flexner had intended.[54]

This is an unusual exchange between a university president and an individual who had been responsible for providing large amounts of funding to the institution. All the more unusual because in his autobiography Flexner recounts an exchange concerning Colonel Isaac M. Ullman, the president of the hospital's board, in which Hadley expressed his reservations about Ullman. According to Hadley, not only was Ullman "not a Yale Graduate," but "his closest friend was a Roman Catholic while he himself was a Jew." Flexner answered that being a Jew himself and having for years been "making [his] way among Christians and working with them," he felt confident of being able to handle Ullman "tactfully, so that prejudice need not be stirred." Hadley is then reported to have said that Ullman was a corset manufacturer, and Flexner, whose father was in the clothing trade, replied, "Now I feel perfectly certain that he and I will get on famously."[55]

There were also building plans afoot for the hospital. Shortly after Winternitz had become dean, the hospital Executive Committee discussed the desirability for the hospital to assume control of the dispensary. Winternitz and the superintendent urged the unification of the hospital and the dispensary in a report to the hospital's board, and an agreement was ratified in September 1920.[56] Agreement was reached on a building program for hospital and dispensary in which the dispensary would occupy a central site (figure 26), and the activities of the dispensary and hospital were amalgamated.

Amalgamation included the assignment of single record numbers so that individuals could be tracked both as inpatients and as outpatients. An appointment system was also inaugurated, a major improvement over the previous arrangement of first come, first served. Under the old system, the patients either did not appear or arrived in overwhelming numbers. With the new appointment system, the number of clinic visits increased, as did both patient and physician satisfaction. Winternitz was impressed enough to devote almost as much space to these improvements in his 1922 pamphlet as he did to the Yale system of medical education.

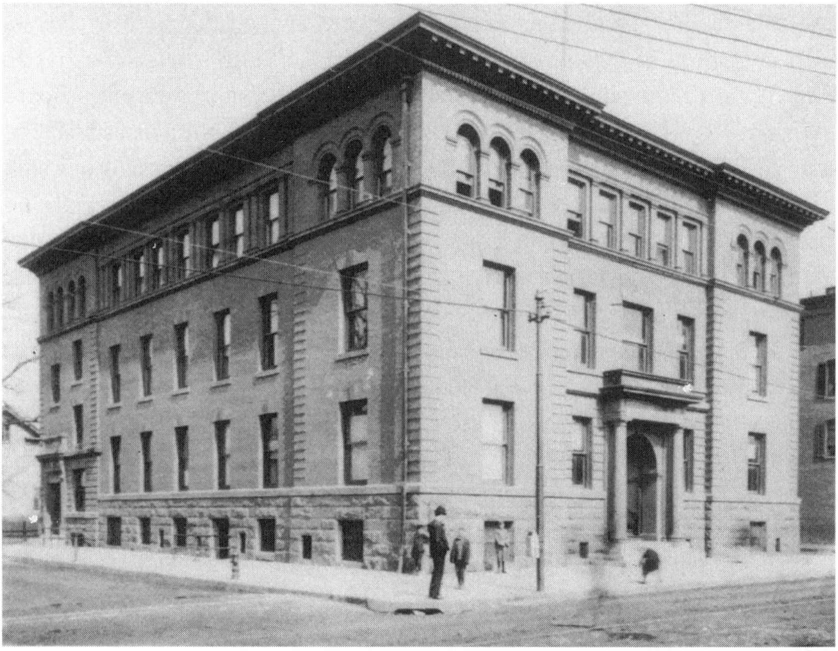

Figure 26. The Dispensary (Hope Building)

The construction that occurred in the 1920s under the guidance of Milton Winternitz required enormous amounts of money. The Sterling Hall of Medicine was a marvelous start. But there were ever more demands, and Winternitz's close relation with Abraham Flexner was of great benefit. Flexner staunchly defended Yale in a 1924 letter to President Wilbur of Stanford, who had provided uncomplimentary material. "As a matter of fact, no medical school in the United States or in any other country, with which I am familiar, has within so brief a period—about six years—made anything like the progress which has been made in New Haven."[57] Winternitz and Flexner maintained a personal and professional correspondence. In January 1925 Winternitz wrote, "All I have to say is that if you are not bothered any more by the deans of other medical schools than you are by me, your life must be one of blissful tranquility."[58] In another exchange Winternitz wrote to ask for the "privilege of a formal interview." Flexner replied with strong words, "Don't ever write me asking for 'the privilege of a formal interview': 'Privilege' and 'Formal' be d———!"[59]

The Sterling Hall of Medicine was dedicated in 1925. William Henry Welch, then director of the School of Hygiene and Public Health at Johns Hopkins University, and Harvey Cushing gave addresses. Cushing spoke first, giving a talk entitled "Experimentum Periculosum: Judicium Difficile." He remarked that both he and Welch had been called upon previously to comment on the medical school. On those occasions, they could only discuss individuals, rather than influences exerted by the school. "In the want of a hospital under university control, wherein the professors might do their clinical teaching lay the crux of the situation."[60]

Cushing went on to pay tribute to the "patience and persistence" of George Blumer and Joseph Marshall Flint, to which could be ascribed the "rescue" of the medical school. Flint had been recruited as chairman of surgery in 1907 when Cushing declined the position. Cushing also spoke to the faculty of the town-gown relationship: "You will long be regarded as interlopers, as cuckoos in a hedge-sparrow's nest. Man is by nature chauvinistic, and the medical man perhaps more than others is prone to look with jealous eyes upon a foreign transplant to his bailiwick." He directed the rest of his talk to the importance of preclinical subjects in relation to clinical medicine, for in clinical medicine rather than in the preclinical sciences, "where normal structure and function is largely dealt with, is experience found fallacious and judgement difficult."[61]

Welch's address followed and, according to Cushing's account, disagreed with everything that had just been said about concentrating on the patient in the preclinical years. "Dr. Welch then arose and tore my proposal to bits."[62] Welch said that with a public-health officer in every community, people would not become ill, leaving "the old-time practitioner twiddling his thumbs." After the talk, Welch reportedly agreed with Cushing that men like Osler and Janeway were not likely to be seen again. Asked why he had not said so in his speech, Welch replied: "Because I'm now a Professor of Public Health."[63]

President Angell formally accepted the Sterling Hall of Medicine on behalf of the university. "It combines in remarkable degree convenience and effectiveness for laboratory training and scientific research. In it there is nothing wasteful, but also there is nothing unworthy, nothing cheap. It will stand for years to come a striking memorial to Mr. Sterling."[64] Reporting on the fiftieth anniversary of the Sterling Hall of Medicine, the *Yale Medical Alumni Bulletin* commented that the building still retained "dignity and fitness of form," and that the subtle tug-of-war between a basic science curriculum and a clinically oriented curriculum continued "not only at the Yale School of Medicine but in medical schools across the nation."[65] The same may be said today.

As the medical school became increasingly active in clinical practice, "creative" tensions arose between the community physicians and the medical faculty. In the fall of 1925 Winternitz, along with Herbert Thoms and Creighton Barker, who were officers of the Connecticut State Medical Society, organized a three-day Connecticut Clinical Congress modeled after similar successful enterprises in the mid-West. In addition to the exchange of knowledge, the congress provided an occasion to build relationships between the Yale faculty and practitioners across the state. The object of the congress was to afford practitioners an opportunity to bring themselves up to date on the latest in diagnosis and therapy through lectures and demonstrations by recognized authorities. This early example of continuing medical education was a huge success. More than 25 percent of all the physicians in Connecticut attended, and a total of twenty papers and demonstrations were presented by eminent physicians from the entire Eastern seaboard.

Whereas clinical practice had burgeoned, psychiatry had long been stagnant at Yale, with virtually no facilities and personnel, and no opportunity to develop a significant program in psychiatry. The absence of a formal department was a definite weakness. A clinic for developmental psychology had been started in 1911 by Arnold Gesell, but it was small and relatively isolated. In 1921 the university had a bill introduced into the Connecticut State Legislature to establish a psychiatric clinic in New Haven that could be used for teaching medical students and physicians.[66] When it became clear that the bill was not going to pass, a substitute bill was introduced that successfully asked for a commission to investigate the need for such a clinic in Connecticut. The commission duly recommended that a state psychiatric hospital be established in New Haven. Accordingly, a bill was placed before the legislature for the 1923 session requesting $250,000 for the psychiatric hospital; it included language indicating that the hospital would be used as a teaching institution. Unfortunately, the bill never made it out of the Appropriations Committee.

Finally, during the 1924–1925 academic year, the General Education Board pledged $15,000 a year for five years to establish the Department of Psychiatry, a pledge that was matched by a Yale alumnus. Arthur Ruggles, superintendent of the Butler Hospital in Providence, joined the Yale faculty for a year to initiate the program in mental hygiene, but it soon became clear that both funds and facilities were inadequate. The need for psychiatric facilities coincided with Winternitz's vision of uniting in one geographical area all aspects of instruction in the science of behavior throughout the university. Not only would the individual disciplines benefit, but the development of the Department of Psychiatry would also be greatly facilitated. The plan called for construction of an Institute of Human Behavior in the vicinity of the medical school that would house the Department of Psychology, the Institute of Experimental Psychology, the Department of Research in Child Hygiene, and the Department of Psychiatry and Mental Hygiene.

As a pathologist, Winternitz was interested in basic data-driven research, but he was equally convinced that medicine should deal with the welfare of the patient throughout his or her life. The promotion of "wellness" was important for physicians to learn and to practice. He also believed that medicine should deal with the psyche as well as the soma. As Winternitz entered his second term, he developed another dictum: "The patient is not only an individual with a mind as well as a body, but an individual living in, and acted upon by, a social environment."[67] This was a bold new concept in medical education. Expanding the study of human behavior to human relations would make the objective a university objective rather than solely a medical-school one. In the 1928–1929 academic year the Human Welfare Group was conceived to bring together the "various available and affiliated units, which are united in devoting themselves to this cause—the well-being of man."[68] This group included the Yale School of Medicine, the New Haven Hospital and Dispensary, the Yale School of Nursing, and—the most controversial component—the Institute of Human Relations.

The concept of the Human Welfare Group was rooted in a number of contemporary developments: the emergence of the social sciences as academic disciplines, the National Research Council programs established during and immediately after World War I, and, finally, the new "social medicine."[69] Prior to his appointment at Yale, President Angell had been associated with the University of Chicago and the National Research Council, both focal points for this concept of how society could be organized to increase "human happiness and satisfying accomplishment" and decrease "human suffering and failure." Angell felt that the need was for a "more penetrating and usable knowledge of human nature."[70]

If such a program were to have an academic home, Yale at this point was ideal. President Angell was interested in social science and in integrating the graduate school across the university. Angell, who was a charismatic speaker, got along well with the corporation but was distant with the faculty and remained an outsider.[71] He was frustrated at not being allowed to appoint deans for the various schools, which remained the prerogative of their respective Boards of Permanent Officers. Aware that he was regarded as an outsider, Angell moved carefully. As a result, the faculty saw a gap between presidential recommendation and administrative action, which was disconcerting. Thus, when Angell found a dean like Winternitz, who was interested in his area of expertise, he was only too delighted to focus his attention on the medical school. Winternitz was committed to the concept of the Institute of Human Relations and to integrating medicine within the graduate programs of the university. The two men were joined by a third committed participant in this plan, Robert Maynard Hutchins, who had succeeded Stokes as secretary of the university in 1923 and a year later became acting dean, and subsequently dean, of the Yale Law School.

Angell found that much of the clinical and research work of the medical school was "correlative" to university departments. Activities in such departments as pediatrics, public health, psychology, sociology, government, economics, and anthropology, in the Divinity School, in the School of Nursing, and in the Division of Industrial Engineering were all relevant to activities in the Child Guidance Clinic and the Institute of Psychology. In the law school Hutchins was planning to focus legal studies on psychology and economics as well as the problems of government as they related to administration and legislation.

Despite the fact that the president of the university and the deans of the medical and law schools were totally committed to it, the concept of the Institute of Human Relations was not immediately embraced. In retrospect, it is amazing how rapidly the reorganization of 1919 occurred in the face of opposition from both the president and the faculty. In his report to the president for 1927–1928, Winternitz commented that the "expected resources for the Institute of Human Behavior have not materialized." The concept of the institute, however, had been strengthened and broadened into an Institute for Human Relations.

There was concern among the medical faculty that the institute would weaken the professional schools. Winternitz conceived of the medical school as part of a larger Division of Medicine, which would include the biological sciences and possibly the natural sciences. The proposed Institute of Human Relations would bring together in "physical contiguity" the fundamental disciplines and their associated applied fields of activity. The lack of funds for the institute meant that facilities for psychiatry were delayed once again. Although Arthur Ruggles had returned to Providence, he continued as chairman of an advisory group that, along with a local New Haven group, was formulating strategies to further the development of psychiatry at Yale.

As active planning for psychiatry had been going on for the previous ten years during the tenure of Dean Blumer, the groups' persistence was commendable. The chairman of the local group, Stewart Paton, stated the case well: "A fully equipped, well-organized psychiatric clinic is urgently needed. Until this clinic exists, the work of the psychiatrist, mental hygienist, and social worker will remain only loosely coordinated—. Until a psychiatric clinic exists, the problem of this department cannot be clearly formulated."[72]

Psychiatry was a major component of the institute but remained a problem despite successes in other areas. The lack of facilities and the insufficiency of funds were certainly major obstacles, but Winternitz was also unable to stabilize the personnel problem; Ruggles continued to direct the program in an advisory capacity while based in Providence. Additional funds did become available when the Commonwealth Fund endowed mental hygiene with $50,000 a year for five years beginning in 1926, and two years later the Rockefeller Foundation endowed psychiatry with $50,000 a year for five years. The decision was made that in addition to training in clinical psychiatry, each senior member of the department would be required to have training in one of the fundamental investigative aspects essential for advancing some part of the field, such as neuroanatomy or neurophysiology.

In 1930, after years of advisory-committee investigations, psychiatry and mental hygiene were finally launched with the appointment of Eugen Kahn of Munich as Sterling Professor of Psychiatry and Mental Hygiene. Kahn was a clinical psychiatrist with an interest in preventive psychiatry and had been invited to come to New Haven as a "guest" of the university for six weeks. The bundling was successful, and the appointment was promptly consummated. A great deal of the mental-hygiene work was conducted in the Department of University Health for the benefit of the students. Under the direction of Everett S. Rademacher, the university also sponsored a network of mental-hygiene clinics in New Haven, Waterbury, and Bridgeport, with a plan to expand the program to include mental-hygiene activities relating to schools, courts, and other public enterprises.

The Clinic of Child Development, begun in 1921 and headed by Arnold Gesell, also was incorporated into the institute, with Gesell becoming a member of the Board of Permanent Officers.[73] Born in a small town in Wisconsin in 1880, Gesell had graduated from teacher's college, taught, and earned a Ph.D. in psychology. He then worked with Lewis Terman at Stanford, developer of the Stanford-Binet intelligence test, before returning to Wisconsin for a year of basic premedical sciences. When he was offered an assistant professorship in the new graduate Department of Education at Yale, he accepted on a part-time basis so that he could also enter the medical school as a student. Gesell even convinced Dean Blumer to give him a room in the dispensary for use in a study of retarded children. He received his M.D.

degree in 1915 and was promoted to full professor in the graduate school at the same time he was appointed school psychologist for the Board of Education. Gesell became increasingly interested in the developmental patterns of behavior during early childhood and was the first to use photography and one-way mirror observations to collect reliable data.[74]

The concept of the Institute of Human Relations came to fruition in July 1928 when a committee of the corporation recommended a general plan aggregating more than $15 million. The plan included funds for the physical and financial rehabilitation of the clinical institutions affiliated with the school, a permanent endowment for the School of Nursing, and the establishment of the Institute of Human Relations. The project was officially inaugurated on February 23, 1929, with speeches by William Welch, President Angell, and Isaac Ullman, chairman of the Executive Committee of the hospital and dispensary. Conspicuously absent was Abraham Flexner, who was opposed to the idea and expressed increasingly strong displeasure. Although a strong supporter of the medical school and a close friend of Winternitz, he believed that universities were dissipating themselves by dispersing their intellectual resources. In his book *Universities: American, English, German*, published in 1930 and based on materials prepared as part of a Rhodes lecture series delivered in 1928, he railed at teachers' colleges and business schools but reserved his special scorn for the Institute of Human Relations at Yale.[75] In 1930, Flexner had told Angell that he had resigned from the General Education Board in order to have "perfect freedom for study and utterance."[76]

Flexner did not think that institutes in American universities (as compared to the German academic and scientific institutes) played a useful role. "The most recent—and to my thinking the most incomprehensible—development in the way of an institute has latterly taken place at Yale. Yale had long possessed an inferior medical school. In recent years the school has under the highly intelligent, enthusiastic and energetic leadership of its present dean, Professor Winternitz, rapidly improved its personnel, facilities and resources. Its development, however, is far from complete." Flexner firmly believed that major advances in knowledge do not occur through collective effort or committee proceedings, and he stated his position unequivocally: "Again, the Institute of Human relations ignores the necessarily individualistic character of genuine thinking."[77]

Flexner had mentioned his concern in a February 1929 letter to Winternitz: "Perhaps too much thought is going into expansion as against production."[78] Winternitz replied that this concern must have come from "some irritation." Flexner responded that his suspicions had been confirmed that the expansion of the medical school was too rapid. In January 1930 Winternitz asked Flexner to suspend judgment about the Institute of Human Relations until it was in operation, but Flexner replied that he could not defer. Winternitz also sent him the floor plans for the institute, which Flexner dismissed as not an institute at all but a "collection of departments."[79] Winternitz was becoming increasingly at odds with Flexner, who told him not to "grow skeptical about the devotion and attachment of your friends, even if they differ from you on matters of policy and opinion."[80]

The final split came when Flexner asked for a news release about the institute and information about the appointment of Mark A. May as its director.[81] Angell had previously offered the position to George Vincent, a Yale graduate, a lawyer, and president of the Rockefeller Foundation.[82] Winternitz refused to send the requested information to Flexner, who responded, "To put it mildly, your note of January 20 floored me." Meanwhile, despite his railing at university institutes, Flexner had become the first director of the Institute for Advanced Studies in Princeton.

Flexner's antipathy toward Yale's Institute of Human Relations continued to grow, and it eventually spread to include not only the medical school but the university as a whole. In an exchange of letters during 1931 with the Reverend Anson Phelps Stokes, who became dean of Washington Cathedral after stepping down as secretary of the university, Flexner wrote: "No human being ever mentioned Yale University to me at all among the real or even the most promising American universities. . . . The Medical School which made so auspicious a beginning while you were at Yale cooperating with Winternitz has gone down, down, down, though its buildings have gone up, up, up. I am sure that you will believe that it gives me no pleasure to write these things and that my sole interest is that of an impartial observer and learner."[83] Stokes's reply was terse: "I am sorry that you are adopting such rather cheap phrases as that the Medical school is going down, down, down. . . . I think the tone of your letters shows a tendency to extreme criticism which is distinctly unfair."[84]

Flexner did not retreat at all. "As to the Medical School I think my letter did it full justice." Winternitz, he wrote, "was originally an excellent pathologist, though I believe, never an original one. . . . He has made one or two good appointments, one or two questionable appointments, some in important posts, so bad that they are little short of scandalous." Flexner went on to explain that the General Education Board had turned down the request for funds for the institute.[85]

The Rockefeller Foundation funded the institute in the belief that it was a way to start psychiatry at Yale. Flexner later maintained that Richard Mills Pearce, who was director of the Medical Sciences Division of the Rockefeller Foundation, said on the day of his death that this award was the only questionable appropriation the foundation ever made, his endorsement of which he profoundly regretted.[86] Stokes replied to Flexner in a more moderate tone: "I am indeed indebted to you for your excellent letter of July 7th and the fine spirit which it manifests. . . . As to Winternitz, I feel with you that he ought not to try to lead two movements—the medical school and the Institute."[87]

On other fronts, comments were generally more favorable. The *Yale Alumni Weekly* offered congratulations and good wishes to the new institute. It mentioned that for many, the institute exemplified the characteristic American belief that advances in technology and physical sciences could be paralleled by development of "human engineering"; "the sense of a common problem will have a stimulating and fructifying influence upon fundamental research in the social sciences."[88] *Science* magazine carried news of the institute in a report on Dean Winternitz's talk to the Yale Medical Alumni Association. "The Institute," said Winternitz, "will serve as a dynamo and assembling plant for those university organizations concerned from the viewpoint of research, teaching or treatment with problems of human well-being."[89]

The *Yale Alumni Weekly* was particularly enthusiastic. "We have here in the making, one of the most interesting and potentially important movements yet inaugurated by any American university, and one that is already attracting national attention. . . . [The institute is] one of the most forward-looking steps that Yale herself has ever taken in her relations to society at large." Winternitz again described the institute in mechanistic terms: "The Human Welfare Group will be an association of divisions concerned with the promotion of human well-being, and the center of the group will be the Institute of Human Relations, the activating agent in cooperative relations and the assembling plant for correlating data in various fields." He went on to state that "As a result of the affinity between the Law School and the Medical School, the Institute of Human Behavior was expanded to include the social sciences." In the words of Robert Hutchins, dean of the law school, "the two oldest of the professions, law and medicine, thus became the youngest of the social sciences."[90]

In 1930 the Clinic of Child Development, an adult psychobiology unit, the graduate divisions of psychology and the social sciences, and a research group in mental hygiene and psychiatry were installed in the new wing of the medical school, known as the I wing. The far end was specifically designed for Gesell's clinic. The five floors of the I wing, although altered over the years, are still used for the Child Study Center, along with the 1999 addition of the Neison and Irving Harris Building.

The decision to implement the plan for the Institute of Human Relations was aided by the initial success in raising funds for the hospital and the nursing school. There was $3.1 million available for the New Haven Hospital and Dispensary from the General Education Board and a gift from Abram Fitkin, as well as another $1 million for endowment of the School of Nursing from the Rockefeller Foundation. However, the gift that most pleased Winternitz, and had so distressed Pearce, was also from the Rockefeller Foundation: a sum of $1.5 million to launch the plan for the Institute of Human Relations. This included funding for the educational program in psychiatry.

The Human Welfare Group was concerned with the "fundamental and applied aspects of biology and sociology, and consisted of the medical school, the nursing school, and the hospital and dispensary."[91] Winternitz also discussed the need for a professor of clinical sociology, but to no avail. The name of the group reflected the long-term aim of the medical school to incorporate preventive medicine in all clinical teaching. Winternitz believed strongly in this integration and was firmly opposed to the *Zersplitterung der Wissenschaft,* which divided medicine and science into arbitrary units. He preferred an "atmosphere inhibiting the production of doctor-technicians but favoring the development of physicians and humanitarians." Thus the Human Welfare Group was dedicated to the "well-being of man."[92]

Although the concept of the Institute of Human Relations was first and foremost on his list of priorities, Winternitz had important distractions.[93] The Anthony N. Brady Memorial Laboratory, which included an addition to the original Brady Laboratory built in 1917, was to be ready for occupancy by the 1928–1929 academic year. The wing extending along Congress Avenue toward Howard Avenue was to be named Lauder Hall, and the wing along Howard Avenue was to be the Farnam Memorial Wing. At the same time Abram Fitkin gave $1 million for the Raleigh Fitkin Institute, half of which was to be used to construct a six-story structure to replace the old Gifford wing. The Fitkin gift also prompted the Yale Corporation to appoint a committee to continue developing plans, under the auspices of the hospital and the university, for an improved medical center.

The hospital was now financially solvent. During the ten-year period following the prospect of bankruptcy in 1919, the operating budget of the hospital increased from approximately $200,000 a year to $775,000, and the hospital's endowment rose from $2.5 million to $3.9 million. Increased revenues came mainly from patients and from a university appropriation; state and city appropriations rose only slightly. The mayor of New Haven thought that Yale should support the city, and the hospital became a bargaining chip. A report said to be issued by the Department of Public Health suggested that the Grace Hospital, formerly a homeopathic institution and now the second-largest hospital in the city, which was in major financial difficulties, should merge with the New Haven Hospital. In fact, the report actually recommended closing the Grace Hospital and adding an equivalent number of beds at the New Haven Hospital.[94]

Winternitz was also concerned about the general welfare of the medical students as well. "Unfortunately recreational facilities are almost entirely absent in the buildings of the school, and the conditions under which the students live vary from inferior to bad." Although this was the Flapper Era, Yale's Puritan background still permeated the culture of the place. In a letter to Winternitz, President Angell commented that the medical-fraternity dances had "elements of scandal to so marked a degree." Angell went on to say in a handwritten confidential memorandum that all three medical fraternities had served hard liquor at parties after both the Army-Yale game and the Harvard game. The girls at the parties were of the "fast type," and couples had occupied rooms behind "closed doors."[95]

With the extension of the Broad Street wing of the Sterling Hall of Medicine, Winternitz was able to report "there are four squash courts and two large halls, besides a number of tennis courts on the grounds. One of the halls was designed primarily as a gymnasium. Below the gymnasium was a hall of similar size for the social life of the students. A series of teas were given in the late afternoons throughout the academic year." During the 1932–1933 academic year, 16,000 cups of tea were served, with an aggregate attendance of 19,543 at a cost of $461.57. "Four hundred and forty medical faculty wives served as hostesses at the teas during the year."[96] Today the teas are no more, and the medical school has only one tennis court and no gymnasium. The squash courts have been sacrificed for departmental space, although there is a fitness center, donated by the class of 1958. The Edward S. Harkness Dormitory is slowly being renovated after forty-five years. Clearly, facilities to improve the social life of the medical students have not kept pace with the growth of the school in academic areas.

The *Yale Medical Journal,* a successful publication involving the medical students, had been discontinued in 1912. During the 1928–1929 academic year, a large group of students formally petitioned the faculty to cooperate in launching a similar publication. As a result, the *Yale Journal of Biology and Medicine* was founded, with George H. Smith as editor in chief and two faculty members as associate editors. A group of students chosen on a competitive basis from both the preclinical and clinical years formed the editorial board. Theoretically, all editorial work was to be performed by the students. The journal was a great success, thanks largely to the efforts of George Smith, and it fostered the broad approach to medical education that was so important to Winternitz. It continues to be published and has been the training ground for a number of distinguished academicians.

Changes in the curriculum, construction of the Sterling Hall of Medicine, and the growing reputation of the school made the Yale University School of Medicine very attractive to prospective students. There was a perception in Yale College that Yale graduates, particularly those from New Haven, were being discriminated against in admissions to the medical school. Winternitz emphatically denied the charges in an April 1927 issue of the *Yale Daily News*, affirming that admissions were based solely on merit. The students had remarked in a previous newspaper article that a "high official" at the medical school had told them Yale College students were not admitted to the medical school because "they were not over-liberal in lending their financial support to the school."[97] In 1927, half of the entering class were Yale College graduates, and this proportion was increasing yearly. According to Winternitz, medical schools across the country admitted about 80 percent of applicants, while Yale admitted only 50 percent.

The relative freedom from examinations was a particularly appealing aspect to many students. In 1930 Yale took a further step toward eliminating formal testing when the National Board Examinations, which also led to licensure, became the only examinations that were compulsory at the end of the preclinical and the clinical years. Freedom from required exams led to greater student autonomy and a more relaxed atmosphere—but also to greatly heightened anxiety at examination time.

About one-fourth of the medical students were candidates for a master's or doctoral degree in 1927, and thus came under the jurisdiction of the graduate school. Winternitz had made funds available for stipends, because he saw an increased opportunity for individuals in academic medicine, in both the "pure sciences and the clinical aspects of medicine." His hope was that after being immersed in the preclinical sciences, a number of students would wish to pursue a Ph.D. rather than an M.D. To his chagrin, however, very few opted to change to a Ph.D. program. On the other hand, a number of Ph.D. students switched to the M.D. program. Winternitz thought that security and finances played a role and suggested the solution was for students in all fields of biology to enroll as Ph.D. students and take clinical courses as needed. Concerned that subsections of the biological sciences and medicine would narrow the medical students' view of the "role they can play in human well-being," he tried unsuccessfully to found a Department of Clinical Sociology to broaden the medical curriculum and the students' outlook.[98]

Despite his emphasis on the "soft" sciences, Winternitz recruited outstanding individuals in the basic sciences. The neurophysiologist John Farquhar Fulton (figure 27) came to Yale in 1929 as chairman of physiology after working with Sir Charles Sherrington. Just thirty years old, he was the youngest Sterling Professor. Another distinguished neurophysiologist, J. G. Dusser de Barenne, was also appointed Sterling Professor of Physiology. These appointments greatly strengthened the Department of Physiology and the flourishing Neurological Study Unit. Fulton established a primate colony early in his tenure. A year spent with Harvey Cushing at the Peter Bent Brigham Hospital in 1927 and 1928 had aroused his interest in the cerebral cortex, and primates were considered the best model for the human cortex.[99]

Winternitz strongly believed that the interdisciplinary association of scholars would result in far greater advances in physiology than if individuals worked alone, and he encouraged informal study units. The first of these formed on its own in 1923 when four members from various departments came together as the Conference Committee for the Study of Neurological Conditions.[100] This committee grew into the Neurological Study Unit as faculty members from other departments joined it, and it became the first in a series of study units that have been instrumental in developing "translational" research at Yale.

The Neurological Study Unit was further strengthened with the appointment of Harvey Cushing as Sterling Professor of Neurology. President Angell played a major role in Cushing's recruitment, which went on for more than a year. Harvard was trying to retain Cushing after his retirement from the Peter Bent Brigham Hospital at the age of sixty-two, but Cushing wrote to Angell that the main reason he was procrastinating about coming to Yale lay in a disability. He had a circulatory problem with his legs but was more concerned about his "increasing loss in powers of sustained application."[101] Angell responded that twice in the previous ten years he himself had been "confronted with the threat of death or crippling disability."[102] Cushing was also concerned about finances, as he had been during Yale's attempt to recruit him twenty-six years earlier, because the Rockefeller Foundation now

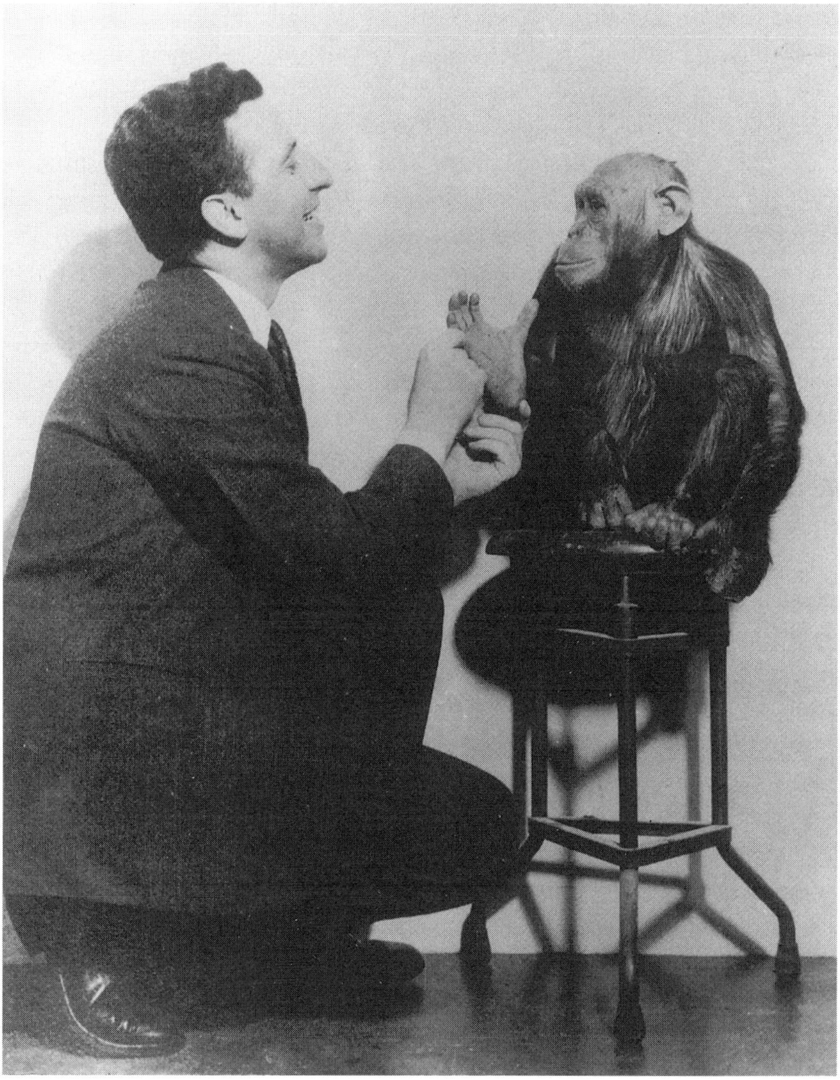

Figure 27. John F. Fulton and "Becky"

refused to support his work on account of his age. The successful recruitment of Cushing not only strengthened neuroscience at Yale but also contributed to the foundation of one of the world's outstanding collections in the history of medicine.

The Sterling bequest is usually thought of in relation to the Sterling Hall of Medicine, but the availability of Sterling professorships allowed the medical school to make a number of outstanding appointments that would not otherwise have been possible. In the 1920s, the chairmanship of physiology and physiological chemistry had been held by Lafayette B. Mendel, one of the pioneers in physiological chemistry.[103] Physiology had traditionally been taught in a didactic fashion, giving little emphasis to experimental method. With the development of chemistry as a discipline, physiological chemistry—later to become biological chemistry—began to flourish. Among his accomplishments, Mendel established a close relationship between the chemical constitution of proteins and their biological value in nutrition. He trained at least 124 Ph.D.s at Yale, of whom forty-eight were women, including Louise Farnam, the first woman admitted to the Yale School of Medicine.[104] When Fulton was appointed to the chair of physiology in 1929, Mendel remained as chairman of physiological chemistry. On the clinical side, there had been the appointment of Daniel C. Darrow to the Department of Pediatrics in 1928. Darrow was a distinguished clinical scientist with an interest in metabolism, which fitted in well with John Peters's interests.

By 1930 there were more programs than ever before laying claim to the resources of the school. Projects involving the Human Welfare Group represented a proposed investment, including buildings and endowments, exceeding $33 million.[105] More than half of the funds had been raised in the prior twelve years, and another $10 million was required for programs already approved. The total amount needed would reach $50 million if all the objectives were to be met. In the aftermath of the 1929 stock-market crash, however, resources were not going to continue to flow as they had in the past. A month after the crash, Fred T. Murphy had told George Day that fund-raising would be a waste of effort "until it has been demonstrated that there is going to be no great unemployment problem, and that industry is really coming back in the spring."[106] As resources diminished, faculty members became understandably concerned about the fate of their own particular interests. The Institute of Human Relations was not the top priority for most chairmen and faculty.

Winternitz was also experiencing a difficult period in his personal life. His wife Helen died in 1930 after five years of a debilitating illness, which may have been nephritis. Winternitz was devastated, but within the year he had recovered sufficiently to fall in love with Pauline Webster Whitney, a prominent New Haven socialite and a widow. Her husband, Stephen Whitney, had also died in 1930, leaving her with four children. Winternitz mounted a campaign, and they were married in 1932. The headline in the *Waterbury Herald* read, "MEDICAL HEAD CRASHES SOCIETY BY WEDDING SMART SET LEADER." Apparently, Winternitz had never informed his five children that he was going to remarry, and the two families did not meld well.[107]

Perhaps because of what was going on in his personal life, Winternitz was beginning to express new concerns in his reports. "Deans often dissipate their energies in futile endeavors to satisfy their critics. . . . Authority and responsibility in particular matters must be delegated to those who have information regarding these matters." He suggested that the educational policies of the university should be determined by a central council composed of outstanding "administrative officers" or deans representing the various divisions, headed by the president. Such a council would in effect replace the various Boards of Permanent Officers, the fundamental structure of Yale University. Winternitz thought a subcouncil on biological sciences would be "what is now nearly represented in the Board of Permanent Officers of the School of Medicine." When Winternitz brought the idea of a subcouncil to the Board of Permanent Officers for discussion, the board voted to remain intact but to reorganize. During the 1932–1933 academic year, the board formed two committees, a Committee on the School of Medicine, which had two subcommittees dealing with preclinical and clinical education, respectively, and a Committee on Biological Sciences dealing with graduate education. A Prudential Committee—in effect an executive committee—was also formed, made up of representatives from the various interest groups.[108]

Although the business slump had not as yet had a significant impact on the university besides the inability to acquire new resources, Winternitz reported "the growing financial support that practically all sections feel that they require," and he made it clear that it is "the prerogative of the administration to determine relative needs. . . . This is not a time for expansion. Indeed, retrenchment must be the watchword throughout the school." These were threatening words to chairmen with their own priorities, which certainly did not include the Institute of Human Relations. Describing the three basic purposes from which the policies of the medical school had developed, Winternitz listed (in order of priority) the advancement of knowledge, the training of practitioners and investigators, and the care of patients. He went on at length about the importance of investigation in limited fields of medicine but also emphasized the need for broad training for practitioners. "Through the Institute, the interests of the School of Medicine have been broadened without interfering with the progress of such disciplines as are included in the traditional and isolated school of medicine."[109]

The *Harkness Hoot,* a student magazine founded in 1930 for "creative writing and fearless discussion," ran an article in 1931 entitled "The Madness at New Haven." Speaking of the Institute for Human Relations, the article said that "no one knows precisely what the function of this great foundation is; but everyone knows how many million dollars it has cost." It said further that "scholarship and science proceeds through individual effort; for Institutes, millions and publicity; for first-class men, not a thought."[110] Flexner himself might have been the author of such reflections.

A joint committee of the Connecticut State Medical Society and the medical school sent out a questionnaire to the members of the society asking for comments about their relations with the school and New Haven Hospital.[111] One-third of the 504 replies were "definitely critical," and thirty-three individuals felt "aggrieved at the treatment received by them." In response, the medical school prepared a leaflet entitled "Opportunities Available for Physicians of Connecticut at the Yale School of Medicine and Affiliated Institutions." Much of the discussion within the committee dealt with patients of community physicians who were referred to the hospital but not subsequently referred back to the physician. In reply to a complaint brought against John Peters for not referring back diabetic patients, he said that nine out of ten patients refused to return to their former physician.

Broad issues involving the responsibility of the medical school to the health-care system also engaged Winternitz's attention. His answer to the question about what constitutes adequate health was "to bring the best available resources of medicine to the individual sufficiently and continuously, to ensure his best development, prevent illness and minister promptly to any indisposition which occurs."[112] He believed that once sufficient data on this type of comprehensive care had been accumulated, a method of distributing the cost of such care would have to be found, although not by the physician.

Winternitz did have time for less weighty matters, too. In 1934 he wrote to John Rice, a friend at the New York City Health Department, about *confiseries* at Henri Confiseur. "The most delectable are those which the Board of Health has now made it impossible for them to make. Am I to be deprived of these?"[113]

A report by the National Committee on the Costs of Medical Care and the Commission on Medical Education in 1937 reaffirmed the sanctity of the physician-patient relationship and the need for general practitioners and for better distribution of physicians. The report called for a plan that would spread the costs of medical care more evenly and would be available to everyone. Whatever plans were developed, physicians should retain their professional independence. A minority of the Committee on Costs had recommended that physicians themselves take the initiative in each community, while the majority supported an organization built around medical centers that would provide medical services to organized groups of individuals.[114]

As a result of the report, Winternitz was asked to write an article on social medicine for *American Magazine* in 1933, but for reasons that are not clear, his piece, "Medicine and the People," was never published. In it he raised questions about the health-care system that could equally well be raised today. He felt that, given the amount of money spent on health care, "good medical care ought perhaps to be more nearly within the reach of all people than it is now." He observed that although there had been real progress in eliminating acute disorders afflicting the young, "ailments which attack people in middle life and old age seem to have increased accordingly."[115]

As the financial effects of the Depression became more severe, Winternitz questioned whether a combined hospital and medical school associated with a university could play a significant role in the organization of health care. The community was already responsible for a significant amount of the costs of health care. He estimated that less than half the costs of health care were paid directly by individuals who were the immediate beneficiaries of care. There was concern, as there is today, about the lack of health coverage for a significant portion of the population, but physicians, too, were in a difficult financial situation. In June 1934 a long article in the *New Haven Register* outlined the plight of the medical practitioner. Physician income was low in general and had decreased markedly during the Depression. Medical schools were turning out too many physicians, and physicians were specializing in order to differentiate themselves. The dispensary at Yale with its free clinics was seen as an additional threat to physicians' income.[116]

Winternitz was concerned about the problems caused by training too many specialists. Medical schools had raised their standards by recruiting highly trained scientists who were specialists and became role models for the students. The family physician had been thrust into the background, and only 25 percent of medical graduates went into general practice. Winternitz wondered whether a Department of Family Medicine should be established in a medical school. No school had one in 1933. In the article he wrote for *American Magazine,* he quoted a verse he had found in a newspaper:

> *For doctors do not doctor as they did*
> *When there's human overhauling to be done,*
> *If you feel in bad condition and you send for your physician,*
> *You discover they have split him ten for one.*[117]

Winternitz proposed that the School of Medicine conduct a practical investigation of family practice in cooperation with the Institute of Human Relations. Families might be divided into three groups: one with no family physician, another with a family physician, and a third cared for by a staff physician in an optimal manner. If the value of family practice were demonstrated, "a chair of family practice might be established in the school." Such an appointment would also help to dispel the artificial social groupings that arose through specialization. Full-time faculty members were "marked in their own and in public estimation as superior because of participation in research and the advancement of knowledge."[118] The creation of a family-practice group would be "a step in the direction of fuller coordination of medicine in the community."

In December 1933, Winternitz sent a memo to the Board of Permanent Officers and a number of influential individuals entitled "A Study of General Practice." He commented that he had intended to include it in his annual report "but, for various reasons, it seemed wiser not to include it at this time."[119]

Winternitz proposed adding family-practice faculty members to a faculty entirely comprised of specialists in the middle of the Depression. His decision not to include this proposal in his annual report is not surprising. Alan Gregg of the Rockefeller Foundation thought the issue of family practice would be better left as "unspoken policy."[120] The New York Life Insurance Company was approached but had no interest in organizing large groups for payment of medical services through insurance. "We insure lives according to prevailing mortality conditions."[121] The members of Yale's Committee on Clinical Subjects, which represented influential chairmen, emphasized that they were sensitive to the social issues but that they were also general physicians with specialized interests. They believed that the "greatest advances in medicine would be fostered by the consolidation of all available resources back of projects already started or contemplated in Clinical Departments."[122] Thus, Winternitz's proposal was shelved through lack of support. Once again, the dean had been ahead of his time. Yale still does not have a Department of Family Medicine.

Although financial constraints were certainly a factor in the proposal's failure, the medical school was not under severe financial pressure. The university had asked for a 5 percent budget reduction, which was accomplished without cuts in salaries or research funds. A dean at another medical school commented on how necessary the students' tuition was for the financial viability of the school. At Yale, after deducting the scholarship and loan funds given to students, tuition accounted for less than 10 percent of the medical-school budget. A portion of the building and endowment funds accumulated over the previous fifteen years had been preserved through the Depression for educational purposes, and money had been made available to provide more financial aid to students.

In general, universities are relatively depression-proof. Salaries were frozen but not cut. No tenured faculty member was dismissed, and a number of junior faculty members were retained even after their appointments ended. The chronic nature of the financial crisis persisting year after year was the real problem. Continuing financial stringency had resulted in the rethinking of a number of ventures and had discouraged any new large-scale ventures.[123] By 1935, President Angell foresaw deterioration ahead for the university unless there was some alleviation. The financial problems persisted, however, until the Second World War erupted in 1939, which was a long time to live under continuous financial pressure.

On the academic front, the freedom that had been built into the medical-school curriculum was causing problems. In his report for the 1933–1934 year, Winternitz commented that "an effort was made to enable faculty members to keep more closely in touch with each student." Of the sixty-five students who took the preclinical examination during that year, four failed. The faculty criticized required-course "creep," which resulted in less elective time. One department suggested that the present system was a "tutorial system without tutors." A more serious criticism was that the "school is not quite meeting its obligations as an educational institution." Faculty members responded to the charge that student-faculty contact was too limited by complaining that their clinical commitments made such contact difficult.[124] The same complaint is still being voiced, even though the Department of Medicine had grown from seventy faculty members in 1934 to 226 faculty members and 186 fellows by the end of the century.[125]

Winternitz's third term ended in 1935, and to his bitter disappointment, the Board of Permanent Officers did not vote to recommend him for a fourth term. There had been discomfort at the direction of the medical school for some time. In 1932 Cushing had told Angell that Samuel Harvey was unhappy and might withdraw. Cushing doubted that Winternitz would give Harvey the necessary support. "The dean whom I know equally well and whose good qualities I admire has his faults like the rest of us."[126] Harvey wrote a five-page letter to the president complaining about increasing "central control" and the uneven implementation of the full-time plan.[127]

Angell was strongly in favor of Winternitz continuing as dean. The Prudential Committee of the corporation had voted to request that the president inform the faculty of the deliberations of the committee that would decide about Winternitz's reappointment. Nevertheless, this did not soften the opposition.[128] The chairs were determined to make a change. C.-E. A. Winslow told Angell that of the faculty members responsible for teaching medical students, eight were opposed to Winternitz and five were in favor, with no likelihood of their arriving at a consensus.

A five-member committee of senior faculty—Edgar Allen, Stanhope Bayne-Jones, Ira Hiscock, Grover Powers, and Francis Blake as chairman—had been appointed to canvass faculty opinion. Angell informed Fred T. Murphy that "to the complete surprise of all of them, including Bayne-Jones himself, the latter was unanimously recommended by the Board to be appointed dean."[129] Angell had also consulted Cushing, who felt that appointing Bayne-Jones was the best course of action. Murphy was not surprised, because there had been "waves of protest" against Winternitz. On December 24, 1934, the committee visited Angell, with Cushing replacing Bayne-Jones. Angell recorded that a slight majority of the Board of Permanent Officers and all the departmental chairs, save one, were opposed to the reappointment of Winternitz.[130] In response to questioning by the president, the committee stated that it had no confidence in Winternitz and did not "regard him as reliable." Cushing later commented that "purely personal animosities and grudges were really the moving causes." Angell informed the committee that he was unhappy to be presented with a conclusion rather than a consultation, but that it did not change matters.

Angell asked Winternitz to state in writing his intention to step down as dean and resume his former duties as chairman of pathology. Winternitz complied, adding that he would return to a position in which, "in your opinion and that of your associates, my training can be most effectively utilized."[131] His granddaughter later wrote that being chair would give him "a clear view of the incompetent Bayne-Jones guiding his trim little ship right onto the rocks."[132]

When his retirement was announced, there was an outpouring of letters filled with praise at the job Winternitz had done. Even Flexner, who had fallen out with him over the Institute of Human Relations, wrote, "I cannot but feel that the progress made in New Haven is well nigh miraculous, and it is all due to your unflagging energy and ability."[133] Winternitz remained chairman of pathology until his retirement in 1950, long after Bayne-Jones had left Yale, and he served as a member of every important committee in the medical school.

Winternitz stayed feisty to the end. A European pathologist reportedly greeted him with a daily "Good morning, Herr Professor." After this had occurred several times, Winternitz took him aside and told him, "The only people called professor in the United States are piano players in whore houses!" Winternitz also retained a strong say in the wider medical community. When the Grace Hospital pathologist retired after the merger of the two hospitals, the director of the new Grace–New Haven Community Hospital wanted to recruit Harry Zimmerman back from New York. Zimmerman had been one of Winternitz's protégés and a favorite of the medical students but was someone to whom Winternitz had taken a dislike, and his appointment was vetoed.

Angell stated in his 1935 presidential report stated that Winternitz's accomplishments had few parallels in American educational history. "He brought a dauntless spirit which could not be discouraged, extraordinary imagination, sound ideals and a capacity for endless hard work."[134]

6

THE BUBBLE BURSTS

The Depression Years

The new dean, Stanhope Bayne-Jones, had been a student and later colleague of Winternitz's at Johns Hopkins. His major interest was in bacteriology, and he happily accepted an offer to head his own Department of Bacteriology at the new medical school in Rochester. In 1932 Stanhope Bayne-Jones, by then dean at Rochester, was recruited to Yale, primarily to be master of Trumbull College and secondarily to be professor of bacteriology and immunology. President Angell was eager to appoint a scientist as master of one of the new residential colleges funded by the Sterling bequest. In May 1930 Winternitz had written a glowing recommendation for Bayne-Jones: "He is a man of the very finest personal qualities."[1] A year later he repeated that "Bayne-Jones is in the first instance a man, clear-thinking, straight-forward, and capable."[2] Bayne-Jones and Winternitz are shown with Blumer in figure 28.

In discussing his appointment as Winternitz's successor, Bayne-Jones commented that because he was relatively new to Yale he was viewed as

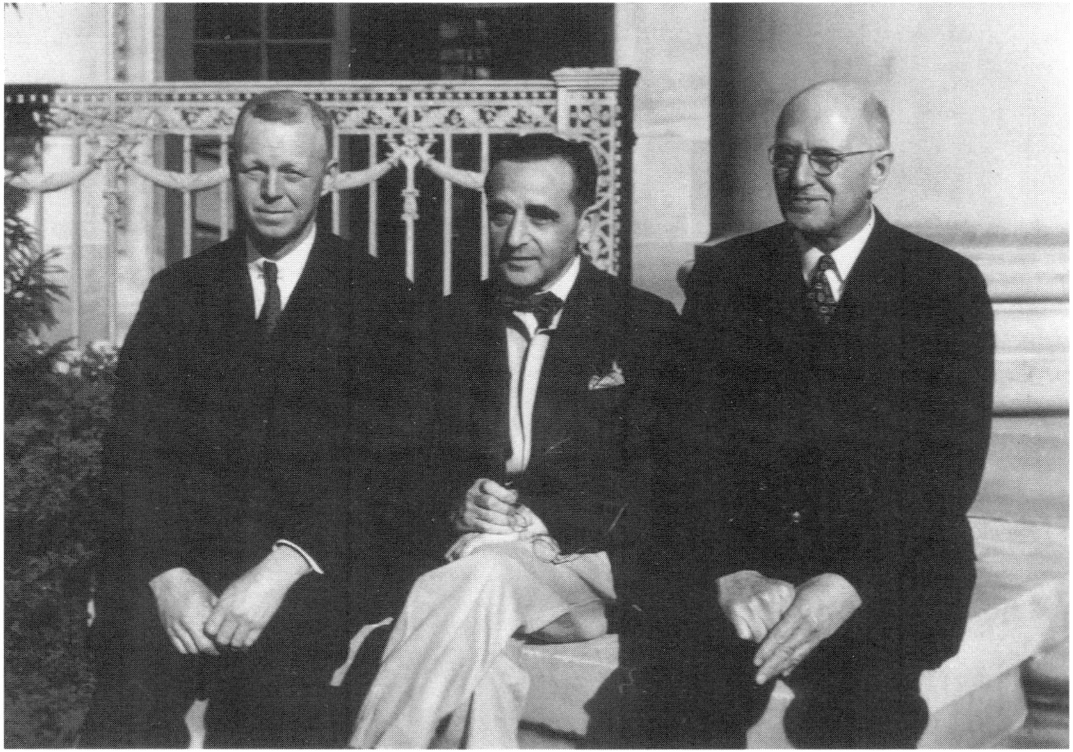

Figure 28. Bayne-Jones, Winternitz, and Blumer

neutral, and that no one else would have been acceptable to Winternitz. "I know definitely that Dr. Winternitz would have fought another nomination very bitterly." When Bayne-Jones told Winternitz that he was letting his name be submitted, Winternitz replied, "B-J, if it's you, it's all right. If it had been somebody else, I would have fought them."[3]

In contrast, Susan Cheever, presumably reflecting her grandfather's views in his later years, wrote that Bayne-Jones "bent all his energy to unseating his difficult benefactor." In the fall and winter of 1934 "Bayne-Jones began secretly lobbying individual faculty members to line up a majority against Winternitz's appointment."[4] The Winternitz family was sure that Bayne-Jones was the arch enemy and expressed surprise that Winternitz did not fight. Nothing, however, in Bayne-Jones's oral history indicates anything less than admiration for Winternitz. "I regarded him as a great man . . . and also had an affectionate relationship because he was never cruel to me."[5]

The son and grandson of physicians, Stanhope Bayne-Jones was born on November 6, 1888.[6] His grandfather, a busy medical practitioner who also held the chair of medicinal chemistry and microscopy at Tulane University, was a lover of books and archaeology, and he exerted a strong influence on Bayne-Jones. Having served in the Medical Department of the Confederate Army, his grandfather had accumulated a large collection of weapons, which no doubt played a part in Bayne-Jones's military interest.

Several members of the Bayne family had gone to Yale, and it was natural for Bayne-Jones to attend Yale, just as it was natural for him as a New Orleans native to attend Tulane University Medical School. Unhappy at Tulane, he wrote to William Welch seeking a transfer to the Johns Hopkins Medical School. He was accepted and by chance ended up living in the same Baltimore rooming house as Welch. Bayne-Jones moved the bed in his room so that it was directly above the bed in "Popsy" Welch's room. Whether thanks to vertical emanations from the room below or to his own native intelligence, he graduated first in his class and was asked to remain at Johns Hopkins in the pathology department.

In 1916 Welch arranged for Bayne-Jones to study under Hans Zinsser at Columbia. The war in Europe reawakened Bayne-Jones's military interest, and he was commissioned as a first lieutenant in the Medical Reserve Corps. When the United States entered the war in 1917, he was sent to England, where his uncle, Surgeon General William Crawford Gorgas, arranged for him to serve with the British Expeditionary Force both in Flanders and, later, on the Italian front. After the war, he returned to Johns Hopkins and in

1921 married Nannie Moore Smith, an X-ray technician at the Johns Hopkins Hospital.

As the new dean, Stanhope Bayne-Jones faced an immediate problem—with his office furniture. Winternitz had furnished the dean's office with oriental rugs and elegant furniture from the Garvin Collection of the Art Gallery. For Bayne-Jones, "it seemed unnatural to have a dean of a hard-working place like that in such rich and gorgeous surroundings."[7] He paid tribute to Winternitz, however, in his first report to the president: "The development of the school under the influence of Dr. Winternitz was of greater and more far-reaching importance than any other events of the past."[8]

Bayne-Jones had certainly inherited problems significantly greater than office furnishings. The Great Depression was causing major financial repercussions at the medical school, which was running a deficit of $400,000, grudgingly subsidized by the university. Bayne-Jones also felt the need to revise the overcrowded curriculum. He realized that students needed to understand the sociological aspects of medicine but, in contrast to Winternitz, who conceived of medicine as embracing all the sciences and part of the humanities, Bayne-Jones considered medicine to have specific objectives in the "prevention and care of disease, and medical education had a task to train men and women for the practice of medicine." Medicine was "not merely a division of social sciences," and the medical school "not simply an administrative and convenient budgetary unit."[9] Bayne-Jones was going to steer the school in a more conservative direction than his predecessor had, a retrenchment that had already been taking place to some extent, because of faculty discontent, before Winternitz stepped down as dean.

Psychiatry and mental health, which had been located in the Institute of Human Relations, would become a department like any other in the medical school. A much sharper distinction would be drawn between the medical school and the institute. The Rockefeller Foundation had remained the funding source of the institute, and a 1936 internal Rockefeller memo had expressed concern about it. The departure of the dean of the Yale Law School, Robert Hutchins, to become the president of the University of Chicago and "the unwillingness or inability of President Angell to assume any firm control, subjected the program to the play of conflicting administrative interests and prevented the Institute from arriving at any adequately integrated program." In contrast, however, to Flexner's comment that the Rockefeller Foundation had supported the program only for the benefit of psychiatry, the memo concluded that "the effective collaboration of the biological and social sciences in research on human behavior has possibilities of profound importance . . . just as . . . in 1920."[10]

Integration of the medical and graduate schools also unraveled, especially after the Committee on the Biological Sciences and the Committee on the Medical School were abolished. The Committee on the Medical School was superseded by a proliferation of medical-school committees, which included the Prudential, or Executive, Committee of the Board of Permanent Officers, the Committee on Admissions, the Pre-clinical Committee, and the Clinical Committee. In Bayne-Jones's view, separating preclinical and clinical education in this manner worked against the "continuity" of medicine.

There were complaints, too, about academic requirements. Twenty-one students out of 229 had withdrawn from the medical school in one year, with eighteen of them leaving because of scholastic difficulties. Concerned, the Board of Permanent Officers abandoned the requirement for students to take the examinations of the National Board of Medical Examiners. Instead, the comprehensive examination was reinstituted at the end of the second year of medicine. Another problem, much more difficult to correct, appeared to be the great variation among departments in their educational philosophy, which marginal students found difficult to handle. Some departments were very specific in their requirements; others gave no direction.

The new dean also had reservations about the full-time clinical teaching system.[11] Lack of sufficient revenues to support an expanding full-time faculty meant that it was difficult to pay adequate salaries and retain good junior-faculty members. Bayne-Jones believed that the full-time system tended to remove physicians from a personal relationship with their patients. The agreement with the General Education Board concerning the full-time clinical system had been changed in 1925 to allow a modified full-time plan. Bayne-Jones was in favor of a modified full-time plan that would allow associate and assistant professors to collect an amount equal to their salaries from patient fees. He had successfully instituted a similar financial plan while at Rochester. With the blessing of the dean, the Department of Surgery—which had been the first department in the school to go to the full-time clinical system—became the first department to adopt the modified system. Professional fees collected under the full-time structure had been considered part of the university budget. Now, after prolonged discussion with the university administration, a Clinical Research and Teaching Fund was instituted to allow faculty members to use their professional fees for academic purposes.

In accordance with university directives, the medical school's annual budget had been reduced in 1933 by $50,000. Always a painful process, the budget reduction placed the incoming dean in an unenviable position. Bayne-Jones commented that further budgetary cuts at the school would damage the departments academically, and that further cost cutting in the hospital would hurt the educational mission.

In spite of the financial pressures of the Depression, almost one-quarter of departmental budgets went to research. In 1935 foundations and commercial companies donated $96,000 for research, although even then there was already concern about the implications of commercial support. "Grants from commercial firms require the most careful scrutiny," commented Bayne-Jones in his 1935–1936 report.[12] The Fluid Research Fund, initiated in 1929, was a particularly successful source of financial support for the medical faculty and is still in existence today. The fund was administered by a committee of the BPO and was used to support numerous investigators in all departments. Initially, Yale and the Rockefeller Foundation shared equally in financial support of the fund, although the foundation's contributions could not exceed $250,000 a year.

To reinforce the concept of continuity in the medical school, the admissions process had been changed in 1935 to allow the Prudential Committee to act as the Committee on Admissions, enabling applicants to be seen by both the clinical and the preclinical faculty. In a distinct departure from previous custom, members of the Committee on Admissions received a list of the applicants from the dean's office divided into three groups: women, Americans, and Hebrews.[13]

Bayne-Jones said in his first report that "much might be written about the intellectual and personal qualifications of those seeking medical training. Both the best types and the poorest are attempting to enter the profession. Among the many problems presented by these applicants as a whole, those relating to Jews and to the economic status of prospective medical practitioners are especially serious." Bayne-Jones estimated that about 45 percent of the applicants to the medical school were Jewish. "This is not a local phenomenon. Men of Jewish origin are crowding towards medical schools everywhere in numbers far in excess of their proportional representation in the whole population of the country. . . . Out of some two hundred Jewish applicants, five or six are accepted for admission here."[14] The total applicant pool in 1935 was 501, of whom 131 were interviewed and 76 accepted, with 51 matriculants.[15]

Bayne-Jones's attitude did not change with time. Four years later, in 1939, he commented that there had been informal requests for admission by a large group of refugees, as well as by "American Hebrew students who were prevented by the war from returning to England to complete their courses at the extra-mural schools." At that time, 204 out of 489 Yale Medical School applicants were Jewish (approximately 42 percent). Bayne-Jones stated that the large number of Jewish students applying to American medical schools "presents a difficult problem for both the medical schools and the applicants themselves. Most of the medical schools appear to have had unofficial quotas, which in the metropolitan areas of the East are about three times the proportional representation of the Jewish element in the general population."[16] From 1935 to 1942, the proportion of Jewish students admitted to each entering class at the Yale Medical School was about 12 percent. During the same period, the proportion of women in each class varied from 6 to 8 percent.[17]

Soon after Bayne-Jones became dean in 1935, a large university Department of the Physiological Sciences was formed as part of the "university concept." It included several laboratories—of physiology, physiological chemistry, primate biology, neurophysiology, pharmacology, and toxicology, as well as the Laboratory of Applied Physiology, chaired by Yandell Henderson. Lafayette Benedict Mendel and John Farquhar Fulton, both Sterling Professors, were appointed cochairmen of the university department. Mendel, who had been professor of physiological chemistry in Yale College since 1903, chaired the original Department of Physiological Sciences when it was formed in 1920; it became the Department of Physiological Chemistry in 1932.

Mendel died in 1935, after less than a year as cochair of physiological sciences. He was succeeded by Cyril Norman Hugh Long, who had been an assistant professor at the University of Pennsylvania, with previous training in organic chemistry, physiology, and physiological chemistry. Although young, Long already had a research reputation in the field of endocrinology and carbohydrate metabolism. He subsequently became the dean of the medical school and chairman of an integrated Department of Physiology.

Within the medical school there were now fourteen major departments and four study units with separate budgets. The departments included seven preclinical departments and seven clinical departments, among them the Department of Public Health and Harvey Cushing's Section for Research. There were also the Atypical Growth, Adolescence, Dental, and Neurological Study Units. When Cushing reached the mandatory retirement age in 1937, he was appointed director of studies in the History of Medicine.

Bayne-Jones oversaw an expansion in cancer research after the medical school received a generous gift in 1937. Clinical interest in cancer had existed in the school, but little research had been done at Yale until Winternitz established the Atypical Growth Study Unit in conjunction with Samuel Clark Harvey and George M. Smith. With financial support from the Anna Fuller Fund, Winternitz recruited distinguished cancer researchers, including Harry S. N. Greene in pathology, Edgar Allen and William Gardner in anatomy, and Francisco Duran-Reynals in microbiology. Harvey Cushing had become aware of the desire of his Yale classmate Starling W. Childs to support medical research, and Childs was invited to visit the medical school. He was particularly impressed with the Atypical Growth Study Unit, and in consequence the Jane Coffin Childs Memorial Fund for Cancer Research was established with a $3.5 million gift from Starling W. Childs and Jane Coffin. Bayne-Jones recommended Winternitz as chairman of the Scientific Advisory Board, but the Childs family wanted the dean himself involved. Winternitz did later become chairman of the board when Bayne-Jones left Yale.

By the time Bayne-Jones became dean, a large proportion of the U.S. population was unable to pay for medical care, as a result of the economic situation. This forced an examination of the entire system of health care. A number of medical educators and politically powerful individuals believed that the provision of health care should be a function of government, and they advocated a variety of reforms ranging from a completely socialized system to one with some form of regulation and government control. These ideas were coupled with "sharp criticism of existing medical practice and a violent attack upon the profession."

A similar debate raged within the walls of the medical school. Bayne-Jones believed that the profession could bring about needed improvements on its own "with the preservation of ideals, standards and behavior proved by long experience to be beneficial."[18] Other faculty members thought that the school was not doing enough to deal with the national health-care issues. In defense Bayne-Jones cited the work of C-E. A. Winslow and Ira Hiscock in public health, as well as the work of Winternitz and that of John Peters, who served on the Advisory Committee of the American Foundation for Studies in Government, which had produced a valuable report on universal health care.

Bayne-Jones realized, however, that there would need to be changes in the medical curriculum in the wake of the Social Security Act and legislation concerning medical care in unemployment relief, as well as the growing awareness that sickness and health were matters of public concern.[19] Bayne-Jones, by nature more conservative than Winternitz or Peters, thought it likely that the United States would administer government control of health care, and that the medical profession would continue to play a prominent role in policy decisions and the provision of care.[20]

The issue of "socialized," or "state," medicine continued to occupy the medical school, with some faculty members strongly believing that Yale should take the lead in introducing the new "medical-social order." Bayne-Jones commented that to "throw the energy" of the school into "social medicine" would be a distraction from its primary mission of teaching and research.[21] To mollify the faculty, who wanted a more activist approach, Bayne-Jones took the time-honored decanal way out by appointing a committee to look into the matter.

The difficulty of meeting medical costs applied as much to students as to anyone else, and the Prudential Committee of the Board of Permanent Officers eventually implemented a voluntary insurance program for the medical students, after much debate. One of the essential features of the plan was that a student could receive three weeks of hospitalization for ten dollars.

Bayne-Jones soon had to deal with a new Yale president. In 1937, after fifteen years as president, James Rowland Angell stepped down and was succeeded by the provost, Charles Seymour. Angell had been much more comfortable dealing with the medical-school faculty than with the Yale College faculty. "The executive has few more discouraging experiences than trying to enlist the interest and support of people who have no real comprehension of what you are driving at."[22] As provost, Seymour had become well acquainted with the problems of the medical school. On the other hand, in contrast to Angell, who had been trained in experimental psychology and was familiar with scientific tradition, Seymour was a historian. Bayne-Jones commented that "it may be necessary for the new President to add to his vocabulary, some of the current jargon of medicine."[23]

Either because Seymour felt the need to be educated or because he was concerned about the medical school's financial status, he presided over the meetings of the Board of Permanent Officers at the medical school. With the school continuing to run significant deficits, relations with the university administration were crucial. The interdependence of the medical school, hospital, and dispensary meant that educational changes affected the hospital and dispensary, while decreases in the hospital budget had an impact on the medical school's educational process.

The role of the Yale University Clinic was debated anew. Most dispensary patients were the "working poor," wage earners who could afford food and shelter but not the cost of medical care.[24] Arthur Dayton, the assistant dean, argued strongly that it should be a general clinic related to the other social and health agencies in the city rather than a specialty referral clinic for patients with difficult problems. Unlike in Hartford, where during 1931 41 percent of clinic visits were made to privately supported clinics, 74 percent of all clinic services in New Haven were provided by the New Haven Dispensary.[25] This amount of unpaid care could not be sustained, and the hospital, which had become financially responsible for the dispensary, wanted the university to provide more financial support.[26]

In an effort to alleviate financial pressures, a President's Committee on University Development was formed in 1938 with George Day as chairman and Harvey Cushing as associate chairman. The committee included a Division of Medicine and Public Health, chaired by Bayne-Jones, which had a goal of raising $10.5 million to support medical education, research and fellowships, psychiatry, and the general fund. The medical committee suggested that the previous hundred years might be called the "Century of Medical Enlightenment while the years to come might be called the 'Age of Health,'" a concept we are still struggling with today.[27]

Bayne-Jones wanted the university to commit to a five-year plan allocating $150,000 annually to the hospital and $350,000 annually to the medical school. "On this [current] basis we have a medical school–hospital institution which is first class in many ways and second-rate or poor in others."[28] In spite of significant financial support from the university, however, funds were still insufficient to compensate the faculty adequately. "The willingness of men and women to lead frugal lives in order to work in medicine is an old characteristic of the breed of medical people. Undue advantage should not be taken of this type of self-abnegation."[29]

Financial problems and underpaid faculty notwithstanding, the reputation of the medical school was growing. A 1934 report by the Council on Medical Education of the American Medical Association had rated the Yale School of Medicine among the top six or seven medical schools in the country except for facilities, faculty salaries, and the condition of the library. A commitment was made by the corporation to improve the library, but prolonged discussions ensued about its ultimate location.

In 1937, the Board of Permanent Officers rejected a proposal from the surgeon general of the army to establish a Medical Reserve Officers' Training Corps at the medical school, even though militarism was on the rise. The board's refusal was based on educational reasons, as it believed that students could better spend their time on the fundamentals of medical training rather than learning military organization.

Meanwhile, the dean's "honeymoon" was ending. Bayne-Jones was "disconcerted by criticism, by some members of the Corporation, that my report though inordinately long showed little evidence that the school was interested in education."[30] Bishop Henry Knox Sherrill, a member of the Yale Corporation and the Board of Managers of the Massachusetts General Hospital, considered himself the resident expert on medical education, according to Bayne-Jones. Another influential corporation member, Fred T. Murphy, was described by Bayne-Jones as "a relatively well-to-do man with little practice and contact with medical schools" who "didn't try to keep up."[31] Howell Cheney, a member of the corporation from Manchester, Connecticut, read Bayne-Jones's reports assiduously and then wrote the dean long letters telling him what was wrong. "I really endeavored to approach your report with a very sympathetic attitude and am sorry to have such a discouraging letter to send," he wrote.[32]

The corporation was particularly concerned about the continuing financial crisis in the medical school. The university appropriation had grown to $400,000 and included $90,000 for the hospital and dispensary, which consumed 40 percent of the total medical-school operating budget. To add to the financial burden, administrative responsibility for the Department of Psychiatry and its clinic was to be transferred from the Institute of Human Relations to the medical school. The Rockefeller Foundation had made a five-year grant, which would cover expenses for the psychiatry department until 1944, but the medical school would then have to find the necessary funds for psychiatry-faculty salaries.

For the first time in the history of the medical school, a consultant was hired to make a preliminary survey of the needs of the medical school and hospital in "collaboration" with the dean. As so often happens, the "needs of the medical school" became a wish list for the faculty, which included increased personnel, raising the level of salaries (particularly for junior faculty and "important" members of the administrative staff), and development of deficient areas (such as the endowment and buildings). In an understatement for a school where the budget deficit amounted to 40 percent of the total operating budget and the effects of the Depression were still being felt, Bayne-Jones concluded, "These needs, translated into dollars and cents, make up a very large sum."[33]

The financial problems continued to affect implementation of the full-time system, holding down the size of the clinical faculty and preventing adequate increases in salary. Also, Bayne-Jones believed that the full-time system interfered with the physician-patient relationship. He thought that having a well-paid nucleus of senior faculty on a full-time university basis was preferable to spreading the budget thinly over the entire faculty, but he realized that most chiefs and clinical faculty members did not share his views. In October 1939, Winternitz commended him for his pragmatism in handling the financial situation: "You have steered the prow of your report with great acumen through the mine ridden sea of full time medicine."[34]

In Europe, World War II had erupted. France was soon occupied, and England's very existence was threatened. Yet the cataclysmic events unfolding on the other side of the Atlantic appeared to have relatively little effect on everyday life at the Yale School of Medicine. Adequate funding remained the major preoccupation.

When Winternitz stepped down as dean in 1935, the Institute of Human Relations lost a powerful supporter, and the faculty was concerned about funds being diverted from the medical school at a time of financial need. Nevertheless, the institute survived. Mark A. May was appointed director in 1938, and the institute was reorganized to operate with a Liquid Research Fund rather than with separate budgets for separate sections. Of the large number of individuals, departments, and schools originally involved in the institute, a group of twenty faculty members from psychiatry, psychology, sociology, and anthropology came together in January 1938 to "formulate some of the basic laws of human behavior and social interaction."[35] A major focus of study was "the process of socialization of the human organism in its culture."[36]

In preparation for submitting a grant-renewal application the institute listed its accomplishments, which included twenty books and monographs and three hundred or more scientific reports and articles. The Rockefeller Foundation, which had provided the major funding for the institute, was sufficiently impressed to award it a further $700,000 over a ten-year period.

Time described the institute in February 1940 as a place whose purpose was "to find ways and means whereby mankind could learn to live together more harmoniously." The magazine reported that its "placid, pipe-smoking" director, Mark May, saw the outbreak of World War II as confirmation of his scientist's theories that aggression is caused by frustration. "The German people are deeply frustrated. At first, they attacked the Jews, and have now turned their attack upon their real frustrators." He explained that because they could not get their hands on the English, whom they really hated, they had turned on the Jews, innocent bystanders. "Since the beginning of the war, we have heard relatively little about the Jewish persecution, for the hatred has now been channelled."[37]

As a measure of university lack of interest in what was happening in Europe in 1939, Bayne-Jones quipped that "Yale was more disturbed about the library than about Poland."[38] Seymour's vacillation on the matter of a site had for years delayed the construction of a badly needed expansion of the Medical Library. The corporation finally decided to add the library to the Sterling Hall of Medicine rather than construct a separate building and recommended to the Sterling Trustees that $600,000 be appropriated for it. The addition would consist of a Y-shaped extension of the present building and house about four hundred thousand books, with the Historical Library as one of the wings of the Y. The completion of the library brought together the collections of Harvey Cushing, John Fulton, and Arnold Klebs, forming an unrivaled history of medicine collection.[39] Kleb's material did not actually arrive until after the war. At the dedication, in 1947, Wilmarth S. Lewis, chairman of the Committee on Libraries and Museums, remarked that "[to] find a moment of equal significance in Yale's history one must go back 240 years to the day when Congregational clergymen placed their books on the table in Branford for the founding of a College in this colony."[40]

In 1938 Charles Wesley Dunn, an attorney for the food industry, had approached Bayne-Jones about developing an Institute of Nutrition at the medical school. The main purpose of the proposed institute was to "develop and practically use the science of nutrition, and thus to protect and to improve the public health." The institute would also serve as a center for instructing students and the public in the science of nutrition. Given the financial state of the country, important efforts were needed to help solve dietary problems for "persons of limited means." The institute would perform tests and studies for the contributing industrial groups and would "aid the food manufacturing industry in the solution of its individual scientific problems."[41]

According to Bayne-Jones, the "food manufacturers were to supply a building, maintenance, and funds for grants-in aid, all of which would be under University control."[42] On May 29, 1939, President Seymour wrote to Clarence Francis, president of General Foods, who represented the Associated Grocery Manufacturers of America, to say that the university would be "happy to cooperate with representative food manufacturers in establishing an Institute of Nutrition."[43] Discussions continued over the next several months with increasing enthusiasm about an industry and university partnership.

The final proposal, approved in November 1939 by Bayne-Jones, Day, and Dunn with the blessing of Seymour, specified that the university would provide a building and upkeep, which would cost about $1,350,000. The food manufacturers for their part would provide a minimum annual income of $100,000 over twenty-five years and grant-in-aid contributions of $100,000 to $150,000. The Institute of Nutrition was to be a separate corporation with its own board of governors, which would include representatives of the university in "equitable proportion."[44] A summary of the proposal was submitted for presentation to the corporation.

A contract drafted in December 1939 by the university's legal adviser Frederick H. Wiggins and submitted to the corporation was almost immediately attacked by Dean Acheson, who was concerned about "the integrity and the independence of the University against possible corroding commercial interests."[45] During the debate, Seymour reportedly never mentioned his approval of the project. A corporation committee was appointed to meet immediately with Bayne-Jones in his office. Bishop Sherrill stated after the committee meeting that the corporation could not allow the university to have this kind of relationship with the food manufacturers. Bayne-Jones felt that if the university adopted the point of view of this special committee, he would not be able to continue as dean of the medical school.

The corporation had already appointed Bayne-Jones for a second five-year term, beginning on July 1, 1940. The Board of Permanent Officers of the medical school had recommended his reappointment to President Seymour, who had agreed to Bayne-Jones's requests for administrative assistance. Seymour had also allocated some funds for the physical plant and a paid physician for student health. After the corporation action, Bayne-Jones told Seymour that "the decision reached involves questions of my judgement and regard for the welfare of the university. It also involves the relation of the dean to the president and other officers of the central administration and my colleagues in the school, and the outcome of further discussion of the committee's action will have a profound effect on my standing and fitness to serve the University usefully."[46]

The food manufacturers were not happy with some of the contract terms and were also aware of the corporation's opposition. They asked that no action be taken.[47] On May 11, 1940, however, the corporation accepted the recommendation of the Committee on Educational Policy that the establishment of a National Institute of Nutrition be approved in principle. A committee including Blake, Bayne-Jones, Long, and Winternitz prepared a memorandum on the proposed institute that suggested a loose affiliation, which was unacceptable to the manufacturers.[48] The food manufacturers ultimately appropriated $1 million for a foundation headed by the president of MIT, in which Yale would play no role.[49]

Bayne-Jones, convinced that Seymour had not supported him, declined renomination for a second term as dean, although he did formally thank Seymour "for all the support and assistance you and the officers of the administration gave me."[50]

A search committee of the Board of Permanent Officers was formed under the chairmanship of C.-E. A. Winslow, and it quickly decided on Alan Gregg of the Rockefeller Foundation as the candidate of choice. In February 1940 Seymour offered him the position, adding that "the University Corporation has decided to make the development of medicine and public health the major aspect of our policy in the immediate future."[51] Seymour suggested that Bayne-Jones visit Gregg, who was on his way back from Europe, but Winslow thought Winternitz should accompany Bayne-Jones, "as B-J might give a somewhat negativistic view of the situation."[52] In the end, Gregg decided that "especially after a visit to Europe in its present condition . . . my duty is to remain with the Foundation."[53]

7

THE MEDICAL SCHOOL GOES TO WAR

After Alan Gregg declined the offer to succeed Bayne-Jones as dean in 1940, the search committee was unable to identify a candidate to whom it could unhesitatingly commit the school's destinies. It recommended that Francis Gilman Blake, the chairman of medicine, be appointed acting dean for the 1940–1941 academic year. Blake was willing but wanted to remain chairman of medicine, and he asked for assistance in carrying out his duties as acting dean. George H. Smith, chairman of the Department of Bacteriology and editor of the *Yale Journal of Biology and Medicine,* was appointed assistant dean, with responsibility for the Committee on Admissions and the Committee on Student Affairs. The medical students viewed Blake as "a fairly stuffy and remote person."[1] "Wrinkle" Smith, on the other hand, short and with lots of facial wrinkles, interacted closely with the students.

In a major administrative change, a Committee on Program and Policy was appointed to replace the Prudential Committee of the Board of Permanent Officers. The new committee was a small, influential group consisting of the chairs of medicine, surgery, pathology, and physiological chemistry and pharmacology—Blake, Harvey, Winternitz, and Long—as well as Assistant Dean Smith. The committee was charged with making "recommendations concerning the future policies and programs of the school."[2]

By 1940, the faculty of the medical school had grown to 242 full-time members, including 26 professors, 24 associate professors, and 36 assistant professors. In addition, there were 179 clinical or part-time faculty members. Winternitz had inherited a mere seven full-time faculty members when he assumed the deanship in 1920. Blake justified the large faculty by emphasizing the need to teach not only 251 medical and public-health students but graduate students and nursing students as well. Similar rationales are given today, at a time when the Yale Medical School has approximately one thousand full-time faculty and about five hundred students. Blake estimated that in addition to the cost of educating medical students, graduate students cost the medical school about $50,000 a year.

At the departmental level, the ten-year search for a chairman of pharmacology ended in 1940 with the appointment of William T. Salter.[3] Salter had studied biochemistry with James Conant, president of Harvard, and had done significant work in iodine derivatives and thyroid chemistry with Sir Charles Harington, the English biochemist who with Rosalind Pitt-Rivers first synthesized the thyroid hormone, thyroxine. At the time of Salter's appointment, pharmacology was split off from physiological chemistry to form a separate department. Henry Barbour, former head of the pharmacology section, had been made a research associate and been relieved of administrative duties, while L. S. Goodman and Alfred Gilman had been reappointed as assistant professors for a three-year term, with no guarantee of future reappointment.[4]

Yale was becoming increasingly popular with medical-school applicants. In 1940, 438 students applied for fifty places in the first-year class. Interviews were granted to 104 students, and seventy were accepted. Despite these statistics, there was concern at the fact that twenty students accepted by Yale went elsewhere. Blake commented, "It is unfortunate that many of these prospective students are today obtaining advice from Yale men, in medicine and otherwise, who still think that the medical school is located on York Street."[5] The social life of the medical school was part of the attraction for students. Highly popular teas were put on by the faculty wives with no complaints about the role. Student and faculty attendance reached 19,663 for the year, at a total cost of $511.18 not including contributions of food and cigarettes from "the many ladies who served as hostesses."

The newly constituted Committee on Program and Policy spent a great deal of time critically reviewing the school's educational program. The school was under pressure to increase the size of its student body in order to accommodate the requirements of national defense. Nevertheless, the committee decided to maintain quality and keep the enrollment steady at about fifty members in each class, and it emphasized that both the thesis requirement and the comprehensive examinations at the end of the basic-science years and the clinical years would be preserved.

Consideration was given to whether subjects are best taught in a "horizontal" manner (for example, the endocrine system taught in anatomy, physiology chemistry, and pathology) or "vertically" (that is, by organ system). It was decided to use elective time to experiment. The proposed changes were adopted by the Board of Permanent Officers, with each department convinced that its courses should be mandatory. The curriculum revision was seen as a reaffirmation and elaboration of the liberalized educational program introduced in the 1920s. Blake felt that the medical student "must learn to pilot his own boat and assume to a large extent the responsibility for acquiring that content of knowledge which is necessary in charting his future professional course."[6]

Restrictive admission quotas had not disappeared entirely. A statement issued by the medical school's Committee on Admissions stated, "It is the policy of the committee on admissions to assure admissions to those candidates who by their outstanding intellectual experience and quality clearly deserve the privilege of medical education. Apart from moral integrity and physical fitness no other factors are taken into consideration. The committee has established no system of 'quotas.'"[7]

The dean of nursing, Effie Taylor, informed President Seymour in May 1941 that neither the medical school nor the nursing school accepted any African-American students. This exclusionary policy was based on the necessity to assign medical and nursing students to a "clinical field where the situation might readily become complicated, and where adjustments might be exceedingly difficult," and, further, where the "difficulty is concerned with harmonious adjustment."[8]

An African-American graduate of Spellman College applied to the Yale School of Nursing and was rejected because of the unwritten policy. "We believe it would be inadvisable for several reasons to admit colored nurses here."[9] The former secretary of the university, now dean of Washington Cathedral, Anson Phelps Stokes, was furious. (Stokes had argued the case for Marian Anderson before the Daughters of the American Revolution in 1938 when they refused to let her sing in Constitution Hall.) In his reply to Stokes, President Seymour raised the question of the "physical fitness of Miss Towns." Rather than comment on her race, he had chosen to comment on her obesity.[10]

Meanwhile, with war imminent, members of the medical faculty were already serving on various government boards involved with national defense, including the Army Board for the Control of Influenza and Other Epidemic Diseases, the Council of National Defense, and National Research Council committees. The amount of time the faculty was spending away from the school to participate in the defense effort made it difficult to maintain the curriculum, a harbinger of things to come.

There was a lack of surgical beds for teaching, because more beds were being used for private and semiprivate patients. To reassign them would take away needed income from a hospital that already had a significant deficit. Hospital admissions had risen from 6,580 in 1930 to 11,186 in 1940, with the medical service more than doubling admissions from 1,200 to 2,473. The hospital had even prepared tentative architectural plans for additional buildings. Blake sounded a note of caution: "The exacting responsibility of meeting ever increasing demands for clinical service can in the end defeat the educational and scholarly interests and obligations of the faculty if the magnitude of that service becomes too great."[11]

The meeting of the Board of Permanent Officers that took place on December 22, 1941, fifteen days after the Japanese attack on Pearl Harbor, exhibited a tone very different from previous meetings. The first order of business was to shorten the medical curriculum to three years, with four eleven-week terms a year, to eliminate most of the clinical electives, and to make the thesis requirement optional. Class size was increased to sixty, and admission requirements were liberalized to admit more students who already had three years of college. The faculty thought that the students were taking too much time studying for examinations in this accelerated curriculum, because most students took both the comprehensive examination as well as the National Board examination. As the results of the two examinations agreed reasonably well, a decision was made to drop the comprehensive examination.

The faculty was faced with the need to produce as many physicians in as short a period as possible while at the same time maintaining the quality of the graduates. Fortunately, both the government and the universities recognized that high standards for medical education were necessary not only for the war effort but also to meet the needs of the civilian population in the postwar period.[12] Despite this recognition, the pressures to accelerate medical education increased as the demand for physicians grew during the course of the war.

The faculty ultimately accepted the idea of admitting students after two years of college, because Blake thought there was no alternative but to accept this "plan for further acceleration dictated by expediency."[13] The implications of the curricular changes were such that a graduate could obtain an M.D. degree just five years after completing a high-school education. Finances, however, were a problem because there was no time for students to earn money for tuition, which had remained at $2,000 for the full course. Fortunately, the Kellogg Foundation provided a grant of $10,000 for scholarship aid, which, when added to other funds already available, provided a substitute for summer earnings.

There were now fewer interns and residents, and their training period was drastically shortened. The educational process was therefore much more intense, while at the same time, fewer faculty members were available to teach because many were taking leaves of absence to serve the war effort.

The Procurement and Assignment Service, which was charged with advising the surgeons general about the availability of physicians for military service, requested a list of faculty that indicated who was available for military service and who was essential for effective teaching. By October 1942, seventy-nine members of the part-time and ten members of the full-time medical faculty had left for service with the armed forces. The former dean, Stanhope Bayne-Jones, left in February 1942 and was assigned to the Office of the Surgeon General for the duration of the war.

Blake received a letter from Frank H. Lahey, chairman of the Directing Board of the Procurement and Assignment Service, criticizing the "unusually high" proportion of Yale Medical School faculty under the age of forty-five who had been listed as essential for teaching.[14] Blake told the Board of Permanent Officers that he thought a reasonable policy had been followed in listing members of the Yale faculty with M.D. degrees as either "essential" or "available." The Committee on Program and Policy of the medical school unanimously agreed that no change in policy should be adopted at the time.

The university recognized the important role the medical school was playing in the war effort. The Faculty of Arts and Sciences promulgated a policy that no promotions would go forward for the current year. President Seymour recommended to the corporation, however, that promotions be implemented in the medical school in view of its contribution to the war effort. The corporation passed a resolution of appreciation for the medical faculty's willingness to teach in the accelerated program during the summer "without additional compensation."[15] The resolution ended on a somber note forecasting a deficit and observing that "the members of the Faculty share with the alumni and students the common task of meeting the demands imposed by the nation at war"—a sentiment similar to President Hadley's during World War I.

Medical-student life changed dramatically during the war. Blake noted in his 1941–1942 report that "the impact of the war upon the students during the past year has largely centered around their relationship to the operation of the selective service."[16] The constantly changing policies fostered in the students a sense of insecurity and a great deal of uncertainty as to their best course of action to finish their medical education. Eventually, both the army and the navy permitted physically qualified students in good standing to be commissioned in the inactive reserve. With the commission, medical students would be allowed to complete medical school and a one-year internship before being ordered to active duty.

Army and navy medical-student training programs were instituted in June of 1943. Medical students who were already officers in the inactive reserve were given the option of either remaining in it until the completion of their medical studies or resigning their commission and attending medical school as enlisted men on active duty with pay, uniforms, and an allowance. On graduation from medical school, they would be commissioned as officers in the medical corps. The majority of students in the reserve resigned their commissions and enlisted as privates.

When called to active duty, the medical students were sent to Camp Devens, Massachusetts, and then returned to Yale for the medical-school summer term. The enlisted men were housed in cramped Calhoun College quarters and were marched to and from meals, which in addition to drilling in the hot weather left them irritable and exhausted. Reveille was at 0630 hours, and meal times were strictly specified. There were daily inspections, and military lectures and exercises were held every two weeks. Eventually—and with difficulty—the medical students adapted to military discipline.

The medical faculty, who felt that much of the military discipline was extraneous and interfered with medical education, duly calmed down, only to be riled by an army directive that medical-school classes would be filled with applicants on a numerical basis without any choice by the school. At the fifty-fourth annual meeting of the Association of American Medical Colleges in October 1943, Major General George F. Lull, deputy surgeon general of the U.S. Army, emphasized that all students in medical school who were under army control should be regarded as being "primarily soldiers, with the study of medicine a secondary consideration."[17]

The general went on to explain the numerical selection process.[18] An unnamed agency would divide premedical students into three groups: superior, average, and below average. The students would then be distributed among the medical schools in proportion to student enrollment. Medical schools would have no choice in student selection. Fortunately, the course of the war was such that the need for physicians subsided before this totally unacceptable directive could be implemented. After the war, General Lull became secretary to the Judicial Council of the American Medical Association, when the Connecticut State Medical Society charged the medical school with unethical practices. After July 1944, students were no longer accepted into the training program and instead became eligible for the draft. If the individual failed to maintain satisfactory standards while on active duty in the training program, he was liable to be assigned to general military duty, possibly as a corpsman, who could administer first aid and rudimentary treatment.

The army and the navy had different approaches to producing the physicians they required. The navy allowed more freedom from military routine. The army, by decision of the First Service Command, demanded a strict military routine, with barracks and mess halls. During the first three weeks of the Army Student Training Program, students were severely handicapped in their medical studies.[19] The Board of Permanent Officers unsuccessfully requested commutation of service for the army students, even though commutation had been authorized in nearly all the medical schools outside the First Service Command.

While the medical students were being trained for military service upon graduation, the order to active duty came on July 15, 1942, for the 39th General Hospital Unit, the Yale University–affiliated unit honoring the 39th Mobile Surgical Hospital, the pioneering Yale unit in World War I. Plans for a medical-school send-off for the 39th were foiled because many of the personnel had been ordered to active duty at various army stations prior to the mustering of the unit as a whole. A message was sent, however, from President Seymour, the deans of the medical and nursing schools, the hospital, and the state medical society: "As you leave for active duty, we are anxious to extend to you, on behalf of Yale and the New Haven Community, our warm good wishes and deep appreciation of the service which you are giving to the nation. University and town are consecrated to that service and all our traditions demand that it should be carried on in whatever field it can be made effective. There is no field more important than that which you enter, where you will bring to the armed forces in the hour of need the science and art of doctor and nurse. We are proud that through you Yale and the New Haven Hospital have the privilege of serving the American people."[20]

Following training at Camp Edwards in Massachusetts and Camp Stoneman in California, the 39th embarked for Auckland, New Zealand, where a thousand-bed hospital was opened, to which another thousand beds were subsequently added for convalescent patients.[21] In 1945 the 39th General Hospital Unit was transferred to Saipan (figure 29), where it helped treat casualties from Iwo Jima. After setting up its own hospital, the unit received large numbers of casualties from Okinawa and was ordered to increase the hospital capacity to two thousand beds, in preparation for the invasion of Japan. Fortunately the war ended before the beds were necessary.

In addition to providing clinical care, the unit conducted research on infectious diseases, psychiatric problems of jungle combat, and atabrine treatment of malaria. Several members of the unit were detached for special duty. Ashley W. Oughterson was appointed surgical consultant to General Douglas MacArthur, and he organized and directed the Joint Commission for the Investigation of the Medical Effects of the Atomic Bomb in Japan.[22] This commission was the forerunner of the Atomic Bomb Casualty Commisssion, on which a number of members of the Yale community served.

Research at Yale took on a decidedly wartime orientation, with departments undertaking projects of military significance funded by the government; much of the work could not be published, because of its confidential nature. Several studies on war gas were carried out, which led to the use of nitrogen mustard for the treatment of Hodgkin's disease. Blake and Bayne-Jones were heavily involved in research under the auspices of the Army Board for the Investigation and Control of Influenza and Other Epidemic Diseases. John Paul was director of the board's Commission on Neurotropic Diseases and was engaged in research on encephalitis. In the Department of Physiology research for the war effort was being done by John Fulton on the effect of altitude on primates.

The Institute of Human Relations, too, was deeply involved in war-related research. The institute had conducted a large anthropological study before the war in the islands of the Pacific, particularly the Caroline Islands. "When this was brought to the attention of the Intelligence Department of the Navy,

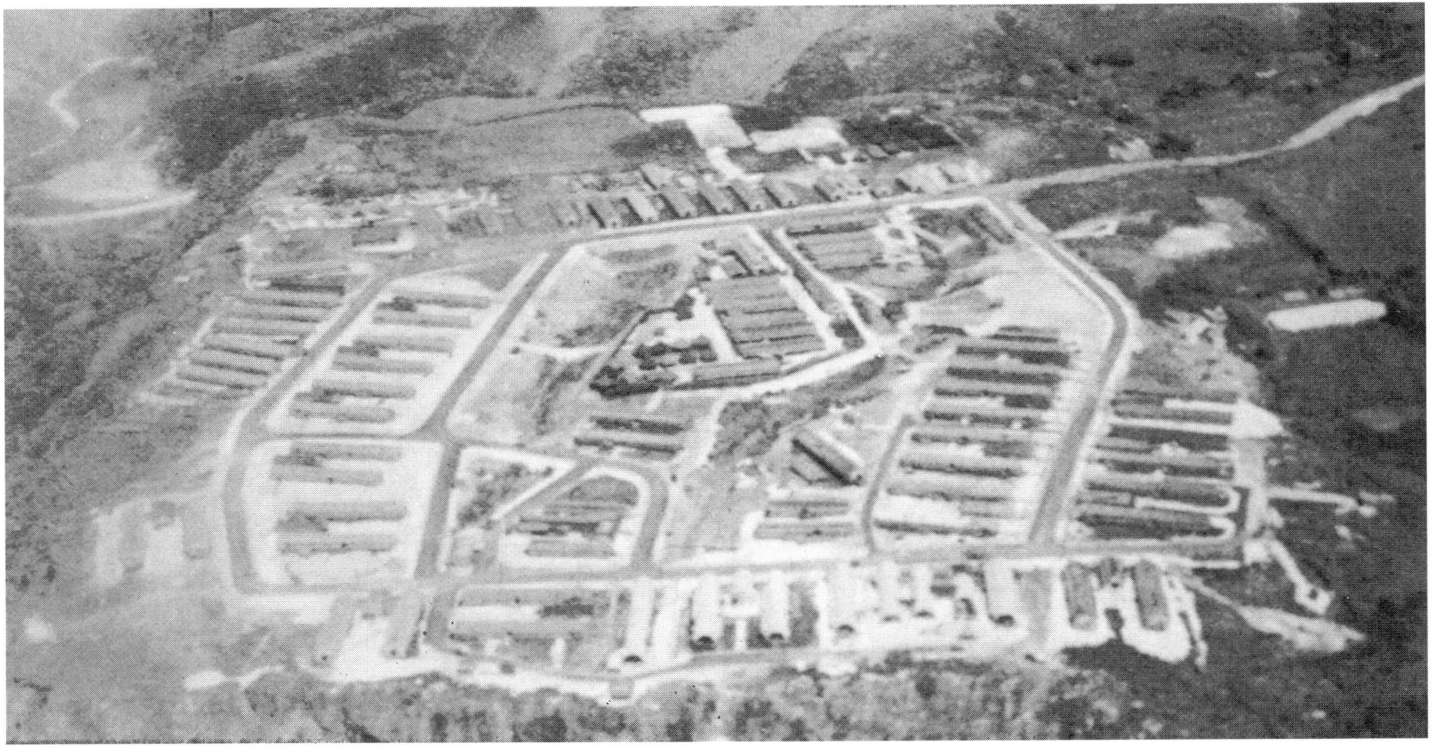

Figure 29. World War II: the 39th General Hospital on Saipan in 1945

it was apparent that this information was of immediate and strategic importance."[23] The Caroline Islands were a key target in the Allies' Pacific strategy and were retaken in 1944.

The accelerated program of medical education had been instituted at the request of the army and navy at the opening of the 130th session of the medical school on June 29, 1942. During the three calendar years—four academic years—of the program, 201 medical students received an M.D. degree and 163 were commissioned as medical officers in the army or navy.[24] The increased enrollment from fifty first-year students to about sixty made additional medical officers available only in the program's last graduating class, whose members would not go on active duty until the completion of an abbreviated internship. Yale's individual contribution as a result of the accelerated program was small but added to the combined effort of all the nation's medical schools.

In the midst of the turmoil caused by the war effort, the Committee on Program and Policy produced a remarkable document in May 1944 entitled "A Statement on Program and Policy of the School of Medicine, Yale University."[25] The concepts underlying the document were similar to those so forcefully advocated in the 1920s by Dean Milton Winternitz, who was a member of the 1944 committee. The statement set out the basic principles of a medical school with high standards and limited enrollment, followed by the more controversial aspects of Winternitz's original proposals. Students admitted to medical school would be undifferentiated and could opt for either an M.D. or a Ph.D. degree. A broad Division of Biological Sciences would include the Department of Clinical Medicine, which would contain departments for medicine, pathology, psychiatry, surgery, pediatrics, obstetrics and gynecology, anatomy, botany, physiology, psychology, and zoology. The budgets of all the constituent departments would be presented to the Executive Committee of the Division of Biological Sciences.

The Board of Permanent Officers approved the statement's concept that the medical-school departments were university departments with educational responsibility for qualified students of the university, irrespective of school enrollment. Although more cautious about undifferentiated M.D. or Ph.D. students, the board did approve facilitating the machinery to change tracks if desired. Dean Blake neatly sidestepped the statement's "Proposal for the Organization of Biological Sciences" by ruling that "the subject needed further clarification."[26]

Unhappiness with the educational process occasioned by the war effort contributed to the general desire to make a clear statement of the goals of the medical school. The 1944 statement was a clear reaffirmation of the 1920 reorganization, which had been in abeyance since 1941. Medical students were mature individuals and should be considered graduate students. The document recommended reinstating the research thesis as a requirement because it had been a mainstay of the curriculum, and there was a desire to educate individuals to become productive scholars in the medical sciences as well as practitioners.

Dean Blake's report for the 1941–1942 academic year pointed out that research in the medical sciences was an important part of the work of the medical school. To accomplish these goals, full-time university departments of clinical medicine were necessary. "The problem of full time in clinical medicine with respect to staff and hospital facilities is the most important and pressing problem confronting the medical school today."[27] A full-time program in clinical medicine required funding, which became difficult with a hospital deficit approximating $188,000 in 1943 and projected to reach $235,000 the following year.

A Joint Committee on Relations of the School of Medicine and the New Haven Hospital was formed, consisting of three members of the corporation and three members of the hospital's board. The medical school required a minimum of 350 teaching beds and approximately eighty thousand outpatient visits a year in order to maintain its teaching program. To compensate the hospital for the teaching requirements, the university would contribute $206,237 in 1945 toward the support of the hospital and dispensary, which was an increase of $50,000 in the annual appropriation.[28]

The joint committee suggested making a new affiliation agreement between the university and the hospital. To determine the amount the university should contribute to support education in the hospital, it was necessary to determine the actual cost per day of ward patients and dispensary patients. In consequence, the costs for various hospital services (such as radiology and laboratory services) that were buried in clinical-department budgets had to be uncovered. This theme of trying to determine the exact costs for each partner in the medical school–hospital relationship has persisted to the present day. Dean Blake added that it would have been better to have had a large endowment but that the sources were "not immediately obvious."[29]

At the same time, the university was "deeply concerned with the whole problem of the biological sciences." After due consideration, the Sheffield Scientific School was reorganized by the corporation to make its functions conform more closely to the original plan for the school, which had been to consolidate and integrate the sciences in a university Division of Natural and Physical Sciences and Mathematics. "Sheff" would now have no undergraduate responsibilities. Medical-school departments would be part of the university Division of Biological Sciences, including bacteriology, pharmacology, physiological chemistry, pathology, public health, and clinical medicine, which would include all the clinical departments. There would be separate Executive Committees for the physical sciences and the biological sciences. Budgets and appointments in the various departments would be under the scrutiny of the division director and the respective Executive Committees.

This reorganization fitted nicely with a "Statement of the Program and Policy of the School of Medicine" prepared by the Board of Permanent Officers of the medical school: "The basic principles of the program and policy of the School of Medicine cannot be divorced from the other science departments of the University."[30] Dean Blake described the reorganization in his 1944–1945 annual report as "a forward-looking step [that] should further the integration of the science departments of the University." He then noted in his report, "At this point in the preparation of this report the whistles have blown, Japan has surrendered and the war is over. It seems appropriate to turn without further ado to plans for the future." Blake ended the report with a prescient comment: "All of this, of course, requires money and doubtless in a changing society new sources must be tapped, including industry and perhaps the federal government, should the Bush Report and recommendation for federal support of scientific research be implemented by properly drawn legislation."[31]

In 1944 President Franklin Delano Roosevelt had asked Vannevar Bush, director of the emergency Office of Scientific Research and Development, to extend the office's work in peacetime. Bush issued a report in 1945, drawing on the reports of four representative committees. The success of the wartime research effort in the medical and physical sciences carried out under the aegis of the Office of Scientific Research and Development was the impetus for the proposed extension of federal support to peacetime research. The findings of the report indicated that such research could best be carried out in universities. The program of federal support would be implemented by a new agency, the National Science Foundation.[32]

Blake himself had chaired a subcommittee for the Yale Committee on Postwar Medical Service that strongly recommended endorsement of the Bush Report, provided academic freedom were protected with appropriate safeguards.[33] Enthusiasm for the report, however, was not universal.[34] A number of competing bills were introduced in Congress, and there was a great deal of jockeying among various agencies to be the principal funding body. Ultimately, legislation was passed endorsing the Bush Report, which became the platform for the tremendous federal support of scientific research at universities.[35]

Over the ensuing year, the medical school returned to a peacetime schedule. The accelerated program of medical education so reluctantly put in place in 1942 was terminated on March 16, 1946, with the graduation of the fifth wartime class.[36] Two hundred and sixty-six medical students had graduated under the accelerated program, during which the school was practically in continuous session. The medical faculty was concerned about shortcomings in the wartime medical curriculum and felt that medical schools and teaching hospitals had a responsibility to remedy any deficiencies.

Rather than teach refresher courses, the faculty decided to offer opportunities for serious postgraduate work in any of the medical-school departments. With the G.I. Bill of Rights making it financially possible for veterans to undertake postgraduate work, fifty-one postgraduate students and fellows enrolled in the 1945–1946 academic year, and eighty-eight in the following year. Postdoctoral education was assuming increasing importance, and the school needed to develop a definite policy as to its responsibility and capacity for advanced education.

Putting the medical school back on a regular academic schedule was complicated by a March graduation in the accelerated program taking place while the other classes were at various stages in their medical education.[37] The fourth-year accelerated class graduated in March as scheduled. Second- and third-year students were advanced into the third and fourth years, respectively, at the opening of the spring term, which provided an extra term at the end for badly needed elective work. The first-year class was not advanced, so there were no second-year students during the spring term. Many of the entering first-year students had received inadequate preparation during their two-year premedical college course.

Despite faculty concern, the students in the immediate postwar classes performed well. Fulton noted that "those who were cut off from academic contacts during the war years appear to have a profound consciousness of what they missed and a desire to apply themselves that transcends anything we have encountered in peacetime."[38] Donald Barron, assistant dean and chairman of the Committee on Student Affairs, was impressed to see how eager the students were to seek additional educational opportunities. He thought that this was due not only to the freedom from wartime restrictions but also to a growing appreciation of the opportunities offered in the "elastic" system of the medical school. Barron was concerned, however, about the quality of the students who applied. Among one thousand applicants the admissions committee was only able to identify 164 who it felt would benefit from attending Yale. To remedy this situation, the school made scholarship aid available to incoming medical students, which it had not done in the past, and recruited alumni to interview prospective students.

Worried about the hiatus in academic medicine caused by the war, the faculty was deeply committed to stimulating the research interests of these postwar students. Although the medical school had major financial problems, the faculty voted to use the $1.6 million in the James Hudson Brown Memorial Fund for the Support of Research, bequeathed in 1944 to establish James Hudson Brown Junior Fellowships, which would allow qualified students to spend a year in research.

Along with the postwar return to academic values, there was firm support for implementing the full-time policy for clinical medicine. Stanhope Bayne-Jones, who had supported the modified full-time plan for financial reasons, had left Yale to become the first president of the Joint Administrative Board of the New York Hospital–Cornell Medical Center. Milton Winternitz, a strong supporter of the full-time system, had remained at Yale as chairman of pathology and continued to play a major role as a senior member of the faculty, chairing many of the key committees. To provide financial support for the full-time program as well as for educational purposes, full-time faculty members were encouraged to see private patients. The professional fees fed the Clinical Research and Teaching Fund, which was modified to allow for the partial support of departments—a decision that was to result in an annual income of $100 million by the year 2000, accounting for almost half of the operating budget of the medical school.

At Blake's request, Winternitz prepared a memorandum on problems confronting the medical school and hospital. Winternitz recommended the formation of a university Division of Medical Affairs to coordinate the activities of the various medical departments, including medicine, public health, and nursing, with a university-appointed director and an Executive Committee representing the various interest groups.[39] This committee aimed to broaden the base of the old committee structure to include junior faculty. Although some of the department chairmen felt the new administrative structure might be too elaborate and time consuming, general faculty sentiment favored it.

Winternitz's memorandum also stressed the crucial need to develop a suitable organization to correlate the different interests of all divisions of the university that dealt with medical matters. A committee was appointed to examine administrative issues, including the role of the dean. Medical faculty of professorial rank surveyed by the committee believed that the faculty should have more input into the formulation of medical-school policy, and that there should be more interaction with other health-related schools and organizations.[40]

Detlev Bronk, future president of the Rockefeller Institute and a distinguished biophysicist, and George B. Darling, a public-health specialist and president of the Kellogg Foundation, were the final candidates for the position of director of the Division of Medical Affairs.[41] The director would be an officer of the university, with responsibility for the budgets of the medical school, the nursing school, and university support of clinical facilities in the hospital. He would also supervise relations among the various constituencies. The choice fell on George Darling, who was appointed in 1946. Some faculty members had worked with him while he was executive secretary of the National Academy of Sciences in Washington, and he was considered to be "a man of broad philosophy, sound administrative judgement and good scientific background."[42]

Blake was willing to be considered for reappointment as dean in 1946 only if administrative assistance were made available to him. There was close to unanimous agreement among the members of the Board of Permanent Officers that Blake should be reappointed for a second term.[43] Blake thought that the reorganization would relieve him of some of the administrative burden, but the load in fact became heavier, and in April 1947 he submitted his resignation to President Seymour. Seymour urged Blake to reconsider, but the loss of several assistant professors in the Department of Medicine convinced Blake that it was imperative he return to the department on a full-time basis. Because of concern among younger faculty members that the financial problems of the medical school were overwhelming, Blake wanted the announcement of his resignation worded carefully, and Seymour duly obliged.

8

PEACE AND READJUSTMENT

During the meeting of the Board of Permanent Officers at which Blake's resignation was announced, President Seymour said that he and division director George Darling had conferred with several members of the board and found that C. N. H. (Hugh) Long, chairman of physiological chemistry, would be favored as the internal candidate. A written ballot was held at the meeting, and Long was unanimously elected dean of the Yale University School of Medicine.

The major problem facing Long as he assumed the deanship was insufficient funds, a problem that had plagued the medical school since its inception. One of the main reasons for the financial difficulties was the support given to the hospital, both direct and indirect, through the budgets of the clinical departments. Unfortunately, the medical-school deficits came at a time when the rapid increase in the university's educational costs far outstripped the increase in income.

At a Board of Permanent Officers meeting in December 1946, President Seymour warned that "the question as to whether the university can afford a four-year medical school must be frankly faced."[1] Earlier that year, Seymour had identified the medical school as a fund-raising priority to the corporation; the school needed additional funding "as provision against the mounting costs of medical education and to strengthen the staff in medicine and nursing."[2] In 1948 the corporation wanted a balanced budget, but Seymour cautioned that "financial economies carried too far will cause educational misfortunes that would stultify the educational purpose of the University."[3] Seymour went on to say that until new funds could be secured, the university would have to dip into its endowment.

The corporation had authorized the president to appoint a University Council charged with improving the entire university's relations with the public and alumni. Alumni were appointed to various subcommittees, including a Committee on Medical Affairs. Prior to the initial meeting of this committee in June 1948, the chairman, Reginald Coombe, chairman of the board at Memorial Hospital in New York, provided an overview of the medical school. He ranked it well within the first ten, and perhaps within the top five, medical schools in the United States.[4] The bulk of his report, however, dealt with the financial burden of the hospital on the university. A member of the Yale Corporation complained that the medical school had a 1945–1946 deficit of about $548,000, whereas the Medical College of Cornell University was completely self-supporting. Coombe explained that Yale would have had a surplus if, like Cornell, the school had received salaries and other expenses from its teaching hospital.

In its December 1948 report, the Committee on Medical Affairs drew the attention of the corporation to rumors that "the School should or may be liquidated or reduced to a strictly pre-clinical basis, because of the heavy financial strain imposed by it, on the University." The committee requested that the corporation reaffirm its interest in continuing the medical and nursing schools, subject to several conditions, including renegotiation of the agreement with the hospital, more teaching, improved public relations, and the inauguration of a fund-raising campaign. The committee recommended that the hospital and medical school develop a logical system of cost accounting, but thought it doubtful that the net cost to the university for the medical school could be brought below $200,000. "Unless the University is to revert to the status of a college, it must be prepared to continue ample support of its graduate schools."[5]

President Seymour said that the corporation wanted no conditions attached to its support of the medical school and had "[reaffirmed] its interest in the continuation of Yale's medical and nursing schools as integral parts of the University, equipping men and women for careers in the health services essential to serve the nation's need."[6] In an effort to create incentives for increasing the medical school's clinical income, the corporation voted that any balance in the Clinical Research and Teaching Fund not needed for expenses would be matched by the university and placed in an endowment fund.

Fortunately, research funds were beginning to become more plentiful, which was both a boon and a source of concern to Dean Long. The majority of research grants were awarded on an annual basis, without any commitment to renewal. Furthermore, the amount of research funding available exceeded the number of trained investigators, creating intense competition among departments and institutions for investigators. There was a growing tendency to judge an individual for promotion solely on the basis of the number of papers published. "The present emphasis on research as the sole criterion for academic advancement is not encouraging to those who believe that a teacher should teach and a clinician be at the service of the sick," wrote Long in his 1947–1948 report.[7]

Long also thought that the national policy of spending constantly increasing amounts of money in the hope of finding cures for diseases like cancer was not sound. Although his concerns about the potential dangers of the research behemoth were well founded and are still valid, universities and humanity have benefited immeasurably from the remarkable scientific advances that have been made. The first ventricular assist device, or "artificial heart," was developed at Yale in 1949 as a research-thesis project by a third-year medical student, William H. Sewall Jr., in collaboration with his faculty adviser, William W. L. Glenn, a cardiac surgeon. The total cost to construct the pump was $28.50, with the motor taken from an erector set made by a company founded by a Yale medical graduate, A. C. Gilbert.

The Clinical Research and Teaching Fund was certainly helping the financial condition of the school, contributing $100,000 to departmental budgets, which meant committing the full-time staff to support various departments through consultation fees. These fees amounted to about 30 percent of the total budget of the clinical departments. Even today one finds discontent among medical faculty members over the disproportion between university salaries and the amount earned by some faculty members, unequal shares of clinical income among departments, and how much private practice should be allowed.

The new dean, although himself a basic scientist, made a powerful statement about the duty of the faculty to do more than impart factual knowledge. Students needed an appreciation that patients are "human beings, subject to all the emotional, economic and social forces that sway the daily existence of us all." He restated the essential features of the Yale system—a minimum of course work and no course examinations, no enforced class attendance, a wide selection of electives, a thesis requirement, and the ability to spend six years in school without extra tuition. Worried about the milieu in which the students were living, Long commented that measurements of their vitamin-C levels had indicated that a significant number of first-year students were vitamin deficient. He also expressed his belief that "in the whole field of medical education, there [was] no more important question than the current value to the first-year medical students of the many hours spent in dissection."[8]

The postwar period produced a growing number of physicians interested in further instruction in the various medical disciplines. The medical school and the Connecticut State Medical Society agreed to joint sponsorship of postgraduate education, which had been very successful in the past. The program offered Yale an opportunity to be helpful to physicians in Connecticut and at the same time have the School of Medicine and its associated hospital be regarded as the "medical center" of Connecticut. There was a perception that the medical school did not favor the applications of Connecticut residents, and the possibility of a second medical school had been suggested.[9] The governor, Chester Bowles, doubted "very much that the state would support a medical school and thought that most of the agitation centered in the 'Hartford medical group.'"[10] President Seymour proposed to increase the medical-school entering class by twenty-five places, which would be allocated to students from Connecticut.

Sentiment for a second medical school within the state grew stronger, however, and in 1949 the state senator from New London asked that legislation for a second medical school be placed on the legislative agenda. The *New Haven Register* reported that "the public also realizes that it is virtually impossible for a Connecticut boy or girl to enter the only medical school in the state."[11] John Davis Lodge, a candidate for governor, made a campaign speech favoring the second medical school, and the university pressed a loyal alumnus, future senator Prescott Bush from Greenwich, into service in an unsuccessful attempt to halt the movement.[12]

In his 1948–1949 report, Long said that medical schools—Yale in particular—were confronting one of the most difficult periods in their history. Decisions about the future of the health-care system, its relation to medical education, and the adverse financial situation held profound implications. In the future, physicians were going to have to be more than simply practitioners of medicine. "Schools will be judged by the degree to which they succeed in articulating their policies and programs with growing social consciousness that adequate medical care for our people, regardless of economic circumstance, must in some way be provided."[13]

One of the ways Yale could respond was to increase the number of physicians it produced. Yale received 1,500 applications but could admit only sixty-five students. A major limitation was the number of beds available for teaching. Sufficient clinical facilities would be available at the West Haven Veterans Administration Hospital for use by an expanded number of students, but part of the problem was financial. Tuition fees covered only about one-quarter of the actual educational cost. In addition, stricter admission requirements made it more difficult for students to enter medical school.

Long was unhappy that medical education was fragmented into four years of premedical courses, four years of medical courses, and often four years of postgraduate education, all under different auspices. In 1950 he proposed that a coordinated program be developed in cooperation with Yale College. The proposal to shorten the period of premedical and preclinical training by instituting a five-year program for premedical and preclinical studies was greeted for the most part with apprehension that the standards of medical education would decline. The specter of medical education during World War II loomed large in the minds of the faculty, and the proposal was not implemented. Comments were made that students were "immature," ill prepared, and tended to be "uncultivated," with criticism directed toward high-school and college education.[14]

Long reiterated his concern about the medical school becoming a research institute rather than a center of medical education. Despite receiving more than $1 million annually for research support, the medical school's deficit was $628,904. Overhead costs for research grants, which covered the expenses of doing research, were reimbursed at a much lower rate than the estimated 25 percent needed. The university had a policy that government agencies should be asked for reimbursement of 50 percent of overhead costs. Private foundations should provide at least 5 percent of overheads, but the university would be willing to accept no overhead reimbursement because such grants would be few in number.[15]

George Darling had summarized the problems of the medical school when he arrived at Yale in 1946. Relations between the medical school and the rest of the university were strained, with a large segment of the university and a significant portion of the corporation questioning the advisability or even the possibility of continuing a four-year medical school in view of its continuing deficit. Morale in the medical school was low because of the general unrest of the postwar period and the inability to plan in the uncertain climate of university policy. No effort was made to increase medical-student enrollment, which in part was responsible for the state's decision to proceed with plans for a second medical school. The school's governing body—the Board of Permanent Officers—was not functioning well, alternating between "rubber-stamping executive actions already taken and furious controversies over inconsequential matters."[16]

A number of factors exacerbated the financial problem. The university's contribution to the hospital had mushroomed, primarily because of the amount of support the hospital required. There was inadequate recovery of overhead and operating costs from grants and contracts. Revenue was constrained by the full-time clinical faculty policy and the small student enrollment. Class size was limited because of the clinical facilities available through a single hospital affiliation. At the same time, large numbers of graduate students were being supported by the medical school without adequate financial reimbursement by the university.

Darling attributed part of the problem in university-hospital relations to the fact that the university played a dominant role in hospital policy. While the hospital administration objected to the imposition of programs by the medical school, there was also an awareness that the university was paying, so it did not really matter.[17] The assumption that teaching beds must be ward beds, and that ward beds were responsible for the financial deficit, had led to the hospital's expectation that it was the responsibility of the medical school to make up the loss. If the hospital closed these beds, the medical school would not be able to support a clinical program, and the university could not afford to have this happen. Therefore, the deficit-financing agreement would continue, giving the hospital no incentive to adjust its rates to costs. Reimbursement from the state, city, and even insurance companies did not reflect real costs. After prolonged discussions between the hospital and the university, the concept that a teaching bed was a ward bed was expanded with an agreement that semiprivate beds also could be used for teaching.

The concept of a group of salaried full-time faculty members collecting fees that were turned over to the school was highly unpopular with organized medicine. The Connecticut State Medical Society decided that the medical school's group practice violated the American Medical Association's code of ethics and referred the matter to the AMA Judicial Council for study.[18] The *Yale Daily News* covered the story with the headline, "Med School System Declared Unethical." In the article—by Gaddis Smith, a future Yale historian—Dean Long denounced the medical society for releasing news of the charges without notifying him.[19] The AMA Judicial Council did not ever bring the issue to the House of Delegates at the next national meeting, from June 11 to 15, 1951.

Financial problems continued to be a major issue for Yale and other medical schools across the country. More than three-quarters of the privately owned schools were operating with a deficit, and even tax-supported schools were having financial problems. The need to expand the physician pool to meet the demands of the Korean War was compounding the problem. Congress was prepared to provide federal aid to education, with the approval of most medical-school deans and leading university presidents, but the political might of the American Medical Association blocked the measure.

The seriousness of the medical school's financial problem can be gauged by the fact that the Board of Permanent Officers, in order to foster group practice, voted to modify the full-time clinical system and allow the dean to use the Clinical Research and Teaching Fund for faculty salaries. The clinical-practice committee recommended incentives, relation of salary to clinical earnings, and similar measures, all of which were anathema to the proponents of the full-time system. It also recommended that clinical services be taken into account at the time of promotion.

Despite the seriousness of the financial crisis, President Seymour had left no doubt in his 1949 Alumni Day address that the university would continue its support of the medical school. "Alumni of a generation ago not infrequently raised the question as to whether Yale could afford a medical school. Today, I am here to say that the school, in its prestige and its service is an essential and vital part of Yale. We cannot afford to omit any effort that would increase such prestige and heighten such service."[20]

In March 1948 Darling, with the concurrence of Long, had outlined the problems that medical schools faced.[21] Costs of medical education were increasing, augmented by the economic crisis in the hospitals and the refusal of the government to reimburse the hospital costs of patients for whom it had assumed responsibility. The evanescent nature of research funding made it impossible for the medical schools to make long-term commitments to investigators, particularly as the school became more dependent on this external funding. The abundance of research funds had created the impression that medical education was doing well even as the financial crisis grew. The danger to the medical school was minimal so long as the educational program was supplemented by the research program and not supplanted by research funding.

The Federal Security Agency administrator, forerunner of the secretary of Health and Human Services, held a meeting in Washington to discuss a program of federal aid to schools of medicine, nursing, and public health. He outlined three possible sources of federal support to the schools, including scholarships, construction programs, and direct aid. The consensus of the attendees was that there was no need to encourage further applications by offering scholarships, and that the idea of construction programs was not timely. Direct aid to schools, however, was considered vital, with only Syracuse expressing concern about accepting aid under a government plan. The federal administrator pointed out that no school would be obligated to apply if such a plan were forthcoming.

When war in Korea broke out in 1950, the medical schools were determined not to accelerate premedical and medical education, which had resulted in the lowering of standards in World War II. In August the Joint Committee on Medical Education in Time of National Emergency, representing the Association of American Medical Colleges, the American Medical Association, and the American Hospital Association, relayed this determination to the government in a statement to the National Security Resources Board. Yale's Board of Permanent Officers wanted to cooperate with the government during the Korean conflict but demanded that every effort should be made to preserve the standards of medical education and that under no circumstances should medical schools be directed in their selection of medical students, which had almost happened during World War II.

There was not much enthusiasm among the medical schools to make significant sacrifices during the "national emergency." The Board of Permanent Officers was only weakly supportive of the emergency; the Korean conflict was never mentioned as a "war" in the minutes. "At the same time, it is deeply essential that schools be in a position to carry forward their programs of investigation." The Association of American Medical Colleges passed a resolution that there be the fullest utilization of nonmilitary federal hospitals. Dean Long thought that academic medical centers should have the "same protection as West Point or Annapolis."[22]

The year 1950 also brought the retirement of the major architect of the modern Yale University School of Medicine, Milton Winternitz, chairman of pathology for more than thirty years, dean for fifteen years from 1920 to

1935, and chairman of virtually every significant medical-school committee. Harry S. N. Greene succeeded Winternitz as chairman of pathology. In response to an inquiry several years previously as to whether Greene would make a good chairman, Long had commented that he had a "dynamic and refreshing point of view." Greene "[was] best described as an individualist," a trait that "has not endeared him particularly to the physicians of this city."[23]

Arnold Gesell, too, retired. Because the Clinic for Child Development had been so closely identified with Gesell, a committee consisting of the chairs of pediatrics, psychology, and psychiatry recommended the clinic be expanded to include child psychiatry. The name was changed to Child Study Center in order to reflect a wider sphere of interest. Milton J. E. Senn, a Minnesotan, was recruited to head the center. Senn, initially interested in the chemical imbalance connected with disease, took time off to obtain formal training in psychiatry. He soon left behind the ideas of behavioral psychologist John Watson and embraced the thinking of Sigmund and Anna Freud.[24] At Yale he recruited a distinguished group of individuals, including his first trainee, Albert Solnit, who later succeeded him as director of the Center. In 1951, when Grover Powers retired as chairman of pediatrics, Senn took over his responsibilities while continuing to head the Child Study Center. Solnit in turn recruited his successor, Donald J. Cohen. As a measure of the center's excellence, all three of its directors were appointed Sterling Professors.

President Charles Seymour also stepped aside in 1950, after thirteen years in office. A. Whitney Griswold, a professor of history, was appointed to become the twelfth president of Yale. George Blumer, who had been dean from 1910 to 1920 and David Paige Smith Professor of Medicine, was concerned enough about the future of the medical school to express the hope to the new president that "Yale University will be able to hang on to its Medical School." At his first corporation meeting, in October 1950, President Griswold suggested that "the whole problem of the School of Medicine, the Department of Public Health, and the School of Nursing and their relations with the Hospital" be taken up.[25] Although there was clearly talk of not "hanging onto" the medical school, a memorandum from Provost Edgar S. Furniss to Griswold in October offered "evidence that the School of Medicine was no longer in a critical stage." Although not all the problems may have been solved, said Furniss, "they have been reduced to manageable proportions and alternative methods of meeting future needs are available for administrative choice."[26]

The corporation supported increasing the class size by fifteen students and allowing savings from financial adjustments with the hospital to be retained by the school.[27] Griswold told a meeting of the Board of Permanent Officers in November 1950 that the administration was attempting to achieve economies in the operating costs of the university and was also trying to increase the endowment.[28] Nevertheless, rumors of the medical school's demise persisted. Walter Winchell said as much during a July 1951 broadcast, prompting George Darling to send him the following telegram: "It is reported you said Yale School of Medicine would close after next semester. . . . Contrary to your report, entering class in the fall will be enlarged from sixty-five to eighty and the school will definitely not close now or in the future."[29]

Unlike Seymour, who had frequently been present at meetings of the Board of Permanent Officers, Griswold seldom attended them, not even for significant announcements. At a November 1951 meeting Provost Furniss, in the absence of President Griswold, "who was obliged to attend a meeting in New York," announced that Dean Long had expressed a desire to give up the deanship on several occasions, and that the president had acceded to his wishes.[30] Long became chairman of the Department of Physiology. In a letter to the president of the University of Western Ontario after his first year as dean, Long had written that the deanship "is not one that one would care to look forward to as a permanent assignment."[31] In addition to a new dean, new chairs were appointed during the course of 1951 in the departments of internal medicine, physiology, physiological chemistry, and pharmacology, and in the new Section of History of Medicine.

Joseph Fruton had been promoted to professor of biochemistry with appointments in both physiological chemistry and chemistry in 1950.[32] With Long's move to physiology, Griswold asked Fruton to become chairman of the Department of Physiological Chemistry. Fruton has written that his appointment was not "welcomed" by either Long or Darling.[33] Fruton thought Griswold had made the decision on the recommendation of E. W. Sinnott, then dean of the graduate school.

John Fulton stepped aside as chairman of physiology to head the Section of History of Medicine. In a draft letter responding to a query from Fulton about resources available to support his new chairmanship, Griswold emphasized that it was "imperative" to act promptly, although the reason for the urgency was not made clear. Allowing Fulton to remain as chairman of physiology for five months until the completion of Long's term as dean, rather than have Donald Barron serve as interim chairman, would have been much simpler. The appointment in History of Medicine would require that Fulton relinquish the chairmanship of the Department of Physiology on February 1, 1951, the date of his appointment to History of Medicine.[34] The final letter from Griswold to Fulton was more gentle than the original draft but asked for the same things and provided funds for two research assistants and a secretary as well as some expenses.

Thus, the era spanning the Depression, the war, and the postwar recovery drew to an end. A new era marked by the ready availability of funds for expansion was about to begin.

9

EXPANSION YEARS

The new dean, appointed in 1952, was not a current faculty member but, perhaps significantly, a full-time administrator. He was Vernon W. Lippard (figure 30), a Massachusetts native who had taken the five-year combined medical course in the Sheffield Scientific School, receiving his M.D. degree cum laude in 1929. One of five students elected to membership in the medical honor society, Alpha Omega Alpha, he was also awarded the Parker Prize, given annually to the graduating student "who has shown the best qualifications for a successful practitioner." During his final year the first issue of the *Yale Journal of Biology and Medicine* was published, and it contained two abstracts, based on articles by faculty members, signed "V.W.L."[1]

After graduating, Lippard remained in New Haven for an internship in pediatrics with Grover Powers at the New Haven Hospital. He then went to Cornell for residency training and was the first chief resident when the Cornell Department of Pediatrics moved to the newly completed New York

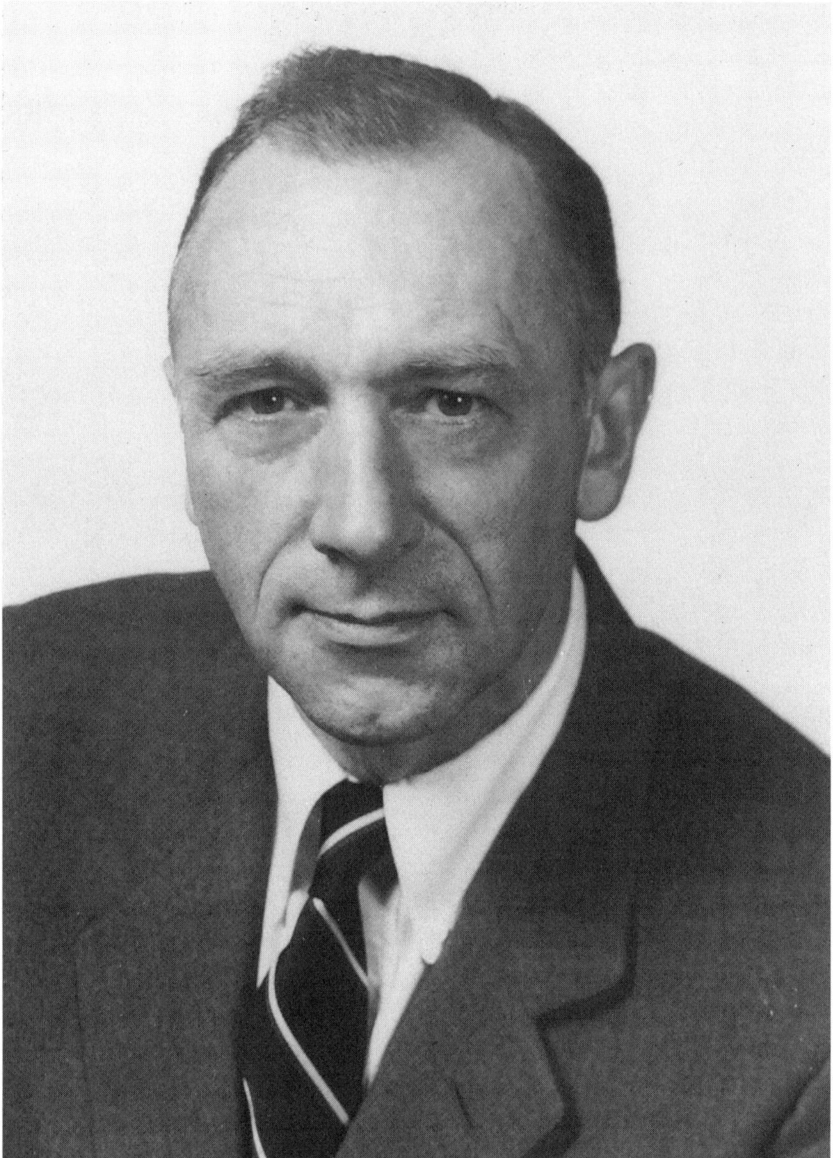

Figure 30. Vernon W. Lippard

Hospital in 1932. After serving as an instructor at Cornell, he entered private practice for a short period and during 1938 and 1939 directed a comprehensive study of the care of crippled children in New York City. In 1939 he was recruited by Dean Willard Rappeleye to be an assistant dean at the College of Physicians and Surgeons of Columbia University and was promoted to associate dean the next year. Rappeleye had been director of the New Haven Hospital in the 1920s but left under pressure when he sought to encourage clinical practice by full-time faculty members to balance the hospital budget.

Lippard entered the army in 1942, serving as executive officer and chief of the laboratory for the 9th General Hospital in the Southwest Pacific. During the last months of the war, he was chief of medical personnel for the Army Forces of the Southwest Pacific. He once remarked that this was one of the most enjoyable periods of his life. After the war, Lippard returned briefly to Columbia, but in 1946, with his interest in administration firmly established, he was appointed dean of the School of Medicine at Louisiana State University in 1946 and then dean at the University of Virginia School of Medicine three years later. The average life span for a dean today is about three years, and Vernon Lippard was to begin his third deanship.

The decision to appoint a full-time medical dean at Yale had been based on the recommendation of a committee of the Board of Permanent Officers, with the realization that this was breaking new ground for the university.[2] Because the appointment of a dean by the Yale Corporation was for a five-year term, an individual who was not already a member of the Yale faculty had to be appointed with a future professorship in some department in mind, in this case pediatrics. As a condition of his coming to Yale, Lippard demanded that the position of director of medical affairs, held by George Darling, be combined with the deanship.

Darling was neither dean of the medical school nor vice president of the university but "something in between with an ill-defined roving commission."[3] President Griswold considered Darling not qualified professionally to be dean, and there was no place for him higher up in the university echelon. With Lippard's concurrence, Griswold tried to convince Darling to become associate dean for financial affairs, with a circumscribed area of responsibility. Darling refused, accepting instead an appointment as professor of human ecology, with the possibility of a program in the subject sponsored by the Commonwealth Foundation. In response to a letter from the search committee for president of the University of Colorado, Griswold described Darling as a man of "great industry, stubborn courage and high principles. . . . His greatest weakness is a rather involved manner of expressing himself. . . . But he is a hard honest worker and a good man."[4] Darling provided an example of his "involved manner of expression" in a final note to Griswold: "No one can appreciate the ramifications and the gravity of the burden of university administration as well as one who is laying down such cares after more or less strenuous years in the administrative vineyard."[5]

Albert Snoke, the hospital director, worried that Lippard would concern himself primarily with the educational and research programs. Although Snoke had wanted Darling to remain in his position, he promised complete cooperation with Lippard in a letter to Griswold.[6] The hospital board had been impressed with Darling's accomplishments over the previous six years and apparently had not been aware that his position was to be eliminated.

In his introductory speech to the faculty, Lippard said that the Yale Medical School justified its existence by providing an intellectual discipline "difficult to achieve when mass production is the primary goal. . . . This institution can continue to grow as an incubator of superior intellectual capacity and ideals," he said, with equally important responsibilities for the advancement of knowledge by research. Lippard went on to ask what he could do to facilitate the development of the school. Having already served as dean at two institutions, he realized that "no one who is effective in administration can satisfy everyone." He stressed the importance of channels of communication from faculty to departmental chairman to dean and on to higher authorities in the central administration, clearly implying that circumventing these channels was not acceptable. Lippard's three years of army experience were embodied in this chain of command. "Effective administration of a medical school depends on active interest and participation of the faculty in the affairs of the school as a whole but within limits which permit them to carry out their primary responsibilities with minimal distraction," through the Board of Permanent Officers. Lippard saw himself as neither the watchdog of the central administration nor the administrator of an independent entity, and he suggested that it was time to break down the artificial barriers among departments, both within the medical school and within the university as a whole. "This institution has suffered by the reputation of being confused internally." When he announced that he was coming to Yale, people had asked, "What future has an institution in which the medical school and hospital must be involved in continuous controversy over their respective privileges and responsibilities?" Lippard ended his speech by reminding the faculty that the primary reason for the existence of the Yale School of Medicine was the education of a highly selected group of young men and women.[7]

The turnover of a number of department chairs gave Lippard an opportunity to put his stamp on the school by recruiting chairmen sympathetic to his views of medical education. The new chairman of internal medicine, Paul B. Beeson, had been chairman of the Department of Medicine at Emory University. William Salter, the chairman of pharmacology, died unexpectedly, and Lippard selected Arnold Welch from Western Reserve University to succeed him.

In his 1952–1953 report, President Griswold commented that annual payments to the hospital from the university had totaled more than $4 million since 1920, but that the new affiliation agreement would not result in any long-term reduction in the cost of medical education, "by far the most expensive of all types of education."[8] The seventy-nine medical schools in the United States at the time had a combined annual deficit of about $10 million, so Yale's medical school was not alone in its financial problems.

Dean Lippard submitted his first annual report after six months in office. "Yale was recognized as one of the leading centers of medical education and research in the world. . . . There are, however, definite weaknesses, and most of them are found in the clinical departments."[9] The continuous turnover with its ensuing loss of promising young faculty members was a major problem, which resulted from the financial constraints imposed by the full-time system during a budget freeze. The subspecialties of ophthalmology, orthopedics, otolaryngology, and dermatology had not been developed in a manner consistent with an academic medical center. The chief of radiology was an employee of the hospital rather than a university appointee, and the radiology service was weak academically. Lippard, correctly believing that the discipline was too important to neglect, founded a university Department of Radiology in 1956.

Lippard was also in favor of a modified full-time clinical system similar to the one Stanhope Bayne-Jones had proposed in 1935. Lippard considered clinical service to be crucial. Arthur Ebbert commented, "This service element in the activity of the full-time members of the clinical departments represents perhaps the most perplexing problem with which this and every other medical school is faced today." To build Yale's clinical reputation, he placed new emphasis on clinical practice, and efforts were made to encourage the referral of private patients. He established a central billing office to collect professional fees with which to pay clinicians and support the activities of clinical departments. Lippard was in favor of a faculty practice plan with its own building, but he encountered considerable opposition from some departments. "They feared they would be regimented by some bureaucracy and lose their independence."[10] Thirty years passed before a faculty practice plan was actually established.

Lippard centralized responsibility in the Office of the Dean with the help of two very competent assistant deans serving in a half-time capacity. Thomas R. Forbes, an associate professor of anatomy, had been appointed by Dean Long as assistant dean for student affairs, dealing with admissions and student progress. Arthur Ebbert Jr., who had been an instructor in medicine at the University of Virginia and had been associated with Lippard in the dean's office there, had the title of assistant dean of postgraduate medical education but did much more. He eventually served as deputy dean under four successive deans, Redlich, Thomas, Berliner, and Rosenberg. The competence of Forbes and Ebbert allowed Lippard to concentrate on the major issues affecting the medical school. By the time of his 1953–1954 report on the School of Medicine, he could state that considerable progress had been made in achieving the balance between complete departmental autonomy and administration by committee, avoiding some of the waste of bureaucratic effort that results from lack of centralized authority. The departmental chairmen, sitting as the Executive Committee, met twice monthly, and the Board of Permanent Officers, which was the mandated authority in the medical school but was considered too unwieldy, met six times a year.

The basic educational philosophy of the medical school was reviewed in a series of meetings of the Board of Permanent Officers, and the Yale system was reaffirmed: no fixed course requirements for qualified students, emphasis on elective courses, no required examinations, and a required research thesis. Students admitted to Yale were expected to graduate. "It is the basic assumption that students are selected carefully, and it is anticipated that failures will be rare."[11] The faculty, therefore, had a responsibility to assist each student to make the most of her or his potential. Because there were no written examinations other than the National Board Examinations, a great deal of pressure was placed on the faculty to evaluate students, and the Board examinations were used to determine students' fitness to practice medicine—a use for which they were never intended.

Changes in the full-time clinical system had been resisted in the past, particularly by Francis Gilman Blake as chairman of medicine, but Paul Beeson supported them: "I am in full accord with the policy of cautious and steady expansion of private practice by full-time members of the faculty."[12] He believed that private practice was necessary not only for generating revenue but also for educational purposes.

The Department of Medicine was greatly aided by the increase in available clinical material with the opening in 1953 of the Grace–New Haven memorial unit and of the Veterans Administration Hospital in West Haven. Beeson liked having a department of manageable size in one location and was reluctant to supply house staff to the VA hospital, but he relented after negotiating permission to appoint the chief of its medical service. The link with the VA hospital in West Haven grew from a grudging affiliation to an important full-fledged partnership, in both education and, especially, research. The VA hospital was an ideal institution in which young faculty members like Patrick J. Mulrow could begin their research careers, as both funding and laboratory space were available. Most of these young faculty members remained at the hospital, providing a cadre of senior academicians committed to the VA. Because of good follow-up, VA hospitals were particularly fertile ground for clinical investigation. The first study showing the effectiveness of antihypertensive therapy in moderate hypertension was done in the VA system.[13] Approximately half of the house staff in the United States has received training at VA hospitals. This relationship of VA hospitals and academic medicine has been perfect in many ways. In return for the teaching and research benefits, the veterans have received a higher quality of care than would otherwise have been possible.

With the end of direct subsidization of the New Haven Hospital by the university, negotiations between the medical school and the hospital rested on "mutual respect rather than financial dependence." The school was to be primarily concerned with teaching and research and the hospital with service. Over the years, the school became increasingly dependent on clinical service for financial reasons. Research grants and income from patients were soon playing a dominant role in clinical salaries. Only 34 percent of the 1955–1956 budget came from university funds, leading Beeson to comment, "I seriously doubt that it is safe to let this proportion become smaller."[14] Today, financial support from the university accounts for less than 10 percent of the medical school's operating budget. This financial dependence, coupled with the medical faculty's belief that the hospital should play a more active role in academic support, has led to increasing tensions between school and hospital.

In his 1955–1956 report, Lippard attempted to define the role of Yale's medical school within the university and among the nation's medical schools. To maintain its position within the university, the medical school had to foster scholarly activity rather than technical training. It needed to continue its emphasis on the physiological and pathological processes rather than on diagnostic and therapeutic methods. The Yale system treated medical students like graduate students, with close faculty contact, avoidance of an examination mentality, and encouragement of special interests and active participation in research.[15]

Lippard entitled his 1955 presidential address to the Association of American Medical Schools "The Medical School—Janus of the University," referring to the need of the medical school to face simultaneously toward the university and toward the community. He contrasted the German system, where the medical school was an integral part of the university, to the British system, where medical schools were associated with hospitals. Lippard thought that there was too great a tendency for the university administration to consider the medical school outside the fold. If the university were to be more than a "holding company," the central administration needed to ensure that the medical school contributed to university activity and took advantage of the university's intellectual riches. Coming back to the Yale system, Lippard defined a university atmosphere as a situation in which "scholars of varying levels of maturity are learning together."[16]

When Vernon Lippard stepped aside as dean in 1967 after fifteen years, Arthur Ebbert was the guest editor for a Festschrift issue in Lippard's honor of the *Yale Journal of Biology and Medicine* on medical education.[17] One of the articles, by C. Arden Miller, vice-chancellor of health sciences at the University of North Carolina, Chapel Hill, was entitled "The Medical School and the University." Lester Evans had remarked that what distinguished the medical school from the university was that the medical school was the only professional discipline that must be practiced in its entirety to be taught.[18] Miller commented that at Yale the medical school paid a price for its differences, because the university never pretended to assume responsibility for the costs of medical education. The two oldest institutions continuously in existence in the Western Hemisphere, dating from the sixteenth century, are both devoted to health and education—a children's hospital in Mexico City and a university in Peru. Miller wondered why, with that long tradition, academic medical centers are so difficult to administer.[19]

At Yale, separation of the university and the medical school was maintained in other ways as well. The medical faculty was frequently not incorporated into the university's academic structure. On the other hand, medical-school funds, unlike university funds, could come from either research grants or clinical income. As a result, rapid scientific growth occurred in the medical school, which assumed the leadership in biological sciences. Although support for medical education came from clinical income, the educational program was not as strong as it should have been. In time, other parts of the university also began developing income streams that made medical education appear less conspicuous in its external involvement.

The Liaison Committee on Medical Education, which is responsible for the accreditation of medical schools in the United States and Canada, surveyed Yale in 1958 and was very positive: "There can be no question that medical education at Yale represents a quality enterprise. . . . The outstanding leadership of Dr. Vernon Lippard was apparent to the committee repeatedly. . . . In our opinion, Yale represents an outstanding example of a medical school where medical students are treated as adults and as graduate students, and in the best sense of these terms."[20]

Richard Light, chairman of the Committee on Medical Affairs of the University Council, in contrast, had told President Griswold in 1957 that the Yale Medical School lacked "any reputation at all outside its own bailiwick."[21] The Committee on Medical Affairs critically reviewed the medical school in 1959. Teaching of the preclinical sciences was considered to be outstanding, but teaching of clinical subjects failed to receive the same widespread approval, which was attributed in part to lack of clinical material. Hartford Hospital had proposed that its clinical facilities become part of the teaching program at Yale. Yale would remain the home base, but a dormitory would be built in Hartford, and there would be frequent interchange between the two institutions. This arrangement would correspond to Harvard's hospital relationships. Dean Lippard replied that the combined facilities of the medical center—the hospital plus the medical school—and the Veterans Administration Hospital were adequate, but the committee persisted and recommended "early and decisive review by the University Administration."[22]

"Hartford Hospital is a plum waiting to be picked off by some medical school."[23] The Board of Permanent Officers rightly or wrongly decided that Hartford Hospital was not a plum. "Members of the Board were unable to see the benefit to the educational program of the School and many disadvantages were mentioned."[24] The Committee on Medical Affairs believed that talk of a new medical school at the University of Connecticut was probably prophetic. Thanks to federal funds, a medical school a year was being founded, mostly by state universities, to keep up with the population growth.

Yale, and particularly George Darling in his role as director of medical affairs, had worked diligently to prevent a second medical school from being established in Connecticut. The Committee on Medical Affairs of the University Council had been reorganized in October 1953 to include greater representation of Connecticut residents as well as several individuals interested in a nursing school, in an attempt to offset the pressure for a second medical school in Connecticut. The committee confidently reported that "the pressing problems of the Medical School have in the main been solved."[25] Yet in 1960 there was still a misperception that Yale's medical school admitted very few Connecticut residents.[26] In 1959 the Board of Permanent Officers had considered increasing the size of the student body. The consensus of the faculty was that the Yale School of Medicine should strive for excellence rather than size, and no expansion in enrollment was implemented.[27] Times change, and when additional federal funds became available in 1966, arrangements were made to increase the class by twenty students over three years, which was the number required for maximal federal funding.[28]

The Committee on Medical Affairs of the University Council also reviewed the School of Nursing and was disappointed with its progress compared to the medical school's. Founded in 1923, the nursing school flourished during the 1930s and early 1940s but then began to decline. The Yale requirement for a baccalaureate degree was unique among nursing schools, and it became a liability as job opportunities grew after the war and new schools of nursing were established. Students wishing to be nurses did not want to spend four years obtaining a baccalaureate degree. Enrollment at the nursing school decreased, and the administration finally terminated the standard nursing program in 1958. The university deliberated about disbanding the nursing school altogether, but a compromise was reached by instituting short graduate courses for nurse practitioners in obstetrical, psychiatric, and public-health nursing. This solution caused the Board of Permanent Officers some discomfort. As the minutes record, "The Dean attempted to allay suspicion that the program constitutes an attempt to produce third-rate doctors rather than good nurses."[29] Although concern on the part of the medical profession about the role of nursing in patient care has not disappeared, nurse practitioners and physician associates play increasingly important roles in patient care, particularly in managed care.

While the nursing profession was becoming more specialized, so was the medical profession. As more and more residents sought postdoctoral fellowships after their house-staff training in order to specialize, the length of residency training increased. Dean Lippard commented in 1959 that the number of postdoctoral fellows had increased from forty-four to 119 during the previous eight years, and he expressed concern at the lack of control over their appointments as well as the increased pressure on facilities available for medical-student research.[30] The problem of the postdoctoral fellow has grown even larger with time, despite the move to primary care. Nowadays the Department of Medicine at Yale has about 220 faculty members and about 185 postdoctoral fellows, all destined to become specialists. There is still little decanal or departmental control over the appointment of postdoctoral fellows, which tends to occur at the divisional level and is based on the availability of funds with little regard for academic manpower requirements.

The status of a division director in the medical subspecialties can be measured by the phalanx of postdoctoral fellows surrounding her or him at the national meeting of a particular academic society. Nor is the problem limited to clinical departments, where the fellows provide care to their supervisor's patients. It is also rampant in preclinical departments, where the fellows conduct much of the supervisor's research, but where insufficient academic positions exist for the number of individuals completing their fellowships.

The Board of Permanent Officers, recognizing the trend toward specialization, raised important questions for extended faculty consideration.[31] Should the Yale School of Medicine declare itself a center for the education of specialists, and if so, was the required background in the basic medical sciences appropriate? A 1963 Ad Hoc Committee of the BPO on educational policy began with the premise that Yale graduates would enter medical careers in specialized practice or teaching and research, and in view of the long training period, the committee questioned the necessity for technical experience during the clinical clerkship.[32] The BPO also wondered whether students would be better prepared for specialization if the internship were included as part of the medical-school curriculum. The overwhelming majority of medical school deans today would incorporate the residency training into a seven-year curriculum if the funding for house-staff salaries were not controlled by the hospitals.

The combination of federal research support and clinical-practice income resulted in a period of financial stability at the school for the first time since its inception in 1813. Throughout the school's history, turbulence was directly connected to the financial state of the school and the university. Although some viewed with alarm the school's dependence on "soft money" from outside income to pay for faculty salaries and operating expenses, in 1956 the operating budget of the School of Medicine was about equally dependent on funds derived from sources within and outside the university.[33] University sources included income from tuition, endowments designated for medicine, and an annual contribution from general university funds. External sources included $1.18 million from research grants and $350,000 from clinical practice. The university support of $400,000 had remained stable, because the faculty salary budget had been frozen since 1947. Half of this support was returned by the medical school as an assessment for central university administration. Arguments still rage over medical-school responsibility for general university areas like the Peabody Museum and the Payne Whitney Gymnasium.

Vernon Lippard was particularly adept at obtaining construction funds from foundations, especially the Commonwealth Foundation, which supplied most of the funds for the Edward S. Harkness Memorial Hall, marking the end of a thirty-year quest to provide adequate housing for the medical and public-health students. In 1952 the assistant dean of the medical school, Thomas R. Forbes, had described the dismal living arrangements available for medical students in three "aged and neglected" buildings at 837 to 847 Howard Avenue. Seventy-three male students lived in two of the buildings, and twenty women students, including ten medical students, lived in the third. Fourteen men students were housed on the third floor of the Hope Building. The interiors of the old buildings were largely of wood, and the danger of fire was real. The rooms were "dingy, bleak and unattractive" and located in a "very poor section" of the city. They offered little respite from the noises of the street, and prowlers lurked around the women's dormitory.[34] Rents were low, however, and the rooms were convenient to the hospital. As there were only 107 rooms available to accommodate 308 medical and public-health students, there was a long waiting list.

Eating facilities were equally unsatisfactory. Men students ate some meals in the hospital, but the number of them was a problem for the hospital administration. Nearby eating places (restaurant was too dignified a term!) were reasonably priced but generally unattractive. Actual dietary deficiency had been discovered in medical students two years earlier.

By 1956 the dormitory, which had been discussed as a real need since Winternitz's deanship in the 1920s, was finally coming to fruition. The Department of Architecture had assigned the medical-school dormitory as a student project in 1949, with the building to be placed in the triangle between York Street, Oak Street, and Davenport Avenue at a cost of about $2 million. When the announcement was made, Dean Long had prophetically said, "We are still a long way from realizing its fulfillment."[35] Students did not actually move into the Harkness dormitory until the fall of 1956.

The Edward S. Harkness Memorial Hall was the first major postwar construction project at the medical school. Arthur Ebbert commented that "comfort and convenience have been emphasized," and that "the completion of the new residence Hall should increase significantly the efficiency and well-being of the able group of young men and women studying at the School of Medicine." A young faculty family lived on the ground floor as a "steadying influence," and unmarried junior faculty members or postdoctoral fellows occupied suites on each floor, serving (at least by title) as counselors. One floor of the eleven-story wing was reserved for women students, the ten-to-one ratio of available rooms reflecting class composition fairly accurately.[36]

As one of the first occupants of Harkness Hall, I can attest to its advantages over a garret on the corner of Park and George streets. When the dormitory plans were considered by the Board of Permanent Officers, all but two of twenty members thought that rooms for single students should be given first priority, with married quarters a distant second, reflecting that generation's view that marriage was not desirable in medical students. Although interns and residents at Yale were free to marry, in the past the house staff at the Peter Bent Brigham Hospital in Boston had to seek permission. As a result of the BPO decision, apartments for married students were in short supply at Yale. Harkness Hall today has same-sex floors with common bathrooms. (One of my first acts as dean was to be shown how inadequate the lighting was in the common shower by one of the female students!) Most medical students now live in apartments near the school rather than in the dormitory.

Funding was also found to construct new laboratory facilities. Dean Lippard continually emphasized the importance of biochemistry in his annual reports to the president; it had replaced physiology as the "anchoring discipline" in the basic sciences. "One of the most striking trends in recent years has been the restatement of biological terms in chemical terms and thus biochemistry has become the most basic of the biological sciences."[37] Lippard repeatedly stressed the need to increase laboratory space in the Department of Biochemistry. The corporation concurred, and a new laboratory was placed among the top three priority building requirements for the university.[38] Joseph Fruton contended in his autobiography, *Eighty Years,* that Lippard did not understand the importance of biochemistry and did not support it.[39] But it was Lippard who finally secured the necessary funds for an addition to the Sterling Hall of Medicine to accommodate the desperate need for more space for biochemistry and anatomy.

In 1956 Governor Abraham Ribicoff proposed establishing a psychiatric research and treatment center. Lippard assured the governor that Yale was decidedly interested in having such a center and would provide heat and food services at cost.[40] The Connecticut Mental Health Center eventually opened in 1966, a state-supported psychiatric facility that included research space and was staffed by Yale faculty psychiatrists.

Discussion about research space in the medical school had concentrated primarily on the expansion of the Laboratory of Medicine and Pediatrics, which did not address the need for more space in the Department of Medicine. Accordingly, the Laboratory for Clinical Investigation was erected in 1965, with funds from the National Institutes of Health and the munificent Commonwealth Fund, to accommodate the increased research needs within the Department of Medicine and the Department of Pediatrics. With the growing emphasis on clinical practice, the faculty required a place to see private patients in consultation, and the Dana Clinic was opened for this purpose in 1964.

There were other changes, too. Past attempts to combine the public-health and epidemiology programs had failed because of personality differences. The retirement of Ira Hiscock in public health and John Paul in epidemiology finally provided the opportunity to merge both programs into a single department in 1961. A decision was also made about the future of the Institute of Human Relations. The institute's unique achievement was the training of personnel in the various branches of the social sciences concerned with the interplay of human behavior, social organization, and culture, and its postwar goal was to strengthen programs in the "behaviorist" sciences at all levels.[41] President Griswold, who was not in favor of institutes in a university, was particularly disturbed by a Ford Foundation grant to the institute for the support of Charles Walker, a faculty member for whom no departmental appointment could be found. Griswold decided an "irregularity such as this causes increasing embarrassment." Walker and the Institute of Human Relations would be terminated with the retirement of Mark May in 1960, when the Ford Foundation grant ended.[42]

More construction occurred at the medical school during Lippard's fifteen-year tenure as dean than under any other dean before or since, with the exception of Milton Winternitz. Lippard's success was due in large measure to a combination of the financial stability of the school, which pacified the university administration, the federal government's perception that more physician manpower was needed, and Lippard's good relations with a number of foundations.

Faculty salaries remained a problem, however, and something had to be done to assist development of the clinical departments. There was agitation for a system, particularly in the surgical specialties, that would allow faculty members to benefit directly from their practice income. But in July 1961

Lippard told the clinical faculty that he and the chairmen had given the topic a "tremendous" amount of consideration and had come to the conclusion that the present system had contributed to the "fine spirit which had developed in the school over the past 40 years and was not to be cast aside lightly."[43]

Lippard stated that Yale was committed to the full-time clinical system, and that each faculty member would have to decide individually whether it provided an enjoyable atmosphere. He went on to say that over the previous ten years, salaries had increased by 35 to 40 percent and would continue to rise. He wished to expand the clinical faculty, which numbered two hundred on the regular staff, but growth could only take place in parallel with facilities and income. Lippard also emphasized that promotions were based on total achievement in teaching, research, and patient care. No one was expected to carry out all three with equal intensity and skill. Good clinical investigation would receive the same recognition as laboratory research. Both the importance of clinical research and the ability to get promoted on the basis of that research are still being emphasized today, if not altogether convincingly.

Three months later, in October 1961, Lippard was ready to modify the full-time plan. In a letter to the provost, Kingman Brewster, he stated that a modification of the plan was necessary, because there was no proper relation between a faculty member's contributions to the Clinical Research and Teaching Fund through practice and the amount of compensation he received.[44] The existing salary scale was not competitive with even the most inferior medical schools. Yale increasingly had to use the private patients of the full-time faculty for teaching. The medical faculty should not be forbidden income from other sources when faculty members elsewhere in the university were permitted outside income. Lippard recommended that the salary scale remain the same but an income supplement be determined for each faculty member, based on his contribution to the Clinical Research and Teaching Fund during the previous year. The formula would be 50 percent of the first $5,000 contributed, 25 percent of the next $10,000, and 10 percent above $15,000, in amounts up to $5,000.

The chairmen of the clinical departments wished to avoid the accusation that they were competing financially with other members of the departments. Their basic salaries would be increased to $28,000, which would place their income close to that of the highest earners. Pressure for salary improvements continued to mount. Lippard and the department chairmen hoped to retain as much of the full-time system as possible with this plan. In his report for 1961–1962 Lippard commented, "Announcement of this program has quelled the unrest which existed a year ago and avoided the necessity of adopting a 'geographical full-time plan.' "[45]

In the same report, Lippard noted that alternating current was being installed throughout the buildings, at a cost of about $1 million, to meet the demands of increasing use of electronic equipment. In 1954 he had informed the Board of Permanent Officers that he wanted to limit alternating current in the medical school, but he finally had to relent. The university had decided in the 1920s that the future lay in direct current, and the entire university and hospital had been wired for it. On one memorable occasion as an intern, I had to place an emergency page for an electrician to bring a long cord in order for me to obtain an electro-cardiograph.

The growth of the departments was making the job of chairman more complicated and more difficult. In 1963 Kingman Brewster, who had become president of Yale, received a letter from an "admired colleague," presumably a university president, who commented that every department seemed to be an exact image of its chairman and that chairmanships seemed to be permanent. Asked to comment, Lippard replied that although chairmanships should not be permanent positions, appointments at Yale were for three-year terms with an expectation of renewal if things were going well. A limited term made it easier for someone to leave problems for his successor, but "the presumption of permanency has made displacement a major diplomatic effort."

The university announced a policy of limiting chairmanship appointments to two three-year terms, which Lippard felt would be good for the medical school if exercised judiciously. He recommended that reappointments be made on recommendation of the dean after he had convened a small committee of senior faculty and had conferred with the president and the provost. For clinical departments, the hospital director should be heard but not have veto power. "Some men best qualified to provide leadership in academic programs and care of patients may be less diligent in their roles as hospital administrators."[46] The chairman of pediatrics, Davenport Cook, wrote Brewster that he would never have come to Yale for a three-year or six-year term and that there would be great difficulty recruiting "temporary department chairmen."[47] Three-year terms were duly implemented, with the expectation in the medical school that there would be a review in the fifth year.

The continuing growth of departments presented renewed financial demands, especially after the university stopped subsidizing the hospital. The mood now was that "financial problems of the hospital are not the business of the University."[48] The hospital, however, did reflect on the medical school. In a 1964 cover story on President Brewster and Yale, *Newsweek* commented that "Yale has a good, if not outstanding, medical school." Physicians at other medical centers said that Yale suffered from the lack of a "truly first-rate, big-city type of hospital affiliation."[49] These same comments had been made fifty years before, when survival of the medical school was in the balance. In contrast, the presidents and deans of the thirty institutions belonging to the prestigious American Association of Universities ranked the Yale School of Medicine third behind Harvard and Johns Hopkins in 1966.[50]

Lippard had commented in 1962 that "relations with the Hospital, satisfactory on the surface, have been a constant source of irritation because of the difficulty in arriving at an equitable basis for division of financial responsibilities." The next year, with new sources of insurance available, he raised the question of the university taking control of the hospital. "There would be enormous advantages to the School if we controlled the hospital," and "the operation of the hospital need not be a financial liability to the University." The community physicians and the hospital board would not easily agree, and the strongest leverage would be to threaten to build a university hospital. He concluded, "Yale would be foolish to procure large sums of money for the Grace–New Haven Community hospital without insisting on control of its administration and policy."[51] The university chose not to control the hospital, which was probably the correct decision in view of today's health-care economics. A new affiliation agreement was signed in 1965, with the Grace–New Haven Hospital becoming the Yale–New Haven Hospital. The university was given greater representation on the hospital board in return for a commitment to joint fund-raising. The community medical service, in which community physicians served independently, was eliminated by consolidating the wards under the chairs of the university departments.

The hospital director was sure a survey would show that the great majority of a resident's time was involved in educational pursuits and that the costs should therefore be borne by the medical school. Lippard noted that only 16.5 percent of a resident's time was spent in either receiving or giving instruction, and as the average work week of a resident was eighty hours, the hospital was more than getting its money's worth.[52] Lippard prophesized that the Medicare program would make adjustments in funding necessary. With the passage of the Medicare Act, the federal government would fund resident salaries and support academic medical centers that provided care for the underserved. The hospitals were more than happy to retain control of the residents along with the funding. With the current cutbacks in Medicare and diminishing clinical revenues, academic medical centers are developing major financial problems.

Whitney Griswold, Brewster's predecessor as president, did not live to see the new hospital arrangement. Sadly, he developed cancer and died in 1963. He has been portrayed as no friend of the medical school, making efforts to rid the university of an "encumbrance." In fact, the school flourished under his tenure. Mary Griswold, his wife, thought that his strong support of science caused him problems, "because he brought so many eminent scientists to the faculty, which cost the moon and got him a deficit."[53] With his recruitment of Vernon Lippard, the quality and size of the faculty improved. Desperately needed facilities were built, and, perhaps most important, the reputation of the Yale University School of Medicine soared. People have said that during his illness, Griswold really came to appreciate clinical medicine and its role in the university.

The memorial to Griswold at the meeting of the Board of Permanent Officers in April 1963 captured the essence of his style: "With a moral rigor and earnestness characteristic of his Puritanical predecessors, he preached and wrote to promote his message of individual striving for excellence."[54] His successor, Kingman Brewster, a graduate of both Yale College and the Yale Law School, had been brought from Harvard by Griswold to be his provost. On President Brewster's recommendation the Yale Corporation appointed a Standing Committee on Medical Affairs.

A number of new department chairmen had taken over at about the time Lippard became dean in 1952. Now, fifteen years later, there was a major turnover in chairmen once again. Paul Beeson left to become Nuffield Professor of Medicine at Oxford and was replaced by Philip Bondy, a distinguished endocrinologist and chief of the Division of Metabolism. Gustaf Lindskog, chairman of the Department of Surgery, and C. N. H. Long, chairman of physiology and former dean, retired and were succeeded by Jack Cole and Carleton Hunt, respectively. The chairman of microbiology, Edward Adelberg, stepped down and was replaced by Byron Waksman. Shortly afterward, William Gardner, chairman of anatomy, also retired. Joseph Fruton, unhappy with the politics, was stepping down as chairman of biochemistry and moving to the Department of Biology, but not without rancor.[55]

In November 1966 an Ad Hoc Committee on Departmental Reorganization chaired by Carleton Hunt, the new chairman of physiology, proposed that the departments of anatomy, microbiology, and physiology be merged into a single department. This evoked much discussion and strong emotions.[56] Fruton and Gardner wrote a dissenting opinion asking that biochemistry be included in the merger.[57] Because the search for Fruton's successor was active, their proposal was tabled. An intense effort had been made to recruit Gordon Tompkins from the National Institutes of Health as chairman of biochemistry. After protracted negotiations Tompkins declined the offer but several months later accepted it, only to decline it again after several months. By this time he had been voted a full professor in biochemistry by the Board of Permanent Officers. Eventually Frederick Richards, who had left the Department of Biochemistry to found the Department of Molecular Biophysics in Yale College, was appointed chairman of a combined Department of Molecular Biophysics and Biochemistry, which has been an enormous success.

Although the proposed merger of anatomy, microbiology, and physiology never took place, the department names were changed. Physiology became the Department of Cellular and Molecular Physiology, microbiology became the Department of Genetics, and anatomy became the Department of Cell Biology. Gross anatomy was made a section in the Department of Surgery. In addition, both anesthesiology and clinical pathology were made independent sections, which do not have the irreversible status of a department.

The new chairman of cellular and molecular physiology, Carleton Hunt, and his newly appointed senior colleagues refused to support two members of the department for tenure. One of the candidates for tenure appealed but in the meantime accepted a position as chairman of physiology at the University of Cincinnati. Whether a sign of Vernon Lippard's waning powers or Kingman Brewster's style, faculty members frequently wrote directly to the president or provost, without copying the dean. Arthur Galston, who was director of biological sciences, told the provost, Charles Taylor, that Lippard, who should have heard the tenure appeal, did not inspire confidence in the "younger and more aggressive faculty." He was viewed by the young faculty as a "builder of buildings and stabilizer of the status quo."[58] Hunt informed Brewster that he would be compelled to resign if the promotion of the other candidate for tenure were approved. "This is a mediocre department, and the majority vote will perpetuate the mediocrity."[59] Arnold Welch wrote to the provost in strong support of Hunt's position.

After reviewing all the material, including seventeen letters of reference, the Joint Committee on Promotions voted seven for and three against the promotion. The matter was referred to the Executive Committee of the Board of Permanent Officers, who returned it to the promotions committee for "careful reconsideration."[60] Because the candidate taught in a preclinical department and was a member of the graduate school, the promotions committee contained representatives of both the medical school and the Faculty of Arts and Sciences. The decision was made more difficult by the cultural differences and tensions that existed between the college faculty and the medical-school faculty. Tenure was ultimately denied, but the decision left raw wounds that were not easily healed, and it weakened Vernon Lippard's position as dean.

In addition to the other tensions among faculty members, the clinical faculty thought that the medical school was becoming too research oriented. In contrast, Philip Bondy, chairman of the Department of Medicine, and Associate Dean Arthur Ebbert thought that Yale should prepare medical students for a career in teaching and research.[61] Both commented that half the Yale medical graduates had some academic affiliation, with about a quarter holding full-time academic appointments. Bondy foresaw greater concentrations on biochemistry, cell biology, and physiology and less on gross anatomy. As cancer and heart disease were eliminated, the delay of death rather than the prolongation of life was going to become a major problem. Surgery would experience an increased emphasis on repair and replacement rather than excision. All these advances depended on medical research.

Lee Buxton, the chairman of obstetrics and gynecology, representing the clinical faculty, thought that Yale should become either a two-year medical school or—preferably—a five-year medical school that educated sophisticated clinicians.[62] E. Richard Weinerman, a professor in epidemiology and public health, stressed the need for primary-care physicians who related to the family as a biosocial unit and coordinated the specialist and supportive health workers.[63] Weinerman, who later died with his wife in a tragic plane accident, pioneered this concept of the physician, which has gained widespread acceptance.

As part of the change that was in the air, the Board of Permanent Officers recommended a major revision of the curriculum. While the Yale system was reaffirmed, the preclinical and clinical years were shortened to one and a half years each, and a final year was devoted to electives. The expectation was that, after ward experience as a clinical clerk, the student would recognize the importance of basic science to clinical medicine and undertake further work in the sciences. Howard Levitin, a member of the Department of Medicine, was appointed associate dean to implement the curriculum change.

The medical school was now affiliated with four hospitals—the Yale–

New Haven Hospital, the West Haven Veterans Administration Hospital, the Yale Psychiatric Institute, and the Connecticut Mental Health Center. A master plan for the Yale–New Haven Medical Center was prepared but never approved. Lippard saw a need to define the "perimeter" of the complex, and that perimeter became a major problem in the school's relations with the surrounding Hill neighborhood. The master plan portrayed the medical center as a castle with a divided road encircling the site and serving as a moat to separate the center from the surrounding neighborhood. Fortunately, the plan was never implemented. The medical center interacted with the Hill neighborhood in a variety of ways. The Connecticut Mental Health Center provided psychiatric care for the medically indigent of the neighborhood, and comprehensive medical care was given to children in the neighborhood with funding from a federal grant. These programs grew into the Hill Health Center, in which the medical school played a significant role without direct responsibility. The school was interested in developing the surrounding area for parking, apartments for married students and fellows, and doctors' offices; as usual, the local neighborhood was not involved in the planning.

Change was also occurring on a regional basis, with the Connecticut Regional Medical Program envisioned as a system linking multiple health services in southern Connecticut, which would facilitate the transfer of patients and the exchange of various services. The program was inaugurated by a steering committee composed of interested individuals, including medical-faculty members from both Yale and the University of Connecticut.

Care provided to students at the University Health Service was unsatisfactory, and the corporation voted to expand the patient base to cover employees and their dependents, which would lead to more services. Community physicians were concerned that they would lose most of their patients, but several of the physicians with large university practices in fact joined the expanded Yale Health Plan. Although relations between the medical school and the health plan have varied over the years, the plan has been a decided success.

By now Vernon Lippard had spent fifteen very successful years as the ninth dean of the Yale University School of Medicine. One of the secrets of a good administrator is knowing when to leave, and Lippard felt the time had come for him to step down. During his tenure Yale had been firmly established as one of the nation's finest medical schools. He had recruited some outstanding departmental chairmen and had provided the facilities for them to recruit outstanding faculty members. Lippard had been fortunate to be dean during a period when federal funding was available and foundations were willing to fund buildings.

The winds of change were blowing hard, and the dean of the Yale University School of Medicine was going to have to spend a lot more time dealing with the community at the expense of education and research. An indicator of growing social unrest was the controversy evoked by an article in the *Yale Journal of Biology and Medicine.* Louis Lasagna, a clinical pharmacologist from Johns Hopkins, had been invited to Yale to participate in a series of lectures on medical ethics, and he discussed the murder of three civil-rights workers in Mississippi. In a resulting piece published by the journal, he described the autopsy of one of the victims and implied that the University of Mississippi pathology department had covered up a severe beating.[64]

Mississippi faculty members angrily responded in a number of letters to the journal. Among them was Robert Q. Marston, dean of the University of Mississippi Medical School and subsequently director of the NIH and president of the University of Florida, who asked J. Edgar Hoover for a statement.[65] The letter was guarded because the case was in the courts, but it strongly implied that the University of Mississippi pathologists had done a good job.[66] Lasagna replied that although he had not meant to incriminate the University of Mississippi, the New York pathologist's findings raised the question of unethical conduct. Arthur Ebbert did not think the journal was at fault, because it had simply published Lasagna's talk.

In any event, unrest was increasing throughout the university. Younger faculty were going to have to be listened to, as were medical students. By the end of the decade President Brewster had issued a strong statement that interference with university activities, by either students or faculty, would be dealt with firmly. Students disrupting such activities would be unlikely to receive a degree, and disruptive faculty members would be suspended. Brewster indicated that if a significant portion of the faculty believed that the president or provost had exercised his powers wrongly, the corporation would ask for the administration's resignation.[67]

It is doubtful that anyone realized how tumultuous times were going to be, but it was an ideal moment for Vernon Lippard to leave the field with honor. Although he had worked to pay his way through Yale College, Lippard had an urbane, patrician manner that would hinder dealings with the community. He found "participatory democracy" increasingly difficult, and this was just the beginning.

10

SOCIAL UNREST

The Turbulent Years

As Vernon Lippard prepared to step aside in 1967 after fifteen years as dean of the medical school, he expressed concern about medical education. The ready availability of research funds and the ensuing dependence on them had diverted faculty attention from teaching. Increasing interest in social-action projects, while important, threatened to divert attention even further from educational goals. What Lippard could not realize at the time was that the medical students themselves would divert their attention from educational pursuits to become heavily involved in community social-action projects and in the governance of the medical school.

Kingman Brewster asked Paul Beeson for suggestions about the next dean. Beeson replied, "I have gone through a medical school directory and do not find a single person on the spot whom I would recommend."[1] But he did mention three possibilities, including John B. Hickam, chairman of medicine at the Indiana University School of Medicine. The search committee for the new dean wrote letters to various individuals in 1966 asking general questions about the selection of a dean. Robert Wagner, chairman of microbiology at Johns Hopkins, wrote that the best he could offer was negative advice. He thought that the day of the professional administrator (to wit, Vernon Lippard) was over, and that Yale should appoint someone who had accomplished something in his own right. But, he continued, "beware of both eager volunteers and reluctant dragons."[2] President Brewster received a number of unsolicited letters about possible candidates. Franklin Epstein, a nephrologist, wrote a prescient letter recommending Robert Berliner, then director of research at the National Heart Institute, stating that his greatest attribute was an "absolutely infallible nose for excellence."[3]

The search committee decided to focus on Fritz Redlich, the chairman of psychiatry. Albert Snoke, executive director of the Yale–New Haven Hospital, acknowledged that Redlich would be a fine academic dean but favored Jack Cole, the new chairman of surgery who had been at Yale for only six months. The chairman of pediatrics, Davenport Cook, told Brewster that he too liked and admired Redlich but wondered if he had the necessary dynamism. Eventually, in January 1967 Brewster extended a "most genuine and unqualified invitation" to John Hickam to become dean of the School of Medicine and associate provost for medical affairs. Brewster went on to say that he had taken the greatest care to consult his colleagues, "lest my own enthusiasm carry me away."[4] The position of associate provost for medical affairs was a new effort to replace George Darling's former position within the academic structure. When Hickam had not accepted the position by February, Philip Bondy told Brewster that Hickam was probably going to turn down the deanship. He recommended Redlich and Cole as possible internal candidates but considered Arnold Welch too emotionally labile.[5]

When Hickam finally declined, Brewster appointed Fritz Redlich dean and associate provost for medical affairs. Redlich's understanding, to which Brewster assented, was that the provostial appointment gave him "authority above all other officers in the Medical Center," including the hospital director and the dean of the School of Nursing.[6] Because the director of the Yale–New Haven Hospital reported to an independent board and not to the Yale Corporation, Brewster was unable to grant this authority. Vernon Lippard was appointed assistant to the president for health affairs. Redlich was comfortable with a fund-raising role for his predecessor but reserved judgment on his other functions.

Time magazine took note of Redlich's appointment, reporting that he was said to run the Department of Psychiatry like the old Austro-Hungarian

Empire—"with absolutism mitigated by sloppiness."[7] The article, in which the School of Medicine was rated among the top six medical schools, also mentioned that Redlich had fled Vienna and Nazism because of his partly Jewish ancestry and had anglicized his name during World War II, as he was told that he could not be named Fritz like "every prisoner of war."

Although Vernon Lippard had ended his deanship on a high note, Fritz Redlich's first report to the president and fellows of Yale University was anything but upbeat. "We were constantly constrained by crises such as seven empty chairmanships, serious cutbacks in federal support, and the emerging strict assumption by the University that the medical school is 'a tub on its own bottom.'"[8] There was a need for major reorganization of the basic-science departments, which was being resisted by many faculty members who liked the status quo. Departments like anatomy, biochemistry, and pathology had been gradually deteriorating for a number of years. In addition, pediatrics, psychiatry, internal medicine, and radiology had leadership problems. Traditional disagreement existed between the basic-science and clinical departments, and there were tensions between clinical scientists and clinical teachers. Student and community activism, not present during Lippard's tenure, was a major problem for the dean. Financial difficulties, empty departmental chairs, and faculty tensions were all part of the normal landscape.

Morale was low among members of the faculty, partly because of their assumption that they were underpaid and partly because of their perception that the school was moving from a research orientation to a practice orientation. The American public had become deeply involved in social issues. Congress became less interested in medical research, and federal funding for research decreased. Lack of funding in turn led to increased faculty unrest.

The perception of movement toward a practice philosophy was shared by community physicians, who were concerned about the development of group health organizations, like the Yale Health Plan, with close affiliations to the Yale–New Haven Medical Center. There was also increasingly direct competition among faculty members for patients. The dean would probably have been happier with even more competition, leading to a better organized, more efficient, and higher-quality practice. In fact, a new faculty track was instituted in which full-time professorships in clinical specialties were created so that outstanding clinicians and clinical teachers could remain in the academic system. Traditionally, an individual was allowed ten years from initial appointment in which to achieve tenure or leave. The new track allowed these valuable clinicians and teachers to remain in academic medicine.

There was increasing pressure for the school to become more active clinically, as a contribution to the new "social contract" and as a source of badly needed revenue. Davenport Cook, the chairman of pediatrics, warned both Redlich and Brewster that the heavy emphasis on clinical practice would interfere with both teaching and research. Brewster agreed in principle but did not share Cook's impression of "current jeopardy."[9] Cook, who had a prickly personality, had let Brewster know during the decanal search that he was not in favor of Redlich. The two men represented different poles of behavior, New England abrasiveness versus Viennese *gemütlichkeit.* Relations between them deteriorated to the point that Redlich sent a handwritten note to Cook in December 1970, with blind copies to Brewster and Taylor, pleading with Cook to "remedy the situation."[10]

Although convinced that hospital relations were among the most complex and least understood of organizational relationships, Redlich was pleased with his personal relationship with Charles Womer, the hospital director. "Fortunately Mr. Womer and I have developed an effective and trusting relationship which was not possible for Drs. Lippard and Snoke." Albert Snoke had written a letter to Redlich and Lippard in 1967 bitterly decrying the medical school's decision that the hospital's executive director should not meet with his clinical chiefs, who also happened to be department chairmen.[11] Snoke was informed that discussing issues about the affiliation agreement was irresponsible and was told to stay away until the hospital chiefs and the dean could consult with Brewster on their position for the future.

The hospital board, with strong university support, subsequently decided that Snoke should step down in favor of his deputy, Charles Womer, who was not a physician. The "team" of Redlich and Womer soon questioned whether the medical center affiliation agreement, over which there had been so much joy only a few short years before, was an effective organizational instrument.

On the educational front, a new curriculum had been instituted in September 1968. It was imaginative but considerably more time intensive for the faculty. Implemented by Howard Levitin, the associate dean, the preclinical years were shortened to one and a half years, as were the clinical clerkships. The final year of medical school was designed to interest the medical student further in basic science after he or she had had an opportunity to grasp how important it was in the practice of clinical medicine. The basic scientists would have preferred compulsory examinations, a topic that was not brought up for discussion. Clinical experience between the first and second years was scheduled to give the students a sense of being a "doctor." The impending clinical experience was a source of great anxiety to the first-year students, who were convinced they would be asked to do open heart surgery. Many of them spent the six-week clinical rotation working in community medical clinics.

Although only a few students in their fourth year immersed themselves in basic science, the curriculum revision was very well received by the students. Redlich forwarded a letter to Brewster from a student who had turned down Harvard for Yale because of the new curriculum, to which Redlich appended the comment, "This is almost as good as winning a football game."[12] Faculty members, particularly in the Department of Medicine, were required to spend more time teaching in small groups but were also being asked to spend more time in clinical practice.[13] Countervailing pressures produced rising discontent among the basic-science faculty members, who continued to push for examinations and required attendance. Despite the changes in the curriculum, students were still not attending their classes more regularly.

Medical-student activism was also on the rise. The Office of Economic Opportunity funded a Student Health Project in which twenty-eight students from Yale were involved in New Haven and New London and (primarily with migrant workers) in Riverhead on Long Island. Although the projects had real educational value, Redlich had to report that "a small number of student activists have strongly sided with radical community groups and have attacked the establishment including their own Yale Medical School." But things could have been worse: "We have had little trouble with our student group in comparison with other schools."[14]

The medical students demanded, and were given, a much more active role in the governance of the school. Student representatives were placed on the Curriculum Committee and on the committee to look at governance within the school. Although pleased with the new curriculum, the students thought that the thesis requirement, a hallmark of the Yale medical curriculum since 1837, was not relevant in the current climate. The student demand to remove the thesis requirement was successfully resisted by the faculty, and the requirement remained (with some cosmetic changes) a condition of graduation.

A Student-Faculty Hospital Committee was instituted and met regularly in an attempt to defuse issues by disseminating information. Convinced that not enough information was being disseminated, the medical students had published their own *Yale Medical Center Newsletter.* According to the faculty it lacked editorial responsibility, and it had a short life span. For political rather than religious reasons, a nondenominational chaplaincy was established at the medical school. The Reverend David Duncombe, a community activist, had gained the respect of the students and served as a defusing agent for the administration.

A special committee for the recruitment of minority students was formed as part of a special effort to recruit underrepresented minority students, particularly African Americans. The committee, which contained representatives from the academic and local communities, generated fifty applications from underrepresented minorities. Courtland Seymour Wilson, an African American member of the dean's staff, actually picketed at graduation to stimulate interest. The admissions committee accepted nineteen of the applicants, with eleven matriculating, compared to the usual one or two minority students in previous years.

The first African American had attended the medical school in 1855, sixty-one years before the first woman was admitted. He was Courtland Van Rensselaer Creed, the son of a Yale College employee and a successful businessman. Creed took the required two courses of lectures and one year of clinical training and, along with ten other members of the graduating class, received his M.D. degree from President Woolsey in 1857. Creed opened a successful practice in New Haven and served as a surgeon in the Civil War. Personal misfortune befell him after the war, and his medical practice never achieved the same degree of success.[15]

Seventeen years after Creed entered the medical school, two African American medical students transferred to Yale from the nation's oldest traditionally African American college, Lincoln University, in Oxford, Pennsylvania, when the Lincoln medical department disintegrated. Bayard Thomas Smith graduated from Yale in 1875 and George Robinson Henderson in 1876. Both did well at Yale. Their class was the first for which final examinations were a requirement, and both passed without difficulty. Eight African Americans graduated from the medical school between 1876 and 1903.

It took forty-five years, however, for the next black student—and first African American woman—to graduate, Beatrix Ann McCleary. Segregation and discrimination had returned with a vengeance. The official admission policy of the medical school in 1935 was "the number of women is restricted . . . as are some racial groups including Europeans, South Americans, Hebrews, and Orientals."[16]

The Hill area in which the Yale University School of Medicine is located had gradually changed from being a predominantly Italian-American to being a predominantly African American and Puerto Rican neighborhood. The medical school and hospital had paid little attention to the surrounding area. Even though the master plan for a road that would serve as a moat around the entire medical center was never implemented, it was viewed as indicative of the center's attitude toward the community.

With social activism rampant, the medical school was forced to include the Hill neighborhood, the Black Coalition, and the junta representing the Puerto Rican population in a "new" set of community relationships. Participation of the dean and other representatives of the school was paralleled by community representation at various levels of the medical center in an uneasy and contentious relationship. As Redlich indicated in his 1968–1969 report, "Cooperation with indigent populations under radical, unskilled leadership or without any leadership is extremely difficult. . . . The urgency of need and the style of the ghetto leadership confront the slow and traditional practices of Yale."[17]

Richard Weinerman, director of the Community Health Program, was asked by President Brewster to plan the health aspects of a program involving Yale and the New Haven community.[18] The university could coordinate an umbrella organization to good advantage, as there were several community corporations or councils in existence, including the Hill Health Council, the Connecticut Regional Medical Program, and the Community Health Care Center Plan, a comprehensive, prepaid health-center program sponsored by the labor-industrial segment, which was to be open to the indigent.

Areas of concentration for the organization would include the development of neighborhood health centers and of programs for training community health workers and environmental safety task forces. Weinerman saw the pattern of community-based and Yale-related health-service activities as three concentric rings: the medical center, then the community and the neighborhood health center, and finally the region.

In a talk given to the American Association of Medical Colleges, Weinerman stated that the goals of the community health program at Yale were to create a "balance" of academic emphasis among the clinical and ecological disciplines, the laboratory, and community health-service settings within which the full spectrum of teaching could be accomplished and research in the preventive and delivery aspects of health could flourish.[19]

The Hill Health Board was formed and was controlled by the neighborhood residents with minority representation from health agencies and institutions. The medical school wished to have opportunities for teaching and research as well as for providing excellent medical care, but the notion was resisted by the community and activist members of the faculty. "Dr. Max Pepper's loyalties probably were in the Hill rather than in the school," commented Redlich.[20] The Hill Health Center opened on December 2, 1968, with plans to transfer ownership to the Hill Neighborhood Corporation. To do so required expansion and continuity of federal funding, which would involve a prepaid health plan, anathema to organized medicine. The Connecticut State Medical Society was also strongly opposed to the medical school's sponsorship of the Connecticut Regional Medical Program.

The medical school was being squeezed by community activists on one side and by the establishment on the other. Governance was the major issue in every venue. The community wanted control. The students wanted more say in the running of the medical school. The medical-school administration wanted more control over the departments, while departmental chairmen wanted to retain their fiefdoms. The faculty as a whole had little interest in governance and wanted to get on with research and clinical practice.

A consultant from the Tavistock Institute in London was engaged to prepare a report on governance and management for both the dean and the hospital director. At the conclusion of the study, Charles Womer was not sure that he had obtained anything helpful, but Fritz Redlich maintained that the consultant had stimulated "thinking" and had made a valuable contribution. In the introduction to his report, A. K. Rice stated, "The institutions are complex, perform complex tasks; and to perform them, have to relate to other complex organizations. . . . There can be no simple solutions." In one sense, this is pure "consultant speak." In another, the statement is profound, and the past thirty years have been spent looking for a simple solution to the problems of the medical school and the hospital. Rice concluded that change in organization alone was unlikely to solve the problems of the medical center. "Too much of the disorganization is motivated."[21]

One of the constraints Rice identified was the effect on appointments and chairmanships of the existing definitions of scholarship and traditions of tenure, which he believed were used to express the ambivalence of the university to its School of Medicine and vice versa. On completion of his six-month survey, Rice recommended that management of the medical school be delineated along the lines of teaching, research, and clinical care, directed by a triumvirate. The triumvirate would be collectively responsible for what occurred across the boundaries. Teaching, research, and patient care require different skills, and the suggestion was not without merit. But the institution was not—and is not—equipped to deal with three leaders wielding equal authority. In fact an academic institution may not be equipped to deal with a single leader wielding authority!

Rice raised the question of developing a school of health professions rather than just a medical school, a concept that is gaining momentum today.

In the course of his interviews, Rice had been told repeatedly that the Yale University School of Medicine was a medical school and must teach medicine. He asked, "Will it teach an enlarged concept of medicine?" If new integrated health-delivery systems were to be developed, then innovative leadership was required. If the medical profession did not take the leadership, others would. In fact, this is exactly what has happened. Whether a school of health professions would have altered the current state of health care in the United States is not clear, but there would probably have been earlier emphasis on primary care. Rice spoke to a social-psychology seminar, and his talk was reported in the activist, student-run *Yale Medical Center Newsletter.* He was described as a former colonial administrator for His Majesty's Government and director of the Tavistock Institute. In response to questions, Rice made the comment, "Moral questions have nothing to do with organization questions." When asked about student power, he answered, "The faculty is paid to run the University." The reporter remarked that Rice was to be commended for "exposing his particular prejudices in public."[22]

Succumbing to student and faculty pressure, the Board of Permanent Officers appointed a Committee on Governance to develop a proposal for governing the school. Redlich charged the committee "to create a pattern of representative governance that will enable all people affected by decisions to be heard and still permit the leaders of the institution to exert their constructive influence."[23] To safeguard the wisdom of experienced leadership, the dean favored a senate model, with separate bodies for faculty and students, but he doubted the students would accept less than complete equality. Standards for admission, promotion, and graduation had to remain under faculty control. For the dean of the Yale University School of Medicine to have to insist that the faculty retain control of admissions, promotions, and graduation in the face of student demands would have been inconceivable to previous deans. Nothing like this had ever before happened in the history of the medical school.

The Committee on Governance produced a draft "Report and Recommendations of the Committee on Governance," which was distributed and discussed over the next several months with the various interest groups. Proposed amendments were discussed at a lengthy meeting of the Board of Permanent Officers. Albert Solnit, director of the Child Study Center and chairman of the committee, had been extremely effective in crafting the first draft of the governance document, and subsequent emendations did not alter the essence of the draft.

Following interminable meetings with a variety of constituencies, the

Medical School Council was formed, composed of both faculty and students. The idea was to have a bicameral arrangement, with interaction between the Medical School Council and the chairs of the departments. The Board of Permanent Officers had delegated to the council its role as the "educational policy-making body of the school." Dean Redlich believed that the council provided broader communication between and participation of faculty and students. "In spite of attacks by chairmen and the Board of Permanent Officers, I hope it will survive."[24] The clinical chairmen were unhappy with the new governance structure, which they felt diminished their power at a time when federal budget cuts threatened their financial stability.

A tremendous amount of time and effort had been devoted to the governance issue, which in the long run did not fundamentally change the way the medical school was governed. However, involving medical students in these prolonged discussions defused student unrest to a large degree. Although the Medical School Council still exists and meets on a monthly basis, its major purpose is to disseminate information rather than to debate substantive issues.

Although student activism had been channeled into constructive areas of governance, the local community still presented major problems. Both the medical school and the hospital were being pressed by insistent demands from the neighborhood leaders for better clinical care. The demands were being supported by other citizens, state and federal agencies, and medical students and faculty. The medical school was under intense pressure to become a service organization rather than an academic one. Attempting to maintain the proper balance between service and academic pursuits in a medical school is a difficult task at any time. It was made even more difficult because leadership in the community was dysfunctional and various demands lacked consistency.

Fritz Redlich's report in his third year as dean was rather pessimistic. The medical school's financial situation, friction with the hospital, and community tensions were all worse. The school had been unable to institute educational and research programs in the community despite tremendous effort to build a health-care system in the Hill. Problems were also caused by "divided and unclear authority in decision-making within the University." On the positive side, the new curriculum had been well accepted by the medical students, if not by the faculty. The summer clinical experience was an "overwhelming success" despite the preceding anxiety. More important, "faculty and student relationships severely tested by the Cambodia invasion, the Kent State incident, and the Panther trial, have been unusually good."[25]

The Committee for Change, a group of eighty health-science students, workers, staff, and faculty spent four months developing a document entitled "Proposals for Change." The proposal demanded that discussions be initiated with community groups in the New Haven area to reconstitute the decision-making boards so that "the community will have the power to influence patient care."[26] To do this, the community would need access to all medical-center information, including salaries. During this particularly tense period in medical school–community relations, the last thing Yale needed was an unfavorable portrayal of the medical center as being primarily interested in teaching and research at the expense of patient care.

The relationship between the social environment of a hospital and medical school and the care of hospitalized patients was the focus of *Sickness and Society,* by Raymond S. Duff, a Yale pediatrician, and August B. Hollingshead, a Yale sociologist. Published in 1968, the book asked whether patients received optimal care and whether the social system enhanced or hindered care. Although set in fictional Eastern University, any knowledgeable reader would immediately identify it as Yale. Fritz Redlich, who had written a study with Hollingshead before assuming the deanship, wrote the foreword. After commenting how exciting the book was, Redlich said: "It is impossible for me to accept the fact that medical teaching and research are not compatible with good medical care. I do not believe that an inherent antagonism exists among physicians, hospital administrators and nurses or that hospitals are run for the benefit of physicians."[27] In his decanal reports, however, Redlich lamented the tensions among the groups and thought that the clinical chairmen were not sufficiently interested in patient care. He certainly described antagonism, even though he may not have believed that it was "inherent."

Duff and Hollingshead were particularly sympathetic to the problems of hospital administrators, who were faced with "many dilemmas" in their relationships with academic physicians on the one hand and community physicians on the other. The two groups of physicians disagreed about the hospital's primary mission, but it was they, rather than the administrators, who determined hospital operations. The authors' findings from a study of 161 families caused the most ire: "Rarely did a physician exhibit an effective skill in using himself and his sponsorship to the patient's therapeutic advantage." Duff and Hollingshead focused in particular on the responsibility that physicians took for patients, which they termed "sponsorship," and which they concluded was related to the socioeconomic position of the patient. The care of ward patients was called "committee sponsorship" with the "committee" composed of medical students, interns, and residents. Their degree of interest in the "impoverished patient" depended on the extent to which his or her disease contributed to their learning or research opportunities. These were sweeping indictments of the medical-education system at Yale!

The authors felt that physicians were separated from the everyday concerns of the patient. Neither community nor academic senior physicians could be effective leaders in the management of hospitalized patients as well as carry out all their other responsibilities of private practice, teaching, and research. "Because of the lack of clarity of medical leadership, there was much ambiguity and confusion on the patient care divisions." The care of hospital patients was not really under the control of the hospital or anyone else.[28]

The solution to these problems was societal and went beyond the purview of the medical profession. *Sickness and Society* raised major concerns about the relation of socioeconomic status and optimal medical care at a time when society was expressing similar concerns. The other concerns then engulfing the medical school and hospital, however, resulted in relatively little attention being paid to the book's conclusions. As someone who was a medical resident and junior faculty member at Yale during that period, I can testify that the "committee sponsors" on the wards were as committed to the patients as "committed sponsors," if not more so. The problem with medical residents in books like Samuel Shem's *House of God* was that they were not "committed sponsors."[29]

Affiliations between the medical school and six community hospitals were established as part of the Connecticut Regional Medical Program. Affiliation with the Hospital of Saint Raphael developed into a much closer relationship. The purpose of the affiliations was to facilitate coordination of health-care services in the New Haven area, as well as to provide clinical clerkships for medical students. As a result of Yale's producing more subspecialists than could be accommodated in faculty positions, an increasing number of Yale-trained physicians had joined the staff of Saint Raphael's and were interested in an academic affiliation. There is a certain irony that the Hospital of Saint Raphael, which was founded to provide places for physicians who were not appointed to the New Haven Hospital staff, was now going to provide teaching to Yale medical students and residents.

Discord with the community reached a high point when Dean Redlich was physically assaulted by a community activist during a discussion at the Connecticut Mental Health Center. On September 2, 1969, a group of about thirty-five Hill residents and leaders met with Morton Reiser, the new chairman of psychiatry, and Louis Kaplan, the dean's representative at the Connecticut Mental Health Center. Redlich was asked to join the meeting. After prolonged, intense discussion and apparent general agreement, he excused himself to attend another meeting but was barred from leaving by Hill residents standing at the doors. A statement was presented to him to sign, which he refused to do. Then "Mr. Harris spat upon the dean, grabbed him by the throat and used vituperative language. Within a brief moment residents controlled Mr. Harris."[30]

Redlich did not press charges against Fred Harris, although urged to do so by Mayor Richard E. Lee and Police Chief Ahern, but Harris was removed from his job as a consultant at the mental-health center. Fortunately the event had a good outcome. As Redlich later explained to the Medical School Council, "The physical assault on me by Fred Harris in September led to an extraordinary amount of administrative and institutional work which moved from confrontation to negotiation."[31] Discussions were facilitated with a broader section of the inner-city black and Puerto Rican leadership as a result of the incident, with satisfactory resolution of the issues.

There were, however, major problems in psychiatry, and not solely with regard to the community. Three major factions existed within the psychiatry department: community psychiatrists at the Connecticut Mental Health Center, "biological" psychiatrists located in the Yale–New Haven Hospital, and the analytical psychiatrists at the Yale Psychiatric Institute. Mort Reiser was caught between the departmental factions and the community problems. Redlich asked Brewster for his strong backing in dealing with departmental strife, indicating that he was concerned about "the interference of inter-departmental turmoil and intrigues in the Medical School."[32]

Meanwhile, as the Vietnam War became progressively unpopular, social unrest increased. At a full meeting of the medical school student body on May 6, 1970, in response to the call for a national academic strike, the medical students voted, 246 to 23, to suspend their normal academic activities and to work for peace and racial equality. Concern was voiced about medical responsibilities, but the comment was made that medical students do not render services that are "essential" to the well-being of patients. The medical students made it clear that this was not a strike against the university, and they asked the faculty to develop academic options that would insure that their professional competence was not impaired by the strike.

The social and political issues came to a head in New Haven in May 1970 during the trial of the Black Panthers. Thousands held a demonstration on the New Haven Green. President Brewster, in a controversial but wonderfully effective move, opened the gates of Yale's residential colleges to the demonstrators. Faculty and students of the medical school played an important role in providing medical care to the participants.

The university and the medical school had entered a dangerous and difficult time in their relations with the community. In October Alvin Novack, a member of the medical faculty who had devoted a great deal of time to the founding of the Hill Health Center, received a letter from Adrienne Davis, chair of the Hill Health Center Board, terminating him as project director of the center. She dismissed him "due to the fact that you are a racist and are dead set on creating havoc, like all devils are created to do." She ended her letter with "Blood to the pork chops ass and woe to those who cannot cook."[33] Appalled, the chairman of the board and the executive director of the Hill Neighborhood Corporation informed all staff members that the dismissal was illegal, unwarranted, and insupportable.

In addition to social turmoil, medical-school finances continued to be a problem, because federal support for research was still meager. University support of the medical school had never been adequate, and the reserve funds had been drawn upon to purchase property for expansion. A financial incentive plan had been instituted to augment clinical salaries, which were unreasonably low.

Despite these problems, faculty size continued to increase and by 1968 had reached 634 full-time members. While acknowledging that the departmental chairmen were opposed to any ceiling on recruitment, Redlich raised the question, in view of the financial crunch, of how many faculty members were actually needed. This question has been asked repeatedly by a series of deans without a satisfactory answer.

Funds were needed for the recruitment of new chairmen, particularly of George Palade, the distinguished cell biologist from Rockefeller University, to head a combined section in cell biology, which would play a major role in bringing the school to the next step of reorganizing the basic sciences, minimally involving microbiology and anatomy.[34] There was universal enthusiasm among the faculty to recruit Palade and his wife, Marilyn Farquhar, a distinguished cell biologist in her own right. "It would be tragic if only capital cost prevented us from bringing one of the most exciting leaders in the field of biological sciences to Yale." Palade was offered an annual operating budget of $205,000 a year for nine years at a time when other chairmen were enduring serious cutbacks in their departmental budgets.[35] The preclinical chairmen made real financial sacrifices in their budgets to attract Palade and Farquhar to New Haven. The investment was well worth it. George Palade was awarded the Nobel Prize in Medicine and Physiology in

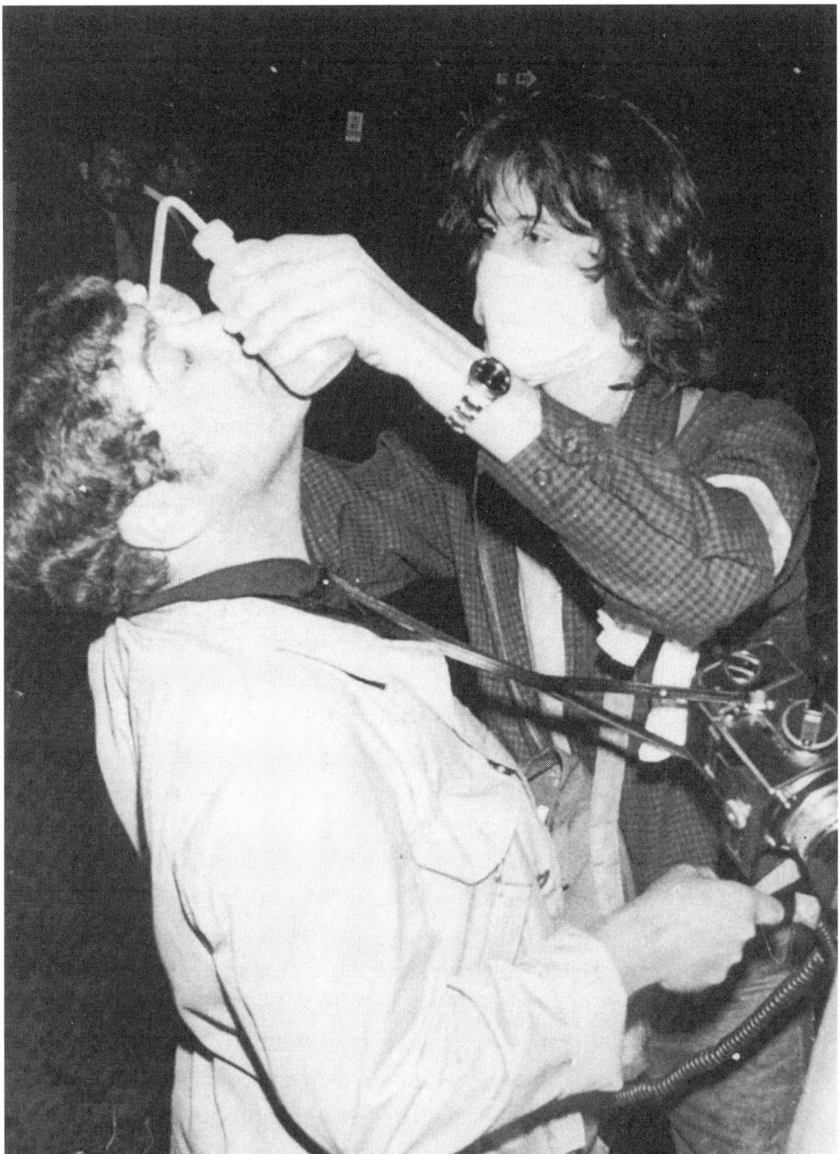

Figure 31. Washing out tear gas: May Day 1970

1974 for his work in cellular biology, which he shared with Albert Claude and Christian DeDuve.

There was also a continuing effort to focus on students and medical education. A physician augmentation grant from the Department of Health, Education, and Welfare enabled the school to increase the size of the entering class by 10 percent, the second 10 percent increase in five years, bringing the class size to 102, where it has stabilized. Redlich felt that without a massive increase in student enrollment, no federal contributions to a building program would be possible.

There was an expansion too of the continuing education program for practitioners. Although medical students spend four years in medical school, they spend forty years or more as practicing physicians. One of the benefits of the regional medical program was the opportunity to extend the continuing education program to affiliated hospitals. During the 1970–1971 academic year, 350 teaching sessions were given by Yale medical faculty members at sixteen affiliated hospitals. A program was also instituted to train mid-level practitioners. Initially using returning Vietnam corpsmen as students, a successful physician's assistant program was instituted under the chairman of the Department of Surgery, Jack Cole. The program had been inaugurated at Duke in 1965 by Eugene Stead, and at Yale it was placed in the trauma section of the Department of Surgery.[36]

Because of the ongoing need for funding, the school commissioned McKinsey & Company to perform a diagnostic review of the relationship between the university and the medical school, with particular regard to financial pressures. Problems identified in the review included a lopsided "three-legged stool" with an increasing emphasis on research "resulting in a mismatch between stated objectives and those implicit in actual operations"; increasing long-term faculty commitments based on "soft" money; and stress on the organization from new thrusts in medical education and expanded clinical practice. The "Osler man" model, patterned after Sir William Osler, assumes the "triple threat"—teaching, research, and patient care—yet promotion was increasingly based on research accomplishments. The growing importance of soft money generated by individual faculty members resulted in loss of loyalty to the institution. The proposed medical-school response to the financial problems was to increase research and clinical income as well as enrollment. In addition, cost sharing by the hospital and endowment income should be increased. A "direct cut in numbers of faculty would be counterproductive."[37] As is often the case with consultants' reports, nothing came of the McKinsey review.

Because of administrative concern about the number of tenure appointments in the School of Medicine covered by "hard" money, the provost decreed that only retiring tenured faculty could be replaced. Barely about a quarter of the school's annual budget for tenured faculty salaries was in fact covered by hard money. The decree meant that a mere five new slots would become available during the next five years. A Committee on Future Tenure Policy recommended that financial commitments for tenure appointments should be assumed by the School of Medicine.[38]

In 1970, President Brewster had appointed a committee to search for a dean for clinical affairs, which was to be combined with the chief-of-staff position to create an efficient clinical organization at the hospital. Robert McCollum, chairman of the Department of Epidemiology and Public Health, recommended Louis Welt, chairman of medicine at Chapel Hill, who was dropped from consideration because of a previous heart attack.[39] Welt was subsequently appointed to succeed Phil Bondy as chairman of the Department of Medicine, and he had a fatal heart attack at his desk about a year later. Robert Chase, a surgeon at Yale, was selected for the position of dean for clinical affairs and chief of staff at the hospital. Before accepting the position, however, Chase wanted to know how long Dean Redlich would remain in office.

Redlich, who had been in the trenches or foxholes for five years, told President Brewster that he did not want a full second term and asked for a sabbatical at the end of his current term. Brewster thought that a short term would make Redlich a lame-duck dean. Before Brewster left for London on a leave of absence during the fall of 1971, he asked Charles Taylor, acting president, to form a search committee for the new dean. This would allow time to appraise possible candidates and to review "the hopes and fears, needs and priorities of the School."[40] The appointments of a dean for clinical practice and a dean for medical science were put on hold.

Fritz Redlich had not experienced a tranquil term as dean of the medical school. A number of the chairmen of clinical departments disagreed strongly with his policies. On the other hand, he guided the school through perilous times without a major conflagration. He was able to keep the ferment of social, faculty, and student unrest below boiling point. On a number of occasions during his tenure as dean, it would have taken very little to plunge the medical school into chaos. The same can be said even more strongly of President Brewster. Both men had handled potentially explosive situations well, but not without incurring the wrath of others.

11

THE DEPARTMENT OF MEDICINE

Ever since Nathan Smith was appointed as the very first professor of the theory and practice of physic in 1813, Yale's Department of Medicine has been propelled by a remarkable cast of faculty members. Smith, who was also responsible for lectures in surgery and in obstetrics and gynecology,[1] was revered as a teacher, in part because he lectured on his cases, making his points with models and illustrations and allowing students to question him, rather than following the traditional didactic manner. Smith emphasized moderation in therapeutics, seldom recommending bleeding, preferring cleanliness and rest, and prescribing drugs only when he had established that they were useful. He often rejected commonly held theories. He disagreed, for example, with Benjamin Rush of Philadelphia, one of the outstanding physicians of the day, who believed in vigorous bleeding and constructed a classification of disease that did not at all impress Smith. "Dr. Rush must be a very interesting lecturer. As to his classification of disease, I do not think it very material."[2] Smith's

1824 classic, *A Practical Essay on Typhous Fever,* opposed Rush's view of typhoid. Smith recognized that typhoid fever was a specific disease rather than a state of fever as described by Rush, but the reviewer in the *New England Medical and Surgical Journal* took issue with the article, believing typhoid fever to be a result of exposure to cold.[3]

Nathan Smith's death in 1829 from the effects of a paralytic stroke came as a hard blow to the Medical Institution of Yale College. Eli Ives, professor of materia medica and botany, succeeded Smith as professor of the theory and practice of physic. Ives had a profound knowledge of botany and was a keen and original observer who gained the affection of his students. Also a respected pediatrician, he occupied the chair in medicine until 1852.

Charles Hooker, who as professor of anatomy was elected the first dean by vote of the faculty in 1845 (although his appointment by the Yale Corporation was not listed until 1853), introduced the newer French medicine to New Haven with papers on auscultation and percussion. Eli Ives and the elder Benjamin Silliman, who had both served on the faculty for forty years, retired in 1853.

Worthington Hooker, Yale 1825 and Harvard M.D. 1829, who had been in practice in Norwich, Connecticut, for twenty-five years and was a second cousin of the dean, was appointed professor of the theory and practice of medicine in 1852 to replace Ives. A talented writer, he exerted considerable influence through his books; his *Physician and Patient* offered one of the earliest discussions of medical ethics. He also wrote a number of well-received elementary textbooks on the natural and life sciences. Hooker died fifteen years after assuming the professorship and in 1868 was succeeded by Charles Linnaeus Ives, Yale 1852 and Jefferson Medical College 1854, who followed in the footsteps of his father, uncle, grandfather, and great-grandfather. Illness forced Ives to resign after five years, to the distress of the medical students, who appreciated his perpetually positive outlook.

Ives in turn was succeeded in 1873 by David Paige Smith, a practitioner from Springfield, Massachusetts, and a grandson of Nathan Smith, who was appointed in response to a letter he had written to President Noah Porter indicating his interest in the position.[4] Smith wished to specialize rather than continue in general practice, although he assumed the job at a financial cost, as Yale medical faculty members were being paid less than $1,000 a year for their educational responsibilities. In 1877 he assumed the chair in surgery and was followed as professor of the theory and practice of medicine by Lucian Wilcox.

Soon after Wilcox's appointment, student access to patients improved.

One of the constant criticisms of the medical school was the scarcity of patients for teaching because of the relatively small size of New Haven. Although the New Haven Dispensary had opened in 1872 as an outpatient clinic for needy patients, its relations with the Medical Institution were distant. Once the patient load in the dispensary had grown to five thousand a year, by 1877, expansion was clearly necessary. When the Yale Corporation acquired property next to the medical school as a new location for the dispensary, the medical faculty was given the right to appoint the medical staff, and medical students selected by the faculty were able to "view" the clinic's medical and surgical practices in numbers not to exceed twelve students a day.

The new charter obtained from the legislature in 1879 allowed the members of the medical faculty for the first time to determine their own curriculum and the number of professors required to implement it. They added courses in the theory and practice of medicine, physical diagnosis, and clinical medicine. Students in the theory and practice of medicine attended three didactic lectures a week. Clinical microscopy was added to the curriculum in medicine, with instruction in chemical and microscopic methods of examining "blood, exudates, transudates, sputum, stomach contents, urine and feces."[5] In addition, weekly clinics in medicine were held at the hospital.

In the early 1880s the professor of the theory and practice of medicine, Charles Lindsley, who was also the dean, gave a clinic, or teaching demonstration, for the medical students on Friday afternoons. A student would examine patients and present his "diagnostic points for criticism" in front of Lindsley and his classmates.[6] He would perform a preliminary examination and present the case to Lindsley, who would explain the symptomatology, make the diagnosis, and give the student general directions. The student would then, "subject to correction," give the patient precise directions in front of the professor. All symptoms and signs would be demonstrated, and bodily fluids, including urine, blood, and sputum, would be examined when required.

Final written examinations in medicine were three hours in length. Each student drew a number by lot, which was used instead of a name. Of the ten questions on the 1899 examination, eight involved infectious disease, reflecting the significant medical problems of the day. Bright's Disease was a perennial favorite, revealing the prevalence of streptococcal disease affecting the kidneys. Questions about cancer and heart disease did not appear on the examination until years later. A practical examination also was given to each student to test clinical skills.

Students in the middle and senior medical-school classes got "free tickets" for the dispensary and were "instructed in the diagnosis and treatment of special diseases" by two of the attending physicians. Dispensary physicians did not have faculty appointments but were nonetheless specialists—Henry Fleischner in skin diseases, Thomas H. Russell in syphilis, Max Mailhouse in diseases of neurology, Charles Park in the digestive system, and Gus Eliot in "rheumatism, malarial and renal diseases." In succeeding years clinics were held in "nervous disease, mental disease, dermatology and throat and ear with personal instruction in the use of instruments."[7] Medical students also attended lectures in sanitary science and public health.

As the dispensary grew busier, medical students shifted from the role of observers to participants, performing useful services. Three groups of three clinical clerks each were assigned twice a week for a month. "While the clinical clerks are appointed primarily for the relief of the assistants in their examination, the students had a chance to learn."[8]

Charles Lindsley, who had resigned as dean in 1885, stepped down as professor of the theory and practice of medicine in 1897 after thirty-seven years of service to the medical school. In his final lecture as a teacher, Lindsley told the students that the practice of medicine has a professional side and a business side. Patients need to be treated in a way that will produce the best results, with reasonable compensation for the doctor's services. He admonished the students to stop smoking, or to take a bath and change clothes before visiting a sick patient. The doctor's office should be appropriately and neatly furnished without extravagant display. The doctor should not permit undignified familiarity from inferiors. "If anyone hails you on the street, 'Hello, Doc.' don't respond." The doctor should send bills regularly, as payment of large bills is apt to be postponed, and a bill should not be itemized, because "you cannot itemize brain products."[9]

A New Yorker, John Slade Ely (Sheffield Scientific School 1881 and College of Physicians and Surgeons 1886), was appointed to the chair in medicine in 1897. Ely was well trained and had a good grounding in science, having taken a year of physiological chemistry with Russell Chittenden and a year of general biology before obtaining his M.D. degree. After studying with Koch in Berlin and Charcot in Paris as well as at clinics in Heidelberg and London, he spent eight years at the College of Physicians and Surgeons as an assistant in pathology under T. Mitchell Prudden. Ely was the first of the "new breed" of professors to come to Yale with extensive formal training. In addition to his medical prowess, he was an avid book collector and expert bookbinder. When his career ended in a fatal horseback accident in 1906, the *Yale Medical Journal* commented, "He was always ready and willing to help his students in any way possible and took a personal interest in them."[10]

Consulted about successors to Ely, William Welch recommended George Blumer, who at the time was an associate professor of pathology at his alma mater, Cooper Medical College, and had previously had a stint as director of the Bureau of Pathology and Bacteriology for the New York State Board of Health while holding the chair of pathology at Albany Medical College. He accepted Dean Herbert Smith's 1906 offer of a position at Yale within days, becoming the first recipient of the John Slade Ely Professorship.[11] Unlike Ely, Blumer was not a college graduate and did not have a strong scientific background but was considered an excellent clinician and teacher.

The professor of the theory and practice of medicine had traditionally been a lone wolf, with sole responsibility for all teaching in the Department of Medicine. When the medical school assumed responsibility for the dispensary, a number of part-time faculty members were appointed as assistants to the medical clinic. By 1895 Louis S. Deforest had been made clinical professor of medicine. When John Slade Ely was appointed chair in 1897, Charles Lindsley became the emeritus professor. Wilder Tileston was hired that year as an assistant professor of medicine. A clinical lecturer and eight clinical instructors and assistants also held appointments in medicine.

George Blumer retained his position as chair of the Department of Medicine when he became dean in 1910. He introduced an "educational advance" in the same year, with the catalogue announcing that he would give weekly demonstrations of "rarer diseases recognizable at sight illustrated by lantern slides." Blumer's 1911 report, "The Relation of a Medical School to a Hospital," stressed that "the student must learn his work by actually doing it himself, under supervision."[12] Blumer noted that medical student education had evolved from following a preceptor to personal contact with dispensary patients to ward rounds by the students.

We recall that when Blumer relinquished the chair in medicine upon stepping down as dean in 1920, transferring from the John Slade Ely professorship to the David Paige Smith professorship, he told Abraham Flexner that "I had no college education, that the instruction which I received in the preclinical sciences [at Cooper Medical College] was a farce, and that I have never been able to fill the gaps in my training."[13] Nevertheless, Blumer was an excellent clinician and teacher who had given much, and still had more to offer, to the Department of Medicine.

When Milton Winternitz, then chairman of pathology, succeeded Blumer as dean, he recruited Francis Gilman Blake (figure 32), a thirty-four-year-old associate in medicine at the hospital of the Rockefeller Institute for Medical Research, as John Slade Ely Professor of Medicine and chairman of the Department of Medicine. This was a crucial appointment. As Alan Gregg, director of medical sciences at the Rockefeller Institute, observed, "The department of medicine is the keystone of the clinical arch and the principal factor in the professional training of the students."[14]

Born in Pennsylvania, Blake was three years old when his father, a mining engineer, died. Francis grew up in Massachusetts and attended Dartmouth College, graduating in 1908 after having taken all the available courses in biology and zoology. A true Dartmouth alumnus, he then spent a winter in a log cabin in the Maine woods to observe nature. He graduated from the Harvard Medical School in 1913 and entered residency training at the Peter Bent Brigham Hospital under Henry Christian. There Blake met Dorothy P. Dewey, a student nurse, and married her in 1916 while a research fellow at the Rockefeller Institute. The following year he was appointed assistant professor of medicine at the University of Minnesota School of Medicine. The United States had entered World War I, and Blake carried out epidemiological research with an emphasis on pneumonia for the army as part of the war effort. In 1919, as a result of these studies, he was appointed associate in medicine at the hospital of the Rockefeller Institute of Medical Research, where, in collaboration with James Trask, he demonstrated that measles could be transmitted to monkeys.[15]

Blake brought Trask and John Punnett Peters with him to Yale in 1921 from the Rockefeller Institute. Peters and William T. Stadie represented the chemical, or metabolic, division of the department. Trask and Arthur B. Dayton represented the biological division. Clinical scientists were being appointed for the first time as faculty members in the Department of Medicine, and Harold M. Marvin headed the work in electrocardiography.

The Department of Medicine was truly becoming a department rather than just a single professor of medicine with a few part-time physicians in the dispensary. Francis Blake worked hard to make it an academic department. Blake commented that he rarely left his desk before midnight four or five nights a week during the first ten years he was at Yale. By 1925 there were eight full-time associate professors, assistant professors, or instructors in addition to Blake, as well as three attending physicians at the hospital, including George Blumer and Wilder Tileston.

The young Blake demonstrated that he was "not only a competent, but an astute, clinician," an essential feature in the days when the old school insisted that science was incompatible with a "bedside manner."[16] As profes-

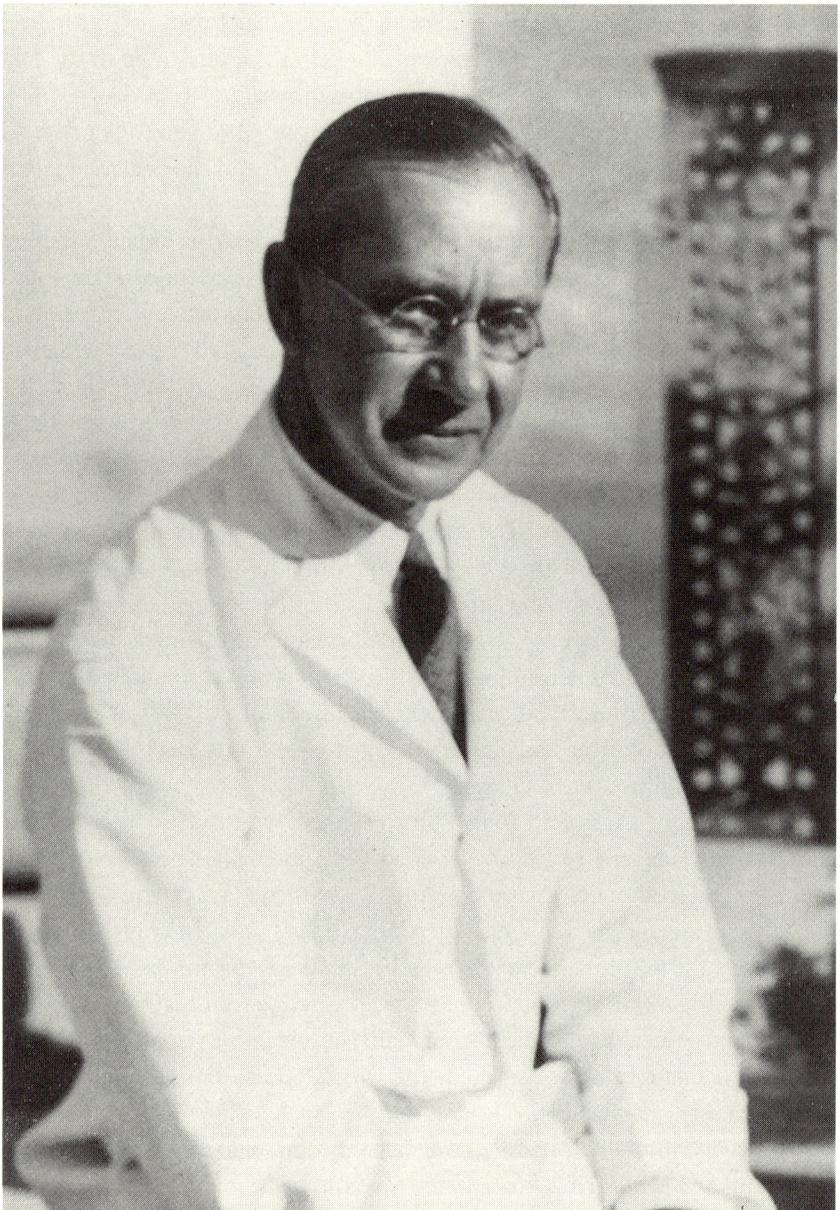

Figure 32. Francis G. Blake

sor of medicine, he participated in regular ward rounds as well as consulting rounds. He was a superb clinical consultant, careful and always displaying excellent clinical judgment. His teaching rounds were not showy but were shining examples of how to present facts in an orderly manner, critically evaluate those facts, and correlate them with other material from the medical literature. Even after he became dean in 1940 during the harrowing wartime years, he usually finished the administrative details of both the deanship and the department by 10 A.M., when he was due to do his rounds on the medical wards.

When a patient's history had been presented to him, Blake would often remain silent and with pursed lips proceed to examine the patient, then go to the X-ray department for the films and to the lab for the blood work, weighing all the evidence before rendering an opinion. His conversations with patients were brief but informative, and he used drugs sparingly.

Blake supported the Yale system of educational freedom, gradually eliminating lectures as the mainstay of the medicine course. He was a leader in changing the sequence of teaching that placed third-year students on the inpatient wards and the fourth-year students in the outpatient dispensary, where they could take more responsibility.

Francis Blake set the academic tone for the Department of Medicine, but his real strength was as a clinical investigator. He viewed the full-time clinical system as an opportunity to carry out clinical investigation. The system was not popular among community physicians, and Blake was labeled a "contract physician" practicing "hospital medicine."[17] Nevertheless, research was very important to him, and he stimulated members of the department with both encouragement and facilities to pursue it. Blake and Trask developed a departmental division for infectious diseases, conducting some of the pioneer investigations on scarlet fever.

Although extremely reserved and even shy in personal conversation, Blake's broad academic background and keen analytic ability made him a powerful figure in American medicine. He was a member of the National Research Council, the Board of Scientific Directors of the Rockefeller Institute for Medical Research, and numerous other boards and organizations.

John Punnett Peters, whom Blake had brought with him to Yale from the Rockefeller Institute, was destined to play an even larger role in clinical investigation than his mentor. If William Osler helped bring the physician to the bedside with the power of observation, then John Peters and his colleagues helped bring the physician to the laboratory chart. Peters was born in Philadelphia in 1887. His father was a clergyman and his mother an accomplished musician. The Reverend Dr. Peters had been rector of St. Michael's Episcopal Church in New York City, where he had had a reputation for delivering sermons that ruffled the feathers of his upper-class congregation, a trait he passed on to his son. He was also a distinguished biblical scholar and archaeologist, with a doctor of science degree from the University of Pennsylvania for his studies in the Holy Land and an honorary degree of doctor of divinity from Yale, his alma mater.[18]

John Peters followed his father to Yale, graduating in 1908 with a major in English. After graduation, he spent a year teaching English and Latin at St. John's Military Academy, where he had been sent as a high-school student to temper "his somewhat incorrigible nature." Peters then entered the College of Physicians and Surgeons at Columbia, from which he graduated with honors in 1913, and completed his house-staff training at the Presbyterian Hospital, where he remained as a fellow and instructor in clinical medicine. When the United States entered World War I, Peters was commissioned a captain in the army and was stationed at a base hospital in France for two years. He served his country well but left the military with a strong aversion to war.[19]

After further fellowship training and research at the hospital of the Rockefeller Institute, Peters initially accepted an offer as an associate professor of medicine at Vanderbilt but then declined it. Even though he had no real position at the Rockefeller he elected to remain there to do research. Clinical investigation was in full bloom at the hospital. Peters became one of the most enthusiastic members of the Van Slyke school, which in addition to Donald Van Slyke and Peters included Baird Hastings, William Stadie, Glen Cullen, and Harold Austins, all of whom went on to play major roles in the biomedical aspects of American medical schools.

Peters's high-school days at St. John's had by no means succeeded in tempering "his somewhat incorrigible nature." In the aftermath of a meeting between Peters and Abraham Flexner, a strong supporter of the medical school, Dean Winternitz apologized for Peters's behavior. "He is very nervous and high strung, and rather argumentative. . . . I am awfully sorry that you had such an unpleasant interview with him."[20] Winternitz went on to say that Peters was very conscientious, a hard worker. When physicians in the New Haven community saw themselves being excluded from hospital practice by the full-time clinical system that the Rockefeller Foundation had mandated, Blake and Peters met with them in an attempt to mollify them. But mollification was not one of Peters's strengths, and these conversations with community physicians were not always helpful. Blake got along well with Peters by letting him complain about various issues. When Blake became Sterling Professor of Medicine, Peters was appointed to the John Slade Ely professorship in 1927.

John Peters was a brilliant clinical investigator with wide clinical interests. He read rapidly and critically, had a prodigious memory, and was a prolific writer. He published more than two hundred articles and books, including *Quantitative Clinical Chemistry,* a definitive work on the analytical techniques applicable to clinical biochemical problems, which he wrote with his mentor Donald Van Slyke.[21] Peters carried out active research in the fields of electrolytes and acid-base balance, carbohydrate metabolism and diabetes mellitus, lipids, body water and edema, thyroid and iodine physiology, nitrogen metabolism, and the social responsibilities of medicine.[22]

Meeting three times a week to discuss the diseases of metabolism informally with each group of students entering the medical clerkship, Peters taught at the level of the best student, believing that the rest of the students would not be worse off. Peters met with the clinical clerks in even smaller groups to discuss their patients, which could be traumatic for the less able student. Lectures he gave to the students in the first two years were written with great care and were made available to the students either through publication in the *Yale Journal of Biology and Medicine* or through Dr. Fulton's library, where Mrs. Peters was curator. If there was nothing new to consider, he saw no reason to repeat the lecture the following year.

His friends described Peters as a "nonconformist and reformer, both scientifically and politically."[23] He was unbending in his principles and absolutely dedicated to those principles. "His uncompromising stands, his stubbornness—his devastating criticism" appear to have been a genetic trait. Mention has been made of his father's ability to disturb the complacency of his wealthy parishioners, but the family trait appears to go back to colonial times: "There is a letter on record of one Abigail Peters written to the presiding judge of the Salem assize, protesting the witchcraft trials."[24]

The Great Depression, which resulted in millions of Americans receiving inadequate or no health care, was intolerable to Peters. Shortly after the American Foundation's health-care study began, he was asked to serve on a medical advisory committee of interested individuals. When in 1937 this committee produced a credo, "Principles and Proposals for Improvement of Medical Care," a committee of physicians formed to promote its tenets. Peters became the secretary and spokesman of this "Committee of 430." Proposals for a system of comprehensive health care in the United States resulted in a furor in conservative medical circles like the American Medical

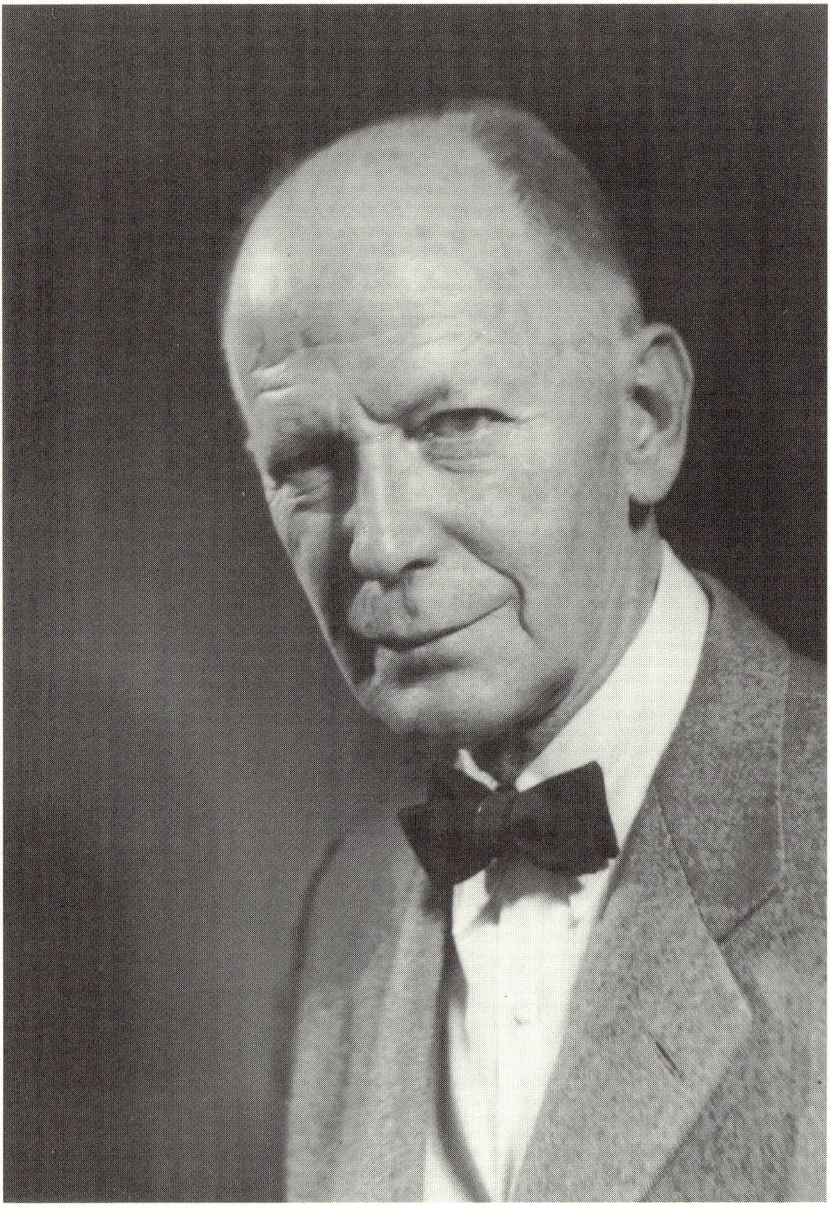

Figure 33. John P. Peters

Association, which blocked any action on the proposals. Morris Fishbein, editor of the *Journal of the American Medical Association,* spearheaded the opposition, and his target was John Punnett Peters.

A memorable exchange between the two men occurred in October 1938 at a medical symposium introduced by the misanthropic critic H. L. Mencken. Peters predicted that federally mandated aid for medical care of the underprivileged and health-insurance coverage for the middle class would be enacted. Fishbein thought that the social experimentation would destroy individual initiative and the stimulus for discovery, and he felt it would be a pity if "the furor over leadership in this battle may make for a time the enemies of man victorious."[25] Peters maintained that medical schools should be supported even by the government in order to maintain and improve the quality of medical care; it was the social responsibility of medicine "to provide all classes of the population medical care of the highest quality."[26]

In the middle of World War II, Peters prepared a thirteen-page report on the status of medical education at the request of President Seymour, with particular reference to the problems at the medical school and the hospital. Contrasting the current practice of medicine with that during Blumer's professorship, he commented that knowledge of internal medicine was no longer within the capacity of one individual. In most departments of medicine, there was a nucleus of full-time salaried men, either heads of departments with professorial rank or junior faculty. Part-time faculty filled the intermediate positions. Peters stated that the part-time individuals were preoccupied with private practice and seldom participated in research. More important, they could not move their clinical practices and so were relatively immobile, which gave medicine a provincial flavor. There were so few full-time positions that research suffered because the younger physicians knew there was almost no chance of obtaining a full-time professorial appointment and did not covet the few positions that were available. "They know that such positions involve economic sacrifice with little reward in opportunity to continue productive activities of teaching and investigation because their incumbents are smothered with administrative duties."[27]

Peters had been on active duty in World War I and came away opposed to war. During World War II he remained at Yale, heavily involved in teaching and performing metabolic research for the war on behalf of the National Research Council and the air force. After the war, Peters's liberal views became increasingly unpopular as the Cold War became more intense. His appointments to the Endocrine and Metabolism Study Section and later the Metabolism and Nutrition Study Section of the National Institutes of Health were challenged in 1949 and again in 1951 with allegations of questionable loyalty to the government. The Board of Inquiry on Employee Loyalty of the Federal Security Agency (now the Department of Health and Human Services), advised him it was satisfied that, on the basis of his written response to the charges, no reasonable grounds existed for the belief that he was disloyal to the government.[28] He was cleared again after a response to essentially the same charges at a hearing in March 1952.

But in 1953 the Loyalty Review Board of the U.S. Civil Service Commission advised Peters that it did not accept the decision of the previous board. The new board judged him to be insufficiently loyal, and his NIH appointment was terminated. He had been charged with, among other things, being a member of the Communist Party from 1939 and signing his name in support of many Communist-backed organizations. In both the 1952 and the 1953 hearings, Peters testified under oath that he had never been a member or supporter of the Communist Party, and that he had signed various petitions and statements because of his profound interest in peace, civil liberties, and a National Health Program.

Acting on principle and hoping to set a precedent to allow individuals accused of disloyalty to face their accuser, Peters challenged the validity of the judgment in the courts with the help of Yale Law School professors Fowler Harper and Vern Countryman. President Whitney Griswold, who almost certainly did not agree with Peters's politics, was nevertheless supportive. "I am sorry that you find yourself in such an uphill fight before you. The statement you have prepared substantiates the confidence I have always had in you."[29] After two rulings by lower courts in favor of the government, the case went to the U.S. Supreme Court (*Peters v. Hobby*, 349 U.S. 331), which circumvented the issue on the technicality that the Loyalty Review Board had not been empowered to hold a hearing. Griswold congratulated Peters on the decision and commiserated that the victory had not been on broad constitutional grounds.[30] The accuser was never identified, and even today the Freedom of Information Act is not applicable in loyalty cases.

One of the few goals that John Peters did not achieve in his extraordinary career was to become the chairman of the Department of Medicine at Yale. Francis Blake retired as chairman in January 1952 and moved to Washington to become technical director of research in the Office of the Surgeon General of the Army, but soon afterward had a fatal heart attack. His successor as dean, Vernon Lippard, appointed the chairman of the Department of Medicine at Emory, Paul Beeson, to be chairman at Yale. This was a bitter disappointment to Peters, but he remained an active—if troublesome—contributor to the department.[31] Beeson discontinued departmental meetings because Peters's response to any suggestion was that it had been tried before and had not worked. Three years later, Peters had a heart attack while making ward rounds and died on December 29, 1955, at the age of sixty-eight, one of the true giants of academic medicine.

The individual who had been appointed instead of him to succeed Blake as chairman was also one of the giants of American medicine, more by leadership than by scientific accomplishment. Paul Bruce Beeson was born on October 18, 1908, in Livingston, Montana, and was delivered by his father, a general practitioner. When Paul was eight, the family moved to Alaska, where his father became the surgeon for the railway and a practitioner in Ketchikan. After three years of premedical studies at the University of Washington, Paul entered medical school at McGill, returning to the United States for a two-year internship at the University of Pennsylvania. He then joined his father and brother in the family practice at the Beeson Clinic in Wooster, Ohio, but soon realized that life as a general practitioner was not his calling, and that he did not have surgical skills.[32]

Through a McGill classmate he learned of a position as a medical resident at New York Hospital and headed there in the summer of 1937. At a party given by another classmate from McGill, he met Thomas Rivers, head of the hospital at the Rockefeller Institute, who offered him a job as a resident, which he accepted, leaving Cornell after four months. Beeson spent much of his time at Rockefeller on the pneumonia ward, which was under the research direction of the brilliant Oswald Avery. Beeson, excited by scientific inquiry, carried out his own research in a laboratory next door to Avery, across the hall from René Dubos. Beeson's later work on the mechanism of fever had its inception in the clinical observations he made at the Rockefeller.

Friendships continued to play an important role in Paul Beeson's career. Through a Rockefeller acquaintance he met Soma Weiss, chief physician at the Peter Bent Brigham Hospital in Boston, who offered him a residency in medicine there. Weiss delegated responsibility to younger faculty and paid attention to the house staff, two lessons Beeson was later to implement so effectively at Yale.[33]

In 1940 Harvard's president, James B. Conant, established the Harvard Field Hospital in Salisbury, England, to show support for the British. The hospital was primarily devoted to infectious diseases, and Beeson was appointed chief physician, leaving in 1942 once America had entered the war. His sojourn in England was rewarding on many fronts. He carried out some important studies in infectious disease, married one of the nurses at the hospital, and developed an affinity for England, to which he and Barbara Beeson often returned.

After his return to the United States, Beeson was appointed assistant professor of medicine at Emory University in Atlanta by Eugene Stead. Stead had known Beeson during their time together at the Peter Bent Brigham Hospital. When Stead left Emory in 1947 to become chairman of medicine at Duke, Beeson was appointed chairman of medicine at Emory. His faculty members included Philip Bondy, who had come from Brigham with Stead as a resident, and Ivan Bennett, a local Grady Hospital resident. The first hint Beeson had that he might be asked to succeed Francis Gilman Blake at Yale came in a conversation he overheard in the men's room during an academic medical meeting in Atlantic City.

Beeson was a fitting successor to Blake, an expert in infectious disease and committed to good clinical medicine. John Peters, however talented, was too abrasive to be chairman. In addition to Peters, faculty members in the department when Beeson arrived included Gerald Klatskin, a superb clinician who had built an outstanding program in liver disease, and Franklin Epstein, a nephrologist, who was part of Peters's metabolism group but appreciated Beeson's concept of a department. Beeson brought Philip Bondy and Ivan Bennett with him from Emory. Bondy, an internationally renowned endocrinologist who provided some balance to John Peters, eventually succeeded Beeson as chairman at Yale, and Bennett eventually became the dean of the New York University School of Medicine. Following Soma Weiss's example, Beeson recruited a number of young individuals to head the various subspecialty sections: Stuart Finch in hematology, Howard Spiro in gastroenterology, and Aaron Lerner in dermatology. Elisha Atkins, who was also interested in infectious disease, came from Washington University in Saint Louis.

Beeson believed that attracting top-notch interns and assistant residents was vital to the success of the whole educational program in medicine, and he devoted an enormous amount of attention to the house staff. In his annual departmental reports to the dean, Beeson emphasized education—particularly house-staff education—while other chairmen discussed faculty recruiting and space limitations. Yale's residency program became one of the most sought after in the country. The highpoint of the residency was the "Morning Report" with Beeson, in which the ward residents would give an account of their patients admitted the previous day. One resident had responsibility for heating the water for Beeson's tea, and despite his nurturing attitude toward the house staff, Beeson was unforgiving if the tea water was tepid!

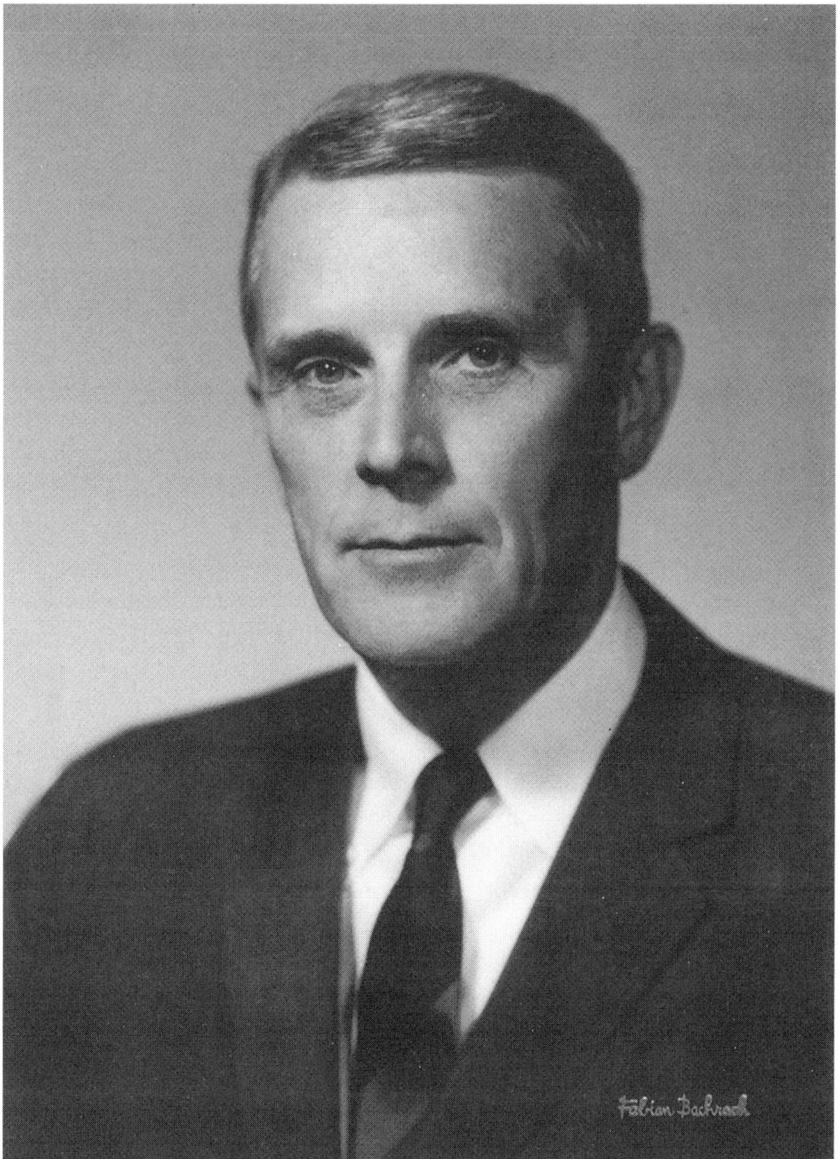

Figure 34. Paul B. Beeson

Beeson thought that the medical students should spend as much time as possible with patients rather than in important but distracting seminars. He stressed the value of postmortem examinations as a way to monitor medical practice, and he put great pressure on the house staff to obtain permission for autopsies. A "Post Derby" was held each year. House officers who had obtained the largest number of autopsy permissions during the year were sent to the academic medical meetings in Atlantic City and taken to Hackney's Restaurant for a shore dinner with Dr. Beeson.

A real commitment to teaching coupled with superb faculty recruitment led to the development of one of the best departments of medicine in the country. These recruitments occurred despite faculty salaries that lagged significantly behind those at peer institutions. Changes in the full-time clinical system that would increase faculty salaries through private practice had previously been resisted, especially by Francis Blake. Beeson, however, declared himself "in full accord" with the planned changes.[34] The revenue was important, but so were the additional patients that would be seen for educational purposes. The department benefited enormously when the memorial unit of the Grace–New Haven Community Hospital opened in 1953, increasing the bed capacity to five hundred. The opening of the West Haven VA hospital provided an additional fifty acute-care beds.

Despite Beeson's initial reluctance to supply house staff to the VA, preferring to keep the department in one place, he finally did provide house staff when he was allowed to appoint the chief of the medical service and, subsequently, the faculty. J. W. Hollingsworth, a young hematologist, was appointed chief, followed by Thomas Amatruda, one of Beeson's first chief residents. Although most of the original VA physicians left, Massimo Calabresi, a distinguished Italian cardiologist and house-staff favorite, remained, and the hospital in West Haven grew into an integral and vital part of the Department of Medicine.

Hollingsworth began a two-year leave of absence in 1958 to become the first chief of the Yale program at the Atomic Bomb Casualty Commission in Japan. The commission had been organized through the National Academy of Sciences to study the long-term medical effects of the atomic bombing in Hiroshima and Nagasaki, but the program was foundering because of lack of continuity. Beeson, concerned about developments in the Sputnik era, decided the program was important and committed the department to supply medical staff. For a number of years the junior staff members at the Atomic Bomb Casualty Commission, myself included, were recruited from the house staff at Yale. When Hollingsworth returned from Japan, he became a rheumatologist and founded a very successful division at Beeson's behest.

The increasing interest in specialization resulted in the Department of Medicine fostering a third group of students in addition to medical students and house staff. Fellows were being recruited at the departmental level as well as by subspecialty divisions. Beeson, recognizing the need for physicians highly competent in the basic sciences, instituted a formal program in clinical investigation under the auspices of the Department of Medicine. The number of postdoctoral fellows has kept growing, even in the age of the primary-care physician. In the Department of Medicine, fellows provide care to the subspecialty patients, allowing the supervisor more time for research.

The availability of funding and the growth in specialities led to continual expansion of the faculty in the Department of Medicine, making the chairman's job more complicated and more difficult. There were eighteen full-time faculty in the department when Beeson arrived at Yale in 1952 and sixty-five when he left in 1965. He commented that being a departmental chairman was like being a juggler who had to keep four balls (teaching, research, patient care, and administration) in the air, one of which was always on the floor. "My intent was to keep all four balls in the air, but to accept the fact that I could not handle any of them with ease and grace."[35] Over the years, the number of balls in the air have increased—and become much heavier.

Beeson had been a chairman of a department of medicine since 1946 and was getting tired of administration. "I was sitting at my desk too much of the time, having less contact with patients and students, and had to abandon research altogether."[36] When Sir George Pickering, then Regius Professor at Oxford, approached him to become the Nuffield Professor of Medicine, he accepted immediately. At Oxford, he led a group with five full-time faculty members and six house-staff members responsible for forty beds in the Radcliffe Infirmary. He recruited his former chief resident, Thomas Ferris, for a year to ease the clinical burden. Beeson remained at Oxford almost until the mandatory retirement age and then returned to the VA hospital in Seattle, where he was a distinguished professor for seven years. A quiet, reserved individual, Paul Beeson, like his mentor Soma Weiss, had an incredible impact on those who came within his ambit, and he succeeded in building one of the world's great departments of medicine.

Beeson was a hard act to follow. The logical internal candidate was Philip Kramer Bondy (figure 35), chief of the Division of Metabolism, whom Beeson had brought with him from Emory. Bondy attended Columbia College and the Harvard Medical School, which he followed with an internship at the Peter Bent Brigham Hospital, where he had clerked as a medical student. Eugene Stead had known him as a student at Brigham and offered him a residency at Emory. Two months after arriving at Emory, however, Bondy was commissioned as an officer in the Army Medical Corps and spent the next three years as a physician in military camps in the South.

After completing the residency at Grady, Bondy spent a year at Yale as a fellow in physiological chemistry under C. N. H. Long but returned to Grady when Beeson offered him a faculty position in endocrinology. Accompanying Beeson to Yale, Bondy succeeded John Peters as chief of the metabolism division, which at that time encompassed both endocrinology and nephrology. The two specialties later separated into two divisions when renal dialysis became a prominent and time-consuming part of nephrology.

Bondy had been a member of the faculty, and as a chairman he was more approachable than Beeson had been. His closeness to the faculty had both advantages and disadvantages, as his colleagues did not ever expect him to say no. Unfortunately, a chairman cannot say yes all the time. The problem was compounded by the fact that the flow of funds from Washington began to dwindle, and the faculty looked to the chairman to make up funding shortfalls. Social turmoil surrounding the Vietnam War was also causing unrest within the department. Despite these problems, the department continued to have a flourishing research program, and it was able to attract excellent house staff.

Five years as chairman under these conditions were sufficient for Phil Bondy. All the reasons that had led Paul Beeson to step aside were still present, with disruptive social unrest added to them. Like Beeson, Bondy moved to Britain, accepting a position as professor of medicine at the Institute of Cancer Research in London.

As the search for a new chairman began, Howard Spiro, director of the Division of Gastroenterology, wrote to Fritz Redlich in March 1971 strongly urging the "re-fashioning of the department. . . . Such a behemoth is, I think, not manageable by any one person."[37] The advice went unheeded, and the department continues to grow ever larger. Bondy was succeeded by Louis Welt, a former Peters trainee and chairman of medicine at the University of North Carolina at Chapel Hill. Donald W. Seldin, the successful chairman of medicine at Southwestern Medical School in Dallas, was also a candidate. Ironically, both Welt and Seldin were disciples of John Peters, who had so desperately wanted to be chairman.

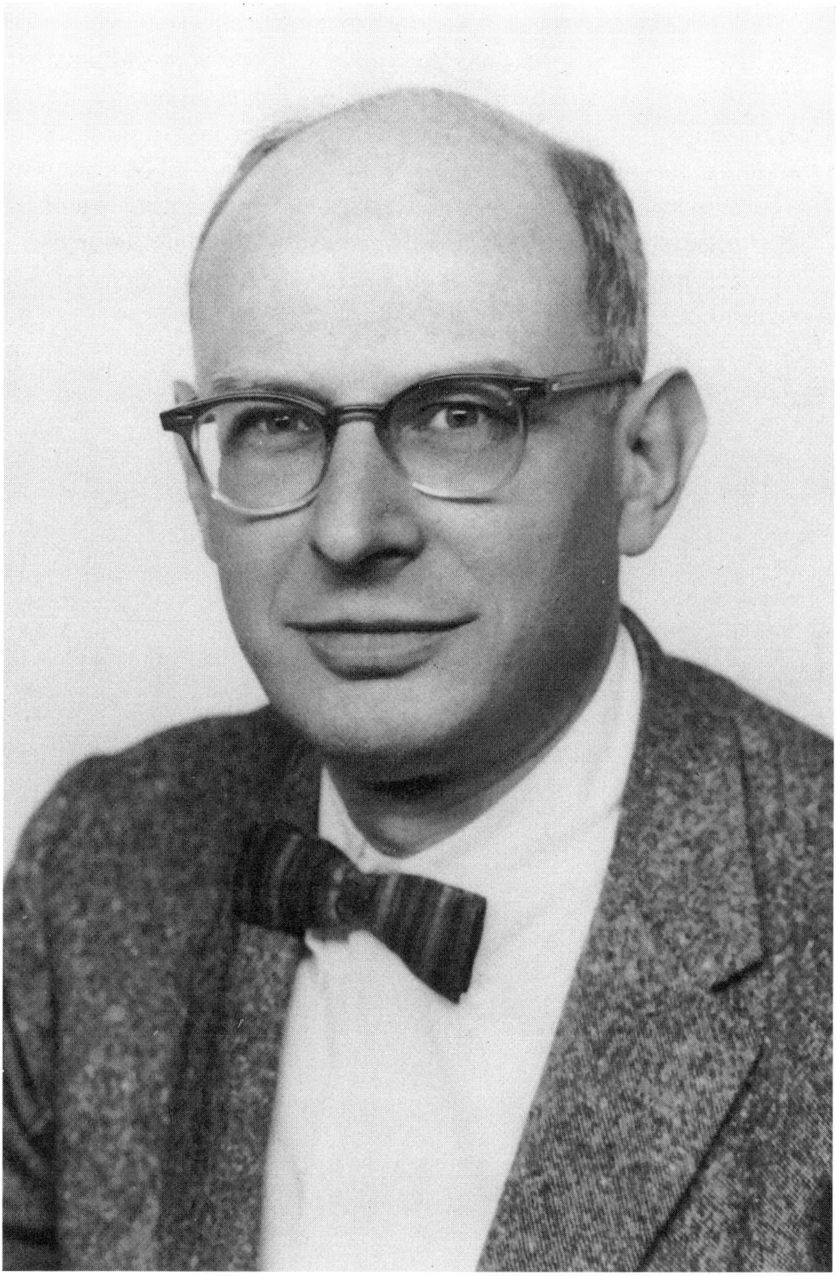

Figure 35. Philip K. Bondy

Sadly, Welt experienced a fatal heart attack in his department office a year later, and he was succeeded by Samuel O. Thier, a nephrologist at the University of Pennsylvania. Thier was an excellent clinician who had done mainly clinical research. When he arrived at Yale in 1975, most of the division directors were Beeson appointees. Perhaps because of his background, or because he saw the future of research becoming increasingly molecular, Thier began to appoint individuals who were outstanding researchers but not necessarily outstanding clinicians. The Department of Medicine, which had reinvented itself under Paul Beeson, began to do so again.

12

PUBLIC HEALTH AND THE GREATER GOOD

Creation of the Anna R. Lauder Chair of Public Health with a gift of $500,000 from the Lauder bequest in 1915 resulted in the establishment of Yale's Department of Public Health. George Blumer had chaired a university committee soon after his arrival in 1906 to consider establishing a department or school to provide education in working with public-health bureaus and philanthropic or charitable organizations.[1] Much of the impetus for the committee had come from Irving Fisher, a political economist at Yale, who was interested in the economic impact of disease on society. He felt that Yale was well positioned to serve the public-health movement, given the combined interests of the medical school, the Sheffield Scientific School, and the Department of Economics. Fisher had become deeply involved with health affairs as a result of his contracting tuberculosis, and he subsequently served on an American Medical Association committee that was looking at medical-school education.[2]

The medical school already offered courses in hygiene and bacteriology, and the Sheffield Scientific School had "already made a reputation for itself in sanitary engineering and dietetics," while the economics department had several people interested in preventive medicine.[3] The committee, consisting of Blumer, Fisher, and Lafayette Mendel, a brilliant physiological chemist at Sheffield, recommended a new department, to be named either "Public Health and Public Service" or "Hygiene and Philanthropy." Graduates of the program would receive a diploma and would be qualified for public-health and welfare positions.[4] The diversity of names for the program and positions for which graduates would qualify was the weakness of the proposal. Yandell Henderson, who was a physiologist at the medical school, thought that the program lacked focus, and the Committee on Graduate Education declared the plan "inoperable," with President Hadley's concurrence.[5]

In 1913 the Rockefeller Foundation became interested in establishing new educational institutions to provide scientific training for a new generation of public-health workers.[6] Three years of conferences and meetings ensued, with the ever-present Abraham Flexner playing a central role. Harvard, Columbia, the University of Pennsylvania, and Johns Hopkins were all interested in having a school of public health, to be supported by the Rockefeller Foundation. Having received the Lauder bequest, Yale was beginning to plan a department of public health and had written to Flexner about possible faculty candidates. He advised Yale to delay any decision until after the summit conference in October 1914 but did not invite Yale representatives to the conference. William Welch dominated the conference and, not surprisingly, the school of public health was awarded to Johns Hopkins. Blumer then told Flexner that Yale planned to develop a school of public health on the Harvard-MIT model, graduating a small number of highly trained health officers.[7]

With the funds provided by the Lauder bequest, the plan for public health at Yale could at last be implemented. The bequest specified that the professorship in public health be held by a physician with experience in public health and sanitary affairs. The department was to "effect changes in the present health laws and organization of the health department of the State of Connecticut."[8] The ultimate choice for the professorship, however, was not a physician. At the time of his appointment, Charles-Edward Amory Winslow was curator of public health at the American Museum of Natural History and director of publicity for the New York State Department of Health. His highest qualification was a master of science degree from MIT.

Born and raised in Boston, the son of a merchant and an English actress, Winslow entered MIT as a student of William T. Sedgwick, the preeminent public-health figure of his day. Sedgwick had begun his career at the Sheffield Scientific School, graduating in 1877, the year Winslow was born. At Sheffield, Sedgwick had fallen under the influence of Russell Chittenden, professor of physiological chemistry. After studying medicine for two years, he decided to pursue general biology and transferred to Johns Hopkins, where he received his Ph.D. In 1883, Sedgwick was invited to MIT as professor and chairman of the Department of Biology, where he devoted his energies to applied biology related to public health.

Winslow decided to switch his goal from medicine to public health, which was becoming defined as a distinct discipline thanks to Sedgwick's inspiration. After graduation, Winslow remained at MIT to obtain a master's degree, which was followed by an appointment as assistant professor. In 1909 he moved to the University of Chicago, then subsequently to the College of the City of New York and Columbia University. Despite his not being a physician, Winslow was well equipped to play a significant role in revising Connecticut's health statutes. In his early days at MIT he had published the first American textbook on water bacteriology and offered the first university course on industrial hygiene. He also understood the significance of voluntary health agencies and their contribution to public health.

Winslow felt that Yale offered a great opportunity to interest medical students in public health. As he told a professor in North Dakota in 1915, in New York there was a great need for physicians trained in public health.[9] Winslow focused his department on "the education of undergraduate medical students along the lines of preventive medicine."[10] This represented a change in focus for him. As a New York State Department of Health representative to the Rockefeller Foundation conference in 1914, he had favored concentration on training the rank and file of the public-health profession.[11]

The Department of Public Health also offered courses in Yale College. A cooperative plan developed in 1908 by the medical school and the Sheffield Scientific School devised a curriculum that would lead to a certificate in public health for individuals who had completed a bachelor's degree or had completed two years of medical study.[12]

The new Yale committee on courses in public health in the graduate school wished to offer a doctorate in public health and thought that the university had adequate resources to support the program.[13] It felt that a conference which included the outstanding public-health figures in the Northeast, such as Welch from Johns Hopkins, Winslow's mentor Sedgwick from MIT, and Milton Rosenau from Harvard, would give the program legitimacy.[14] Winslow had wanted to reimburse the attendees for their travel expenses, but President Hadley, wishing to save money in any way possible, turned down the suggestion. Attending the conference at their own expense, the distinguished experts unanimously agreed that a bachelor's degree was required for candidates to receive a certificate in public health, while the degree of doctor of public health would be granted to graduates in medicine after two years of further work.

Finances for graduate education at Yale were limited and jealously guarded. If Winslow had tried to develop a separate school of public health, "he would very likely not have been hired."[15] The Department of Public Health at Yale consisted of Winslow, one instructor, and two assistants, with a departmental budget of $8,000 a year. Winslow kept a tight hold on the Lauder bequest and refused to share it, despite ardent requests by President Hadley, who was under financial constraints and considered the medical school, including its public-health department, a drain on university resources. He resisted Hadley's suggestion that the Department of Bacteriology and the Department of Public Health be amalgamated with physiology and physiological chemistry for budgetary reasons, maintaining that departments without reserves should undergo reductions to balance the budget.[16]

The university wanted to treat Winslow like a clinician by recommending that he supplement his salary with his outside remuneration from the American Museum of Natural History and Columbia. Winslow responded to Blumer, "It seems most unfortunate to assume that professorial salaries are to be fixed on eleemosynary principles in proportion to need."[17] A week later, Winslow wrote to President Hadley on the same topic, realizing "the great sacrifice the university is making for the medical school as a whole" and offering to maintain his salary at the same level.[18]

Despite being unwilling to share his endowment, Winslow was able to co-opt other members of the medical-school faculty to teach in the public-health program. He felt that the real advantage of the Yale program was that sciences ancillary to public health were taught by men interested in them "primarily as fundamental disciplines rather than in their application to the administrative health field."[19] Winslow's main goal was to co-opt the medical student, because control of communicable diseases and the environment was becoming less important to health in the United States than early detection and prevention of disease, which required physician involvement. Unfortunately, according to his biographer, Arthur Viseltear, "Winslow found a subtle but real prejudice against public health even at Yale."[20] Prejudice is too strong a word. Medical students were simply too involved in the excitement of acute medicine to pay serious attention to chronic disease and prevention.

A reduction in hours allotted for public-health teaching in the medical school came as a major blow. "Driven" by Milton Winternitz, the Board of Permanent Officers concluded that the school's stuffed curriculum allowed no time for independent study, and it drastically reduced the number of classroom hours for all the courses, including public health. Winslow was surprised that he had not been given a chance to criticize the plan. (As a former dean, I am astonished that the curriculum committee was able to implement this reduction across the departments without a revolution, for every department chairman is convinced that his or her complete curriculum is absolutely necessary for the education of a physician!)

Blumer and Winternitz had a strong interest in preventive medicine and public health, and the reduction in hours was not directed specifically at Winslow and his department. Lectures were reduced in all the clinical courses, with the hours saved allotted to hospital wards and clinics. Unfortunately, extra time on clinical service did not benefit public health. Winslow stressed to Hadley that "the public health aspects of medicine are of immense and growing importance."[21] A compromise was reached, with ninety hours of formal classroom time allotted to public health as well as another ninety hours of elective time throughout the last three years.

Although he was not a physician, Winslow more than fulfilled the intentions of the Lauder bequest. He played a leading role in public-health reform in Connecticut, spearheading a successful campaign in 1917 that culminated in the creation of the Connecticut State Department of Public Health. Health surveys carried out by Winslow and his students led to significant improvements in the organization of public health in the state. He also played a major role on the national public-health scene as the first chairman of the Committee on Administrative Practice of the American Public Health Association, which defined the mission of official public-health agencies.[22]

Locally, Winslow was an active participant in the Board of Permanent Officers and a close friend of Winternitz, who became dean in 1920. Winternitz, like Blumer before him, had a keen interest in preventive medicine and public health, and he considered the dispensary to be the key to attracting students to preventive medicine. Winternitz and Winslow thought interest in preventive medicine would be increased by having the Department of Public Health conduct "health" clinics side by side with "disease" clinics in the dispensary. Winslow strongly supported Winternitz in the development of the Human Welfare Group that metamorphosed into the Institute of Human Relations in 1928. The concept of the institute fitted with Winslow's interest in wide collaboration among university departments. In a letter to President Angell he explained, "Public health . . . is really a social science since its uniquely characteristic problems are problems of social organization."[23]

Winslow was convinced of the need for public-health officers with medical training, rather than having sanitary engineers as public-health officers. He envisioned clinicians providing diagnostic, therapeutic, and preventive services in a health center or public-health department. The evening seminars held in Winslow's home were a memorable feature of the public-health program, bringing graduate students and faculty together.[24]

Despite Herculean efforts, Winslow was unable to convince Yale medical students to take up careers in public health, although he was very successful in training nonphysicians. He concluded that the reason medical students did not pursue careers in public health had more to do with how health services in the United States were financed and organized than with the medical-school curriculum. An organized national health program in which the public-health officer and individual physician would practice in a group funded by health insurance or the government was the solution to a preventive-medicine program. Having decided the health-care system was the problem, Winslow joined a group of health professionals who had formed a Committee on the Costs of Medical Care, and he became involved in medical economics and medical-care organizations.[25] The recommendations of the committee made almost no reference to the responsibilities of public-health departments but did sound a clarion call for medical care to be delivered through prepaid group-practice organizations, a concept that was anathema to organized medicine and was roundly attacked.[26] "We have, for example, been charged in supposedly serious scientific quarters of advocating socialism and communism and of 'inciting to revolution.'"[27]

The medical-school faculty was divided over the issue of "socialized medicine." Stanhope Bayne-Jones, who had replaced Winternitz as dean, was more conservative and not a strong proponent of the proposed changes in the medical system. Accusations were leveled that there was little liberalism in the school's attitude.[28] In rebuttal, Bayne-Jones cited the work of Winslow and Hiscock in public health. The opposition of organized medicine to socialized medicine was intense. Replying to a 1938 letter from Winslow that the fight for prepaid health care was almost won in a lawsuit by a federal-employee HMO in Washington, D.C., Thurman Arnold, then U.S. assistant attorney general, wrote, "The officials of the Medical Society have been in to see me, and their attitude is that there has never been such an outrage as this suit since the crucifixion of Jesus Christ."[29]

Winslow had difficulty appointing faculty in public health and felt that he was not receiving adequate support from President Angell. When he wanted to recruit Edgar Sydenstricker as Sterling Professor of Vital Statistics in 1927, Angell said that the Sterling professorship would not be viewed favorably by the corporation, but he would be glad to consider the matter when the endowment campaign was over.[30] Winslow persisted in a flurry of letters to Angell, but to no avail.

Although Winslow focused on issues of medical care, his broad interests covered the entire field of public health. He championed the concept of public-health nursing and from 1919 to 1923 served as chairman of the board of the New Haven Demonstration Health Center, which clearly established the effectiveness of public-health nursing. Along with Winternitz, he was an avid proponent of a school of nursing at Yale. Winslow was instrumental in establishing the Connecticut Department of Mental Health and supported Clifford Beers in the development of the Connecticut Mental Health Association, which was the pioneer mental-health association in the United States. In later years, he conducted important studies on human physiology and heat loss at the affiliated Pierce Laboratory in New Haven. In the best puritanical Yale tradition, Winslow congratulated Angell on stamping out vice in New Haven, commenting that the university ought to clean its own house and control "objectionable conduct due to intoxication in the Bowl."[31]

There is little wonder that the foreword to the reprinting of his 1923 book *The Evolution and Significance of the Modern Public Health Campaign* said that "Charles-Edward Amory Winslow was the leading theoretician of the American public health movement during the entire first half of the twentieth century." In addition to the brilliance of his vision, he was "gracious and humane," with a charismatic personality. Haven Emerson, a colleague who often disagreed with Winslow, noted that "his engaging and quizzical smile, critical and challenging, brought hope and assurance."[32]

Winslow, participating in a symposium entitled "The University and Public Health Statesmanship" in 1940, said, "The contribution of the university to the statesmanship of the future will depend on its will to educate as well as to train, on the vision with which it perceives new problems, on the courage with which it applies the tools of science and of scholarship to these problems. . . . The university can train health officers to do statistics, but it can educate those individuals only by widening their vision and stirring their imagination." He went on to discuss the issue that is becoming one of the great problems in medical care: our ability to delay death almost indefinitely without being able to prolong meaningful life. "'Health' is something much more than merely staying out of a coffin, it should mean vigor and fullness and efficiency and satisfaction in living."[33]

As World War II spread across Europe, Winslow addressed totalitarianism in the context of the university. The university had a responsibility to fulfill the functions of teaching and research, but it also had to correlate human knowledge into "a philosophy of human life and living." Science had produced the technology to wage unimaginable war but had ignored how it might be used. The university had to be sure to instill awareness of those uses. Despite his abhorrence of war, Winslow was not a pacifist. In 1935 he stated that "a good deal of the present-day pacifist propaganda seems to be thoroughly unsound and demoralizing."[34] He congratulated Yale's President Seymour for speaking out against the United States remaining neutral and evoked the passage in Dante's *Inferno* where individuals neither good nor bad would not be admitted into Heaven and their presence in Hell "would give the damned something to look down upon."[35]

In 1940 the public-health faculty consisted of Winslow, Ira Hiscock, one full-time statistical colleague, and a number of visiting lecturers. Winslow was sixty-three, with thin white hair, wrinkled face, and stooped shoulders, but he represented the epitome of the broad vision of public health, and his energy and ability to express himself remained undampened.[36] Francis Gilman Blake, chairman of the Department of Medicine and soon to be dean, was intent on "reorganizing" public health when Winslow retired. Blake had recruited John R. Paul (figure 36) in 1928 from the University of Pennsylvania, where he was director of the Ayer Clinical Laboratory. Paul's research in poliomyelitis and other infectious diseases, which he termed "clinical epidemiology," was flourishing at Yale, and he wanted to head a separate section of clinical epidemiology. He was being courted by the New York University School of Medicine to become the Herman Biggs Professor of Preventive Medicine and chair of the department. Blake thought Paul's section could be a "liaison between medicine and public health" and provide "more of the experimental method in Public Health."[37]

Dean Bayne-Jones had more pressing priorities with pharmacology than with preventive medicine, but there were no pharmacology candidates in the offing. Therefore, John Paul was recommended to the Board of Permanent Officers, supported by Winslow, who said the board "would be remiss if it did not make an attempt to retain Dr. Paul."[38] John Paul was appointed

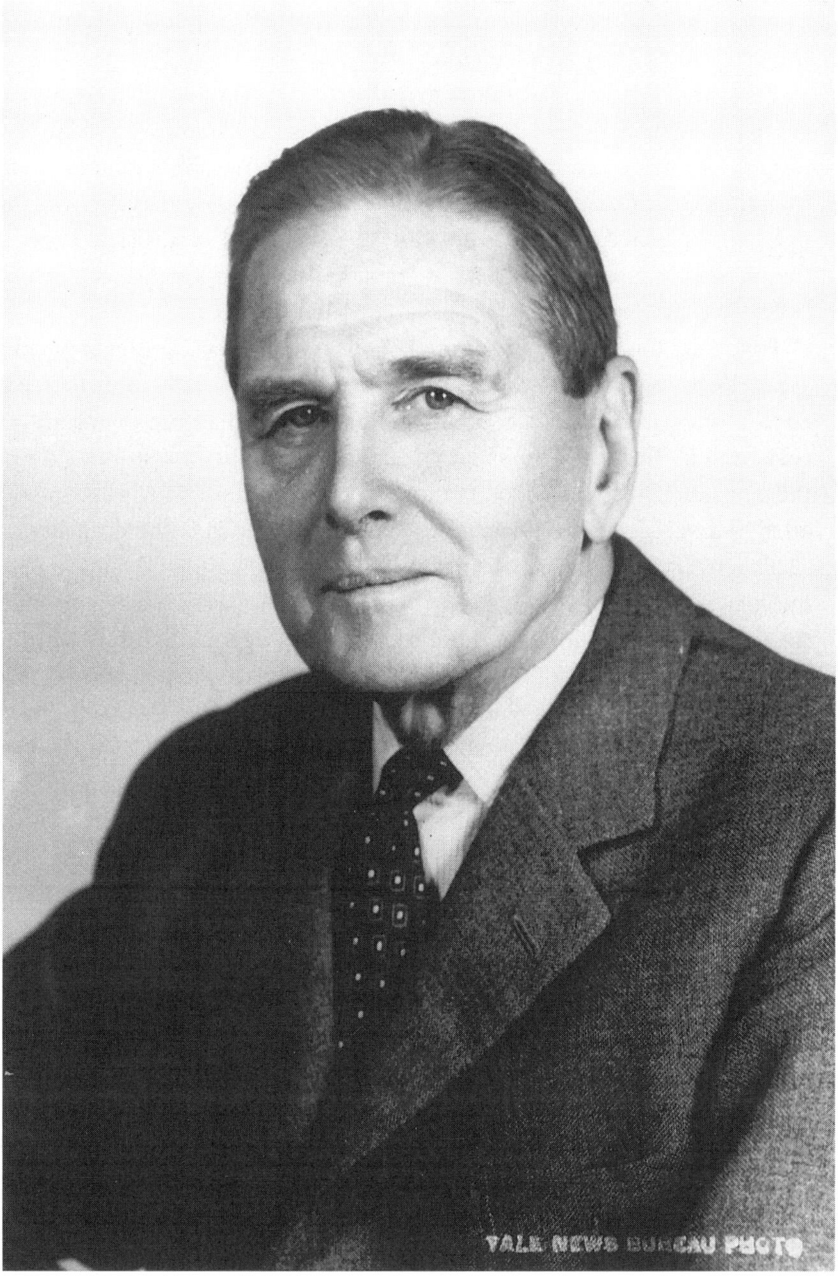

Figure 36. John R. Paul

as a professor of preventive medicine, rather than of public health, in the Department of Internal Medicine.

Paul and Winslow had fundamentally different philosophies about preventive medicine. According to Paul, Winslow's definition of public health used community action and the development of social machinery rather than the medical profession to reach its objectives. Although there was some overlap, a physician's talents did not lie in the field of social welfare. For the physician, disease registered as "positive" and the absence of disease as "negative," while in public health the opposite was true.[39]

Following the entry of the United States into the war, President Seymour asked Winslow to chair the search committee for a new dean to replace Bayne-Jones, who had left to join the war effort, as had John Paul, Ira Hiscock, and all the part-time faculty members in public health. Winslow and the committee recommended Francis Blake, who was serving as acting dean after Alan Gregg of the Rockefeller Foundation declined the deanship.

The inevitable clash between traditional public health and clinical epidemiology occurred in March 1944 at a BPO meeting, when Blake announced the formation of a medical-school committee to study the future of public health at Yale in view of Winslow's mandatory retirement in 1945.[40] Blake recommended that John Paul serve as chairman, and that Blake himself should serve on the committee as well. Winslow expressed regret that the committee was so narrowly focused on the medical-school aspects of public health, and he suggested that broader public-health aspects be examined also.[41] Winslow was invited to meet with the Educational Policy Committee of the Yale Corporation to discuss plans for the development of a university program in public health. As a result of the meeting, President Seymour formed a second committee, which would look at the broad issues of public health. Winslow told Seymour he was happy that "the University is approaching the matter on the broadest lines and with eyes open to all possibilities."[42]

Meanwhile, the medical-school committee chaired by John Paul had completed a draft that acknowledged the great debt the university owed to Winslow but recommended that the "social aspects of public health" Winslow had emphasized should be integrated into the clinical departments, "so that disease prevention, as well as health promotion could be developed simultaneously."[43] The medical-school committee recommended the formation of a university department of public health rather than a separate school or a medical-school department. The public-health faculty should teach preventive medicine as well as public health and social medicine. To upgrade the program, the master of public health degree would be awarded only to holders of B.N. or M.D. degrees.

President Seymour and the provost, Edgar Furniss, were disappointed with the school's report. Furniss considered its recommendations "too simple and obvious." Paul went back to the committee, which now included Winslow, with instructions from Furniss to "amplify" the report.[44] The university committee Seymour had appointed was chaired by Lowell Reed, dean of the School of Hygiene at Johns Hopkins. The members of Paul's medical-school committee thought this subsequent committee was advisory to it.[45] But Seymour emphasized that the university committee was to look at the "whole problem of the development of a Public Health program here."

Winslow commented on the medical-school committee's report in a four-page letter to John Paul.[46] He was particularly disturbed about the possibility of eliminating college graduates from training in public health. Lowell Reed used the questions raised by Winslow as the outline for discussion, which was incorporated into another revision of the medical-school committee's report.[47] John Paul presented the report at a meeting of the BPO, where Winslow commented that the report was "essentially the opinion of the Medical School."[48] The final report was distributed on October 20, 1944, and evoked interesting comments. John Peters, professor of medicine, who had been an outspoken champion of social medicine and the universal health program, which Winslow had promoted, seemed to come down on the side of the "experimental method" in public health.[49] The Committee on Program and Policy of the BPO concluded, "It seems essential to the Committee that real scientific research be developed in the department."[50] Even though Winternitz, a friend and colleague of Winslow's, was an important member of the BPO's committee, it dismissed Winslow's contributions. President Seymour told Blake that he was surprised at the verdict, as the negative comments had come from members of the committee who had produced the favorable report.[51]

Despite attempts by Blake to influence the selection, the corporation appointed Ira Hiscock chairman of public health—an unalloyed victory for Winslow. John Paul wanted to give public health a more clinical and scientific direction, while Winslow wanted an emphasis on administrative and social medicine. Paul, in his role as a clinician, was convinced he could bring the medical students back to his brand of public health, and he classified most schools of public health as "trade schools."[52] Public health had become less popular in the 1950s with the increasing excitement—and increasing funding—of laboratory research.[53] Coupled with the attractions of private practice, the result was fewer highly competent individuals embarking on public-health careers. Even the introduction of polio vaccine was seen as a triumph of medical research rather than as a public-health success.

The Department of Public Health did not thrive during the 1950s. Although a number of students came from abroad, enrollment was down. In all, 620 degrees in public health had been awarded by 1959. Medical students were not particularly interested in the public-health curriculum, and space was inadequate for working and teaching. In 1954, President Whitney Griswold received a long, unsolicited report about the hospital-administration course in public health from the Commission on University Education in Hospital Administration, funded by the W. K. Kellogg Foundation. The report lamented the absence of a business school at Yale, because hospital administration was basically a "form of business enterprise organized to achieve certain social goals."[54] The commission thought too much emphasis was placed on public-health issues at the expense of the business side of hospital administration. Griswold scrawled, "Pay no attention to this" in a note to his executive assistant, Catherine J. Tilson.

With the retirement of Ira Hiscock in 1960, and the impending retirement of John Paul, Griswold was forced to pay attention to public health. Dean Vernon Lippard chaired a committee, which included Gerald Klatskin, C. N. H. Long, Milton Senn, and Henry Treffers, to evaluate the program of study and research in the field of public health. The committee concluded that the public-health faculty was so busy with teaching and administrative responsibilities at local, state, and national public-health organizations that there was no time for significant research. Furthermore, the one-year program for a master's degree in public health was too short to go into subjects in any depth. The Section of Epidemiology and Preventive Medicine, on the other hand, had concentrated on research, particularly the epidemiology of viral diseases like polio. The committee recommended uniting the epidemiology section with public health rather than either continuing along the same traditional path or abandoning public health. "In public health, there has been increasing emphasis on organization and administration, official standards and duties, while medicine has become more scientific. Epidemiology provides an area of common interest."[55]

The corporation approved the proposal of the Board of Permanent Officers in 1959 to combine the Department of Public Health with the Section of Epidemiology and Preventive Medicine. The new department would concentrate its efforts on "education of personnel and research in causation and distribution of disease in large population groups."[56] The decision was not universally popular, particularly among members of the public-health faculty, and was viewed as downgrading the public-health component. Combining the two sections made space limitations a critical issue. A building for the new Department of Epidemiology and Public Health became a major priority—one of several critical priorities the medical school had at the time. When asked by the NIH to rank the school's building priorities, Lippard tergiversated: "It is not possible for me to give a simple meaningful answer to the question of absolute priority between the Public Health and the Biology facilities."[57] The bulk of the funding for the new Laboratory of Epidemiology and Public Health was secured from the Rockefeller Foundation and the Public Health Service. In January 1962 the Committee on Medical Affairs requested the University Council to recommend to the corporation that the university appropriate the remaining funds if they could not be found elsewhere.[58] Success in getting the new building was important, because if Yale could raise the funds, the Laboratory of Virus Diseases, which was the world's premier arbovirus research group, would move to Yale from the Rockefeller Institute.

While the search for the chairman of the new department was being conducted, Edward M. Cohart served as interim chairman, a position he would occupy repeatedly during the next several years. Perhaps because of the longstanding tensions between the Department of Public Health and the Section of Epidemiology and Preventive Medicine, the search committee decided to go outside the university and recruit someone who was in neither camp. It selected Anthony M. M. Payne, who came from the World Health Organization rather than from a traditional academic background. The search committee commented that the widespread interest in international health heightened the prospects of generous support, a vital issue for the new department. Payne was interested in revamping the department along international lines, which would be the "perfect complement" to the work of the Rockefeller group. Perhaps because of Payne's WHO connections—but attributed by Payne to John Paul's achievements—the department was designated by WHO as the World Serum Reference Bank, further building its international character.

At the same time the new department was formed, Dorothy M. Horstmann (figure 37), a member of the Section of Epidemiology and Public Health since 1942 and one of the pioneers in polio research and the first woman to achieve tenure in the medical school, was promoted to professor of epidemiology and pediatrics. John Paul had made the decision to concentrate on virology, perhaps to differentiate himself from Francis Blake, who

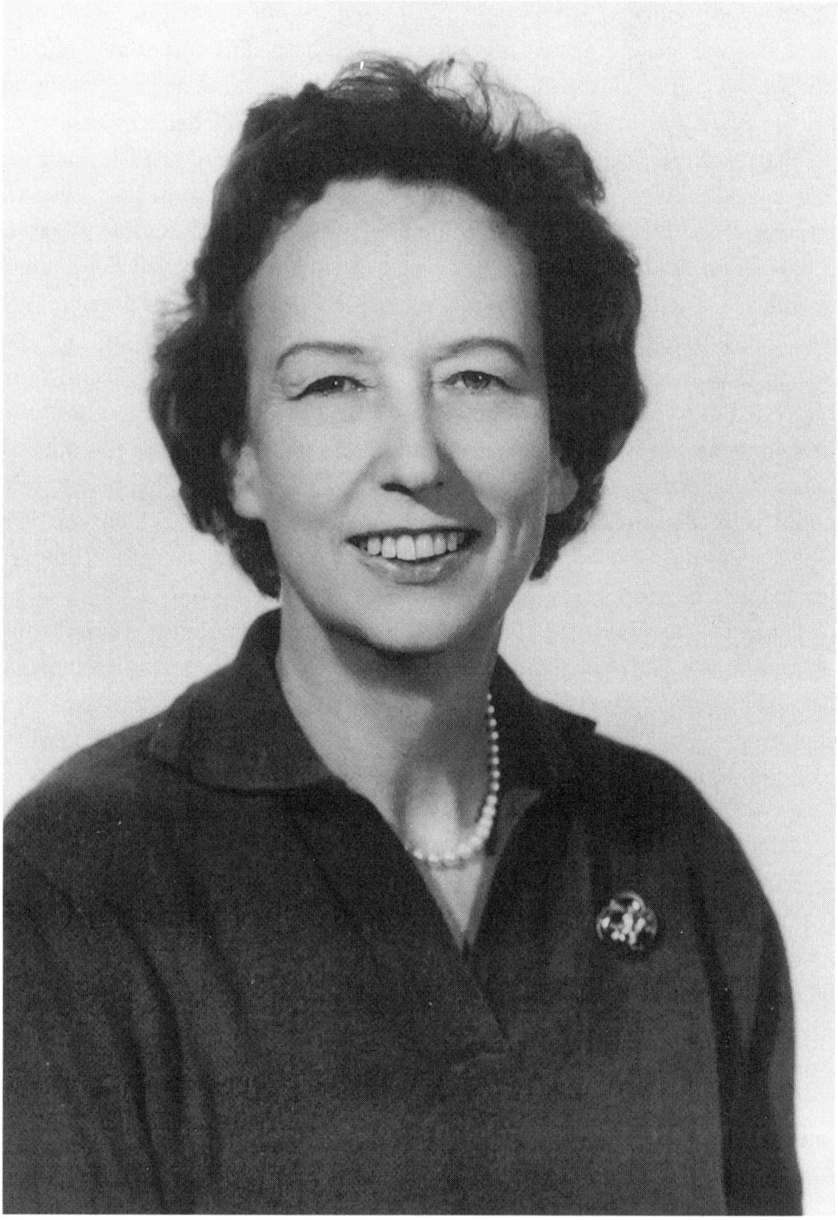

Figure 37. Dorothy Horstmann

was interested in bacterial disease. Paul had recruited Joseph Melnick, a biochemist who had received his Ph.D. at Yale in 1939 and after a fellowship in preventive medicine in 1941 had worked in virology. Melnick was a brilliant recruitment and opened up new areas in virology.

The new Laboratory of Epidemiology and Public Health, designed by Philip Johnson, was ready in 1964. The arbovirus group from the Rockefeller, now the Yale Arbovirus Research Unit, moved in first, followed by the Yale faculty. Unfortunately, financial constraints had resulted in space limitations. The new building was too small from the beginning, and the WHO serum reference bank had to be accommodated elsewhere. The two-year M.P.H. program was instituted, and the added year led to a significant drop in applications. The fourth-year course in public health for medical students was reorganized, with some success, under the direction of Roy M. Acheson, professor of epidemiology and medicine.

After six years as chairman, Anthony Payne was granted a two-year absence to take up the post of assistant director-general of the World Health Organization, never to return to Yale. He was appointed to create a new research division within WHO that would look at the social-science aspects of medicine in relation to disease—the source of bitter disagreement between Winslow and Paul. In the 1960s Richard Weinerman had introduced courses in social and community medicine that had touched on these areas. Having decided to remain in Geneva, Payne relinquished his chairmanship of epidemiology and public health, and Edward Cohart once more stepped into the breach as acting chairman.

The social unrest around the country was generating increased interest in health-care policy and health-care delivery. The nation's first fully qualified health-maintenance organization (HMO) was founded in New Haven as the Community Health Care Center Plan. Isidor S. Falk, a major figure in health economics and medical care, was brought in to develop the plan in 1961. Falk was also given a faculty appointment as professor of public health for medical care. Winslow had brought Falk, a sixteen-year-old high-school graduate, with him to Yale from New York to be a laboratory assistant, although technically he was listed as a janitor.[59] Falk eventually earned his Ph.D. in public health at Yale in 1923, working in bacteriology and immunology, and was recruited by the University of Chicago, where he was eventually promoted to professor. In 1929 he switched careers, joining the Committee on the Costs of Medical Care.[60] Falk entered federal-government service in 1936, ultimately serving as director of the Bureau of Research and Statistics of the Social Security Administration, where he played a major role in formulating government strategy on national health insurance. In the emerging Cold War, he became the object of scathing attacks by the extreme right as a symbol of socialized medicine.

John Thompson also played an important role in the field of health-care delivery. Trained as a nurse, he received an M.P.H. from Yale and was appointed research associate. He subsequently became director of the program in hospital administration. Thompson was one of the very few individuals at Yale to become a professor without an M.D. or Ph.D.

When Payne decided to remain in Geneva and Cohart again served as interim chairman, the effect on the department of the search for a new chairman was "uncertainty and also, undoubtedly, some anxiety."[61] The choice fell on an outsider, Adrian Ostfeld, who was appointed chairman on September 1, 1968. He was immediately faced with funding difficulties. During this period, the Pierce Foundation and the Department of Epidemiology and Public Health joined to offer a course in environmental physiology. Ominously, however, there were cutbacks in Public Health Service funding of research and training programs, which a department with few reserves could ill afford. Things became even worse when, six months after becoming chairman, Ostfeld was forced to resign because of illness. Robert McCollum, who had trained with John Paul and had joined the department after a year at the London School of Tropical Hygiene, replaced him as chairman. One of the problems McCollum faced was proliferation of programs within the department. There were seventeen identifiable subspecialty areas under the umbrella of the M.P.H. degree, which McCollum reorganized into four divisions, each with a director, in biometry, public-health practice, environmental-health sciences, and epidemiology.

The Rockefeller Foundation, which had been supporting the Yale Arbovirus Research Unit under the chairmanship of Wilbur Downs, announced that the appointments of Rockefeller staff members assigned to the Yale unit would be terminated on December 31, 1972; eventually a compromise was reached that extended the fiscal life of the unit for two more years. Downs had started his career as a syphilologist in the preantibiotic era and became intrigued with the mosquitoes used to induce malaria for the fever treatment of cerebral syphilis. The very high fever would kill the malaria parasites, which could not withstand the high temperatures, before killing the patient. Downs went on to become interested in the viral diseases carried by the mosquitoes and founded the arbovirus group at Rockefeller.

In a department heavily dependent on federal support, decreases in government funding led to a large departmental deficit and raised persistent issues about medical-school responsibility for the Department of Epidemiology and Public Health. The loss of federal support of training grants also bred uncertainty about enrollment.

A new medical-school dean, Robert Berliner, was about to arrive, and he would have to deal with two schools. A still unsolved problem is that the Department of Epidemiology and Public Health functions both as a department of the medical school and as an accredited school of public health. The dual role has some definite advantages but also creates problems that are not easily resolved. Some independence has been afforded by naming its chairman the dean of public health within the School of Medicine. Even though there are advantages to integrating the health of the individual and the health of the public, a separate school of public health is probably inevitable.

13

THE STATE HOSPITAL

Dating back to the nineteenth century, the relationship between the medical school and the hospital has been one of mutual, although frequently strained, interdependence. Access to patients would be crucial to the success of the new Medical Institution of Yale College, "because theory without practice in this, as well as everything else, is comparatively of little use."[1] Of the ten incorporators who proposed the State Hospital in 1826, eight were physicians, including four professors at the Medical Institution: Nathan Smith, Eli Ives, Jonathan Knight, and Thomas Hubbard. The fifth Yale representative, Benjamin Silliman, had received an honorary M.D. degree from the Connecticut Medical Society but was not a physician. The solitary layperson, William Leffingwell, became the first president of the General Hospital Society of Connecticut. The New Haven Medical Association formed a hospital committee, which resolved that "the hospital shall be a charitable institution and no physician or surgeon shall receive any compensation for his services."[2]

New Haven in the 1820s was a town of fewer than ten thousand inhabitants, who had little desire (or wealth) to support a hospital. Hospitals did not play a part in most people's lives, as patients remained at home with their illnesses. We recall that the incorporators had applied unsuccessfully to the Connecticut Legislature for funds to found the hospital, and they turned to the U.S. Treasury. Under federal law, sailors were required to pay part of their wages into a fund that entitled them to free hospitalization when sick or injured. New Haven, though small, had an excellent harbor, visited by sailing vessels engaged in active trade with the West Indies. The hospital incorporators appealed to the treasury to use taxes collected for the care of seamen in New Haven to found a marine hospital, but this request was also rejected. A Mr. Swan was hired as a fund-raiser and toured Fairfield County for sixty-eight days, but he met either "systematic opposition or disgusting indifference."[3] With a determination characteristic of the Yale medical faculty, the incorporators again approached the state legislature, indicating what funds were available.

To demonstrate their sincerity and commitment, Smith, Knight, Hubbard, and Ives promised 10 percent of their annual income, or a minimum of $100 a year, to the hospital for the next five years. The incorporators still lacked $5,000, which the legislature duly supplied, and on May 26, 1826, an act was passed to incorporate the General Hospital Society of Connecticut. The State Hospital would be the fourth voluntary general hospital in the United States after Pennsylvania Hospital, New York Hospital, and Massachusetts General Hospital.[4] The hospital was to be a charitable institution, with preference given to Connecticut residents. In addition to the directors, there were to be six "visitors," two of whom would visit the hospital periodically to "enquire into the economical and moral concerns of the Hospital, suggest improvements and designate abuses."[5] Sufficient funds were raised to purchase seven and a half acres of land between Cedar Street and Howard Avenue and erect a hospital, designed by Ithiel Town, that could accommodate seventy-five patients.

Because of the cholera epidemic that broke out in New Haven in 1833 just as the hospital was opening, the Board of Health wanted the new hospital to treat cholera patients. But the hospital directors claimed that their charter forbade admission of patients with communicable diseases. This was not strictly true; the charter merely gave the directors the right to exclude patients "who are not proper subjects for Hospital privileges." The refusal angered New Haveners and slowed popular acceptance of the hospital. With so few patients occupying beds in the early years, the hospital rented out rooms as living quarters. When the number of patients increased, the rooms were needed for them. Dr. James Gates Percival, a Yale graduate and a poet, had occupied his hospital quarters for eight years and was unwilling to leave. A hospital committee was appointed to evict him, as well as a Miss Bunnell.

During the Civil War, it was proposed to the surgeon general that the hospital provide medical care for soldiers at $3.50 per week per soldier. In 1862 the hospital was leased to the government. It was turned into a 1,500-bed military hospital and renamed the Knight Hospital. Jonathan Knight, the professor of surgery, was still active clinically when the first contingent of 260 soldiers arrived in 1862 from the battle at Fair Oaks, Virginia. During the summer of 1864, so many casualties arrived that tents had to be erected on the hospital grounds.[6]

During the three-year existence of the Knight Hospital from 1862 to 1865, some 25,340 soldiers were hospitalized, with a mortality rate of less than 1 percent. Patients had frequently spent four weeks in transfer from the battlefield, which contributed significantly to the low hospital mortality rate. The hospital was staffed with a number of contract surgeons. Among them was William C. Minor, an 1863 graduate of the medical school, who published a series of postmortem examinations.[7] He subsequently killed a man in England and was incarcerated for the rest of his life in the Broadmoor Criminal Lunatic Asylum. He became one of the most prolific contributors to the *Oxford English Dictionary* and was lauded by its editor, James Murray.[8]

During the military occupation of the hospital, civilian patients were cared for in temporary quarters on Whalley Avenue. When the Knight Hospital reverted to civilian status in 1865, the number of beds was inadequate to handle the influx of patients. East and west wings were added with funds derived in part from forcing the federal government to pay accrued rent on the remaining lease.[9] The newly enlarged hospital opened in 1873 and was able to accommodate 525 patients during the year as well as a new Connecticut Training School for Nurses (figure 38). The name of the State Hospital was officially changed to the New Haven Hospital in 1884, but the medical staff of the hospital continued to serve in an entirely voluntary capacity.

Hospitalization during this period in history could not have been an entirely unpleasant experience. During 1877, thirty-one gallons of sherry, whiskey, brandy, and other spirits were consumed in the hospital, along with

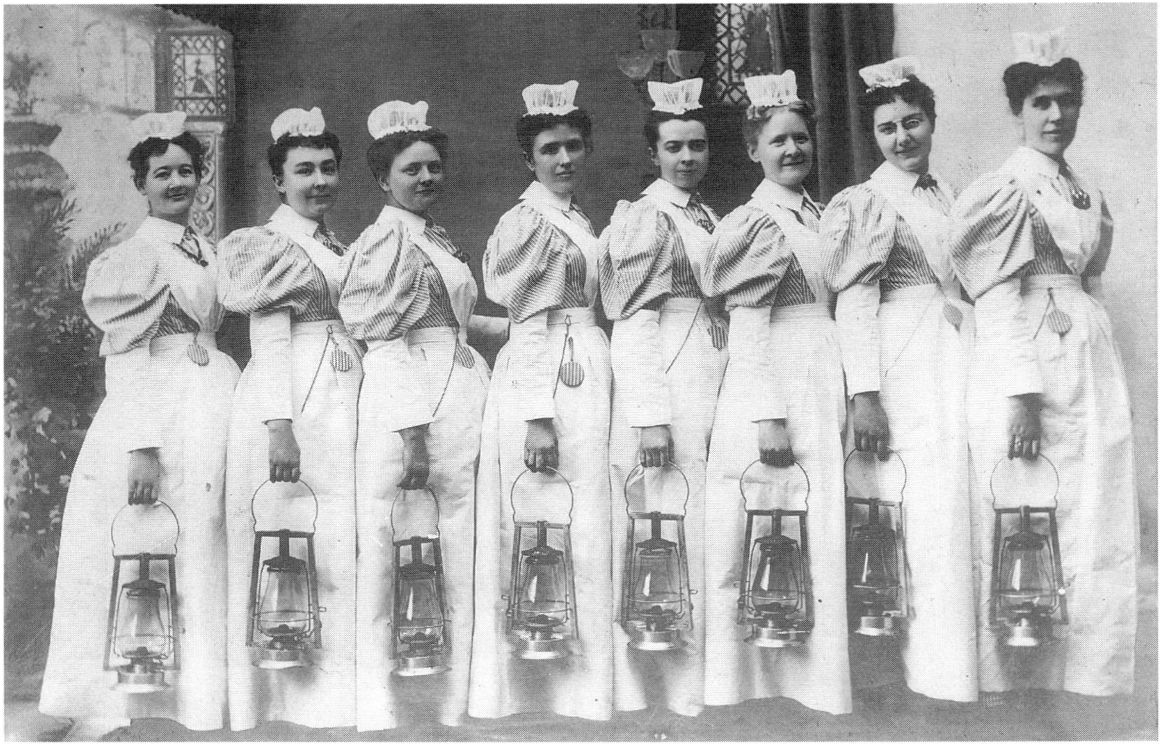

Figure 38. Connecticut Training School for Nurses: Class of 1899

251 barrels of ale. If all this alcohol was divided only among 525 patients, the intake of alcoholic beverages must have been astounding! The following year, William Carmalt, the professor of surgery (figure 39), called attention to the "loose way" beer was given out, especially to the young patients.[10]

The Farnam Operating Amphitheater was built in 1888 with a gift from Mrs. Henry Farnam in memory of her son, George Bronson Farnam. The original operating room had been located in the hospital attic; it was poorly lit, cramped for space, and had minimal washing facilities.[11] The Farnam amphitheater, in contrast, had washrooms and dressing rooms for the surgeons, sterilizing apparatus, and conveniently located etherizing rooms. Banks of seats for students could be accessed without entering the operating theater.

A chronic-disease ward, the Ellen M. Gifford Home for the Incurables, was built over a three-year period beginning in 1889, along with the Gifford Chapel. Simeon E. Baldwin, executor of Ellen Gifford's estate, was responsible for the bequest. He was a long-serving hospital director, twice governor of Connecticut, and former president of the American Bar Association. Both the chapel and the ward were later subsumed by the constantly changing architecture of the hospital; only a small plaque was left as a memorial.

In 1892 a mild case of smallpox went unrecognized in a hospitalized sailor until the patient in the next bed developed the classic symptoms of the disease. Thirteen people, including one member of the house staff and two nurses, developed smallpox, resulting in three deaths. The hospital and its grounds were quarantined for a month, and an emergency hospital was established on Orange Street with a house staff recruited from the fourth-year medical-school class. The Spanish-American War in 1898 brought the arrival of 202 military patients from Connecticut and Long Island. Half of these patients had typhoid fever, and fourteen died. The isolation pavilions, a ward, several tents, and the Gifford Chapel were all used for their care.[12]

The New Haven County Anti-Tuberculosis Association was incorporated in 1902, reflecting a major public-health problem. Among the association's founders were several individuals active within the hospital and the university, including Henry W. Farnam, Irving Fisher, Francis Bacon, and Henry Swain. In 1903, the association bought farmland in Wallingford from the Gaylord family for a nominal price in order to establish a nonprofit sanatorium for the treatment of tuberculosis that was "susceptible to amelioration."[13] Gaylord Sanatorium, now a rehabilitation hospital, opened in 1904. It could accommodate twenty-two patients, and it attracted patients from all over Connecticut, including the playwright Eugene O'Neill, who was ad-

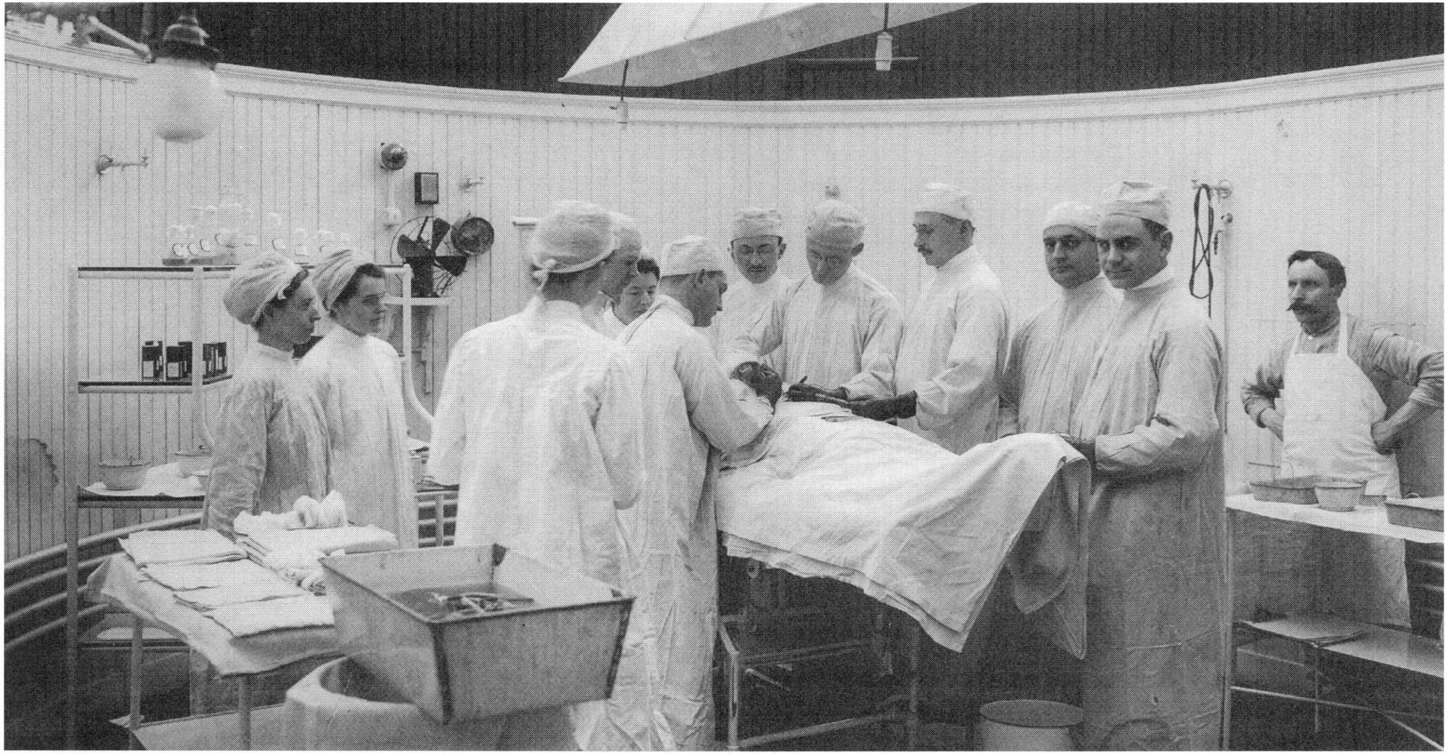

Figure 39. William Carmalt (*center*) in the Farnam Operating Amphitheater

mitted in 1912 and stayed for several months. Gaylord Hospital is no longer a sanatorium, but it has continued to have an important relation with the medical school.

Advanced cases of tuberculosis not "susceptible to amelioration" were admitted to the New Haven Hospital. There was a great demand for a proper place to treat advanced tuberculosis. The open wards of a general hospital were unsuitable because of the danger of the disease spreading, so the TB patients were housed in a tent on the hospital grounds.[14] In 1905 Eli Whitney, president of the hospital, received an anonymous gift of $300,000 to establish a hospital for the care of patients with tuberculosis. The William Wirt Winchester Hospital was built in West Haven on the future site of the Veterans Administration Hospital, with plans for a hundred beds for patients in the advanced stages of tuberculosis. Before the buildings were completed, World War I broke out, and the government leased the buildings for the treatment of tuberculous soldiers. Mrs. Winchester, the anonymous donor, died in 1922, having given more than $3 million, which has grown into a fund worth $30 million for research on and treatment of respiratory disease.

As medical treatment in general improved, more and more patients were being hospitalized rather than remaining at home. In 1905 the Prudential Committee recommended expanding the number of beds once again.[15] This need for more beds at the New Haven Hospital was occurring despite the opening of hospitals in Waterbury, Meriden, and Bridgeport, as well as the establishment of the Grace Hospital and, in 1907, the Hospital of Saint Raphael.

Some small private hospitals also sprang up in New Haven. Dr. Skinner's Sanatorium opened in 1912 with fifteen beds: six private beds, six female-ward beds, and three male-ward beds. Clarence Skinner's aim was to provide a "home-like atmosphere," the best nursing care, and good food, and to render every possible assistance to the physician. In the first four months of operation of his hospital, twenty-five physicians admitted 103 patients. Fifty-two surgical procedures were performed, with no postoperative mortality.[16]

The acutely ill still went to the New Haven Hospital in emergencies, and there was a need for better horse-drawn ambulance service (figure 40), which required placing a phone call to the livery stable where the ambulance was housed. The line was often busy or the horses were not available. The Prudential Committee concluded, "We need a stable of our own with a quick-hitch arrangement."[17] In response, Frederick P. Brewster, a wealthy carriage

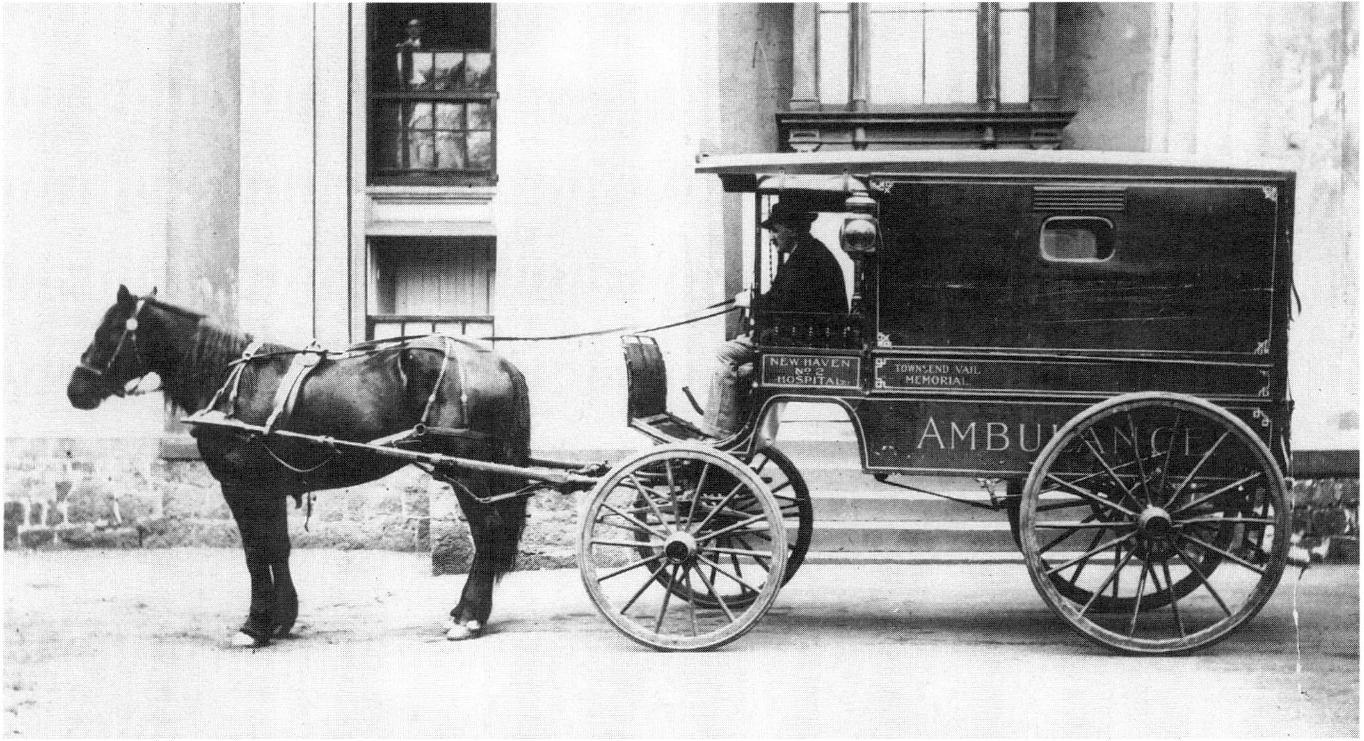

Figure 40. Horse-drawn ambulance

manufacturer, provided funds for a brick stable accommodating three ambulances and a truck as well as two horses.

During the last twenty years of the nineteenth century, the hospital directors and medical staff were indifferent or antagonistic toward the use of the hospital for medical education, even though the hospital had been founded in part for that purpose. Despite the indifference, the medical faculty, convinced that the medical school had to be closely affiliated with the hospital, recommended that the university purchase land opposite the hospital on Cedar Street for educational facilities.

The New Haven Dispensary, founded in 1872 and located on the grounds of the medical school on York Street after 1879, was still the main source of patients for teaching medical students. In 1901 the dispensary moved to the corner of Congress Avenue and Cedar Street into what is now the Hope Building, named in memory of Jane Ellen Hope, wife of Oliver Fisher Winchester. The agreement, which gave the university control, set the stage for the administrative unification of the dispensary with both the hospital and the Connecticut Training School for Nurses.[18]

In 1906, with the impending retirement of William Carmalt, a new professor of surgery was needed. We recall that President Arthur Hadley wrote several letters in an unsuccessful attempt to recruit the neurosurgeon Harvey Cushing. Although Hadley had been concerned that the clinical enterprise in New Haven was too small to compete with New York and Boston, Cushing did not think this made much difference. The major obstacle deterring Cushing from accepting a position at Yale was the fact that the university had charge of the wards for only three months, "a condition almost unheard of in other civilized countries."[19] After intense efforts by Carmalt, President Hadley, and Secretary Stokes, the university concluded an agreement with the hospital that gave the professor of surgery control over one-quarter of the surgical service and the professor of medicine control over one-sixth of the medical service, for the entire year. The university would pay the hospital to engage a pathologist. Even so, Cushing decided not to return to his alma mater.

There would soon be another hospital in New Haven. In 1907, a group of the town's physicians led by William F. Verdi raised a million dollars and founded the Hospital of Saint Raphael. Verdi was an unusual and accomplished individual. Born in Naples, he had come to the United States as an infant. He became the first native Italian to graduate from Hillhouse High School in New Haven, and with the encouragement of the principal went on to study at the Yale School of Medicine, where he received his M.D. in

1894. Verdi studied with Virchow in Germany during the following year and began to practice in New Haven in 1895. He was first listed as attending surgeon at the New Haven Hospital in 1907.[20] His appointment to the hospital staff resulted in a bigger headline in a New Haven paper than the appointment of Joseph Marshall Flint as Carmalt's successor.

Verdi was a consummate surgeon, and prior to his staff position he would join Carmalt in the operating room on Saturdays during Yale football games, when other surgical staff members were occupied elsewhere, to operate on difficult cases.[21] It is not clear whether Verdi founded Saint Raphael's in order to have more operating time or because he lacked hospital privileges at the New Haven Hospital and had to be spirited into the surgical suite.

Abraham Flexner's report to the Carnegie Foundation in 1910 describing the condition of medical schools in the United States and Canada was also an instrument of change for the New Haven Hospital.[22] Flexner had recommended Yale and Harvard as the only two medical schools in New England capable of being first-class schools. Swayed by Flexner's report, the Yale Corporation made a commitment to support the medical school, and a committee of the hospital board was appointed to look at future relations with the school in view of the report.[23] George Blumer, who was a board member and dean of the medical school at the time, wrote a report entitled "The Relation of the Medical School to the Hospital," which outlined the way the two entities should interrelate. Blumer's model has prevailed, with a series of hospital divisions, each under a chief responsible for patient care and divisional policy. Blumer hoped that a fine teaching hospital would result. "Would it be possible to alter the character of the New Haven Hospital to that of an institution ultimately to be of the teaching type without serious friction? With the understanding that none of the present incumbents on the medical staff should be displaced against their will and none of their privileges curtailed, we believe that the hospital could be so reorganized and greatly to the patients' benefit."[24]

Although the Yale administration had discussed building a separate university hospital, funding was scarce and there were already several hospitals in New Haven. So in January 1912, a unanimous committee recommendation was made to the General Hospital Society "that closer relations be established between the Yale Medical School and the New Haven Hospital."[25] Blumer commented to Stokes that the only real criticism of the plan was that some patients would refuse to enter a teaching hospital.

The hospital board accepted the recommendation that the medical school be allowed to nominate the attending physicians and surgeons and to use the wards for teaching. In return, the university agreed to build a clinical and pathological laboratory and to establish an endowment for maintaining it, a total cost of $600,000.[26] The agreement between the hospital and the Yale Corporation would expire if the money was not in place by July 1, 1914—little more than a year away.

The hospital agreement did nothing to remove the Corporation's concern that the medical school might become a permanent drain on university funds. Support came from the Rockefeller Foundation, which was crucial to the success of raising all the necessary money. The full-time clinical program, which was the condition of Rockefeller support, heightened community physicians' anxiety that they might be excluded from the hospital staff.

The clinical faculty now had academic control of the hospital but was unhappy with the way it was managed. Winford Smith, superintendent of the Johns Hopkins Hospital, was asked to review the hospital in 1918. His conclusion: "The New Haven hospital at the present time, judged by modern standards is a poor hospital."[27] Smith considered the organization and administration of the hospital to be weak, and the wards poorly equipped and poorly designed. His recommendations included the formation of an Executive Committee, with university representation but without physicians, and the formation of a separate Medical Board.[28] The full-time faculty members were to have complete control of the public wards, and the "mediocre" house staff was to be replaced with a formal resident training program. The Training School for Nurses should become a department of the university.

The new arrangement, in which the Medical Board reported to the Executive Committee of the hospital's board, caused problems. "Blumer warned that "the assumption of arbitrary powers by the laymen with lack of consideration for the opinion of the Medical Board and want of sympathy with the teacher can only result in loss of efficiency and impaired morale."[29] He also said that faculty members were concerned that they had no assurances their annual hospital appointments would be renewed. Still, the Medical Board was not in favor of building a separate hospital. It felt that the Yale Corporation and the directors of the New Haven Hospital had to operate the school and the hospital as a single institution.

Both Blumer and Dean Winternitz after him considered an excellent nursing program vital to the success of the hospital and believed that the university should sponsor a school of nursing. Although the shortage of nurses was clearly a motive, there was dissatisfaction with the level of nursing care. In May 1918 the Yale Corporation approved the plan for the proposed school, provided the university would be relieved of all financial obligation.

In 1923, the fiftieth anniversary of the Connecticut Training School for Nurses, its successor, the Yale School of Nursing, opened its doors, with Annie Goodrich as founding dean.

Community physicians had relinquished control of the wards unwillingly and, in retaliation, were referring their patients to Saint Raphael's. The hospital became a target of an informal boycott. The average daily census fell from 210 in 1919 to 186 in 1920, although part of the decrease reflected the large number of influenza patients hospitalized in previous years. During the three-year period of the influenza epidemic between 1918 and 1921, the hospital admitted 1,451 cases of influenza, with 388 deaths, a mortality rate of 27 percent.

The decrease in the number of patients was sufficient to push the hospital toward bankruptcy. During the twenty-year period from 1876 to 1896, the hospital had been self-supporting. The weekly cost of a patient in 1880 was $6.55, and the ward rate charged to patients was $7.00 a week.[30] The Connecticut Training School for Nurses was not an expense, because after a year's training, the nurses agreed to work at private nursing for five months and turn their earnings over to the hospital! But the operating deficit kept mounting in concert with the rising weekly patient cost. By 1918, the weekly cost per patient had risen to $18.00, yet the ward rate was only $10.50 a week. The large number of "free beds," which had increased from three in 1876 to thirty-six in 1916, was also a factor. A gift of $5,000 would allow a donor to nominate a patient to a free bed in perpetuity, but the income from the gift did not cover the cost of the patient. The hospital's financial plight, aggravated by wartime inflation, was being met by dipping into endowment funds.

Concerned about the future of the hospital in view of these financial problems, Anson Phelps Stokes, the university secretary, raised the question of the university assuming control of the hospital. The university counsel saw danger in trying to introduce legislation that would give the public the impression of a university takeover (which would be the case). The medical faculty was in favor of the university assuming control of the hospital, but Dean Blumer thought the appointment of a hospital superintendent sympathetic to the university would improve the situation more than university control of the hospital would.[31] A committee of the Board of Permanent Officers eventually proposed "a change whereby complete responsibility is taken over by the Corporation of the University, so that the New Haven Hospital becomes a part of the University."[32]

At a meeting of the hospital board on January 17, 1919, the financial crisis came to a head with the announcement that the general fund was exhausted and that there was an unfunded debt of $60,000. Current operations of the hospital were being financed by the Union and New Haven Trust Company. The hospital's board voted on May 7, 1920, to hold a special meeting to consider what action to take if financial conditions made it impossible to continue operating the hospital under the existing contract with the university.[33] No meeting was held, and the situation remained serious. The treasurer of the university, George Parmly Day, pleaded with the General Education Board of the Rockefeller Foundation for assistance. Unless relief for the hospital could be found in the near future, said Day, "a serious curtailment, possibly an entire breakdown may occur in the clinical opportunities of the school."[34]

As we saw earlier, the General Education Board fortunately obliged and appropriated $1 million to ease the immediate financial crisis, provided Yale raised a further $2 million. The board could not support the hospital directly, because its mandate was medical education.[35] But it did allow $50,000 a year of the interest on its gift to the university to be used by the hospital for education.[36] The funds made possible extra house officers and nurses, ten to fifteen free beds, and utilities and animal care at Brady Laboratory.

Bonds were issued for $1 million, of which the university took half, and $233,000 was raised in a fund drive chaired by Colonel Isaac M. Ullman, whom we have already encountered as president of the hospital's board. Although the acute problem had ended, financial problems persisted during the "roaring twenties." In 1926, William Carmalt, emeritus professor of surgery, lamented, "It is practically impossible for a hospital which is up to date in its medical and surgical services to meet its operating expenses out of its operating revenue."[37]

When Milton Winternitz, who was professor of pathology, succeeded George Blumer as dean in 1920, he ushered in an era of unprecedented progress for the medical school. The scathing review of the hospital by Winford Smith had resulted in the arrival of Willard C. Rappeleye as the new superintendent of the New Haven Hospital in 1922—an appointment that was met with great enthusiasm by the medical school. Rappeleye was recruited for the hospital by George Vincent of the Rockefeller Foundation, who had been impressed by his role as executive secretary of the commission appointed by Rockefeller to investigate the training of hospital administrators. Vincent wrote that Rappeleye would be interested in the New Haven job provided "the hospital trustees are looking for someone who would have an opportunity to participate actively in the development of a University teaching hospital. He would rather not assume the rather conventional and restricted duties which heretofore have been regarded as the functions of a hospital superintendent."[38] The university created a term appointment in hospital administration for Rappeleye, who became a member of the Board of Permanent Officers.

Rappeleye, a well-trained physician, had been responsible for reorganizing the University of California hospitals. His appointment as professor of hospital administration and his broad experience with university hospitals boded well for future relations between hospital and medical school. Finding the hospital finances in a precarious state, Rappeleye calculated the costs of operating a teaching facility and sent Winternitz a bill for hospital expenses attributable to education. Rappeleye told President Angell that the full-time men were not doing enough surgery to maintain their surgical competence and should expand their clinical practice. Community physicians were doing more surgery elsewhere, with fewer referrals to the hospital.[39]

This was not the type of behavior that Winternitz had expected from his new faculty colleague. Their dispute was ultimately referred for arbitration to Angell, who in turn sought the help of Abraham Flexner. Flexner replied that teaching hospitals do cost more, but the difference is really between a good and a poor hospital rather than between a teaching and a nonteaching hospital.[40] Armed with this advice, the university refused to pay the indirect costs suggested by Rappeleye, who soon resigned. Winternitz mentioned the "important loss" in his annual report and stated that Rappeleye had left to become chairman of the Commission on Medical Education.[41] Rappeleye subsequently became dean of the College of Physicians and Surgeons at Columbia at the age of thirty-nine, a position he held for twenty-nine years.

The medical school had won the battle, but the hospital's financial problems had not been solved. Henry Farnam, president of the hospital, invited Angell to dinner at the Taft Hotel to discuss hospital finances. "We should be prepared to remain all evening—can I count on your presence?"[42] Worsening the financial situation was the fact that the hospital had lost part of its subsidy from the state. With the realization that the medical school needed a viable New Haven Hospital to carry out its educational mission, the university promised a subsidy of $25,000 for two years, representing indirect costs for medical education. Little did anyone realize that the university would continue to subsidize the hospital until 1952! After the brush with bankruptcy, the operating budget of the hospital increased over the next ten years, from approximately $200,000 a year to $775,000 a year, and the hospital's endowment rose from $2.5 million to $3.9 million.

The affiliation between the hospital and Yale's medical school had caused a number of community physicians to join the staff of the Grace Hospital, resulting in a loss of clinical material for the medical school as well as financial difficulties for the New Haven Hospital. The Grace Hospital had been founded in 1889 by a group of physicians from the Homeopathic Medical Society of Connecticut who were unable to obtain privileges at the New Haven Hospital. Homeopathy was becoming popular at the time as a form of medical practice but was totally rejected by "allopathic" physicians, who controlled the hospital.

By 1925 the Grace Hospital, too, was having major financial difficulties. Its Board of Directors approached the New Haven Hospital in 1926 about a merger. Winternitz discussed the possibility with Abraham Flexner, who agreed that a merger would provide the medical school with needed clinical strength.[43] In a Yale memorandum prepared to obtain financial support for the merger from the Rockefeller Foundation, the Grace Hospital was said to be "favored with the sentiment" of the community while the New Haven Hospital had its confidence.[44] In June 1927 the Connecticut General Assembly passed the act "Authorizing Grace Hospital Society and the General Hospital Society of Connecticut to Unite and Merge."

The Grace medical staff, particularly physicians who had earlier left the New Haven Hospital staff in protest, were violently opposed to the union.[45] Dr. Burdett Adams said in the *New Haven Journal-Courier,* that "the merger would mean that the city has lost another institution to Yale University."[46] Under pressure, the entire Board of Directors at the Grace Hospital resigned, and the twenty new directors rescinded the intention to merge. Union was inevitable, but it would not happen until 1945. New Haven was not large enough to support three hospitals.

The collapse of the merger heightened the need to ensure sufficient patients for teaching. A possible solution was to offer complete medical and hospital services to university faculty and staff and to employees of the telephone company and other commercial organizations. Health coverage would be provided to 4,500 subscribers and their families, a total of some ten thousand individuals.[47] Subscribers would be protected against additional outlay for health problems, and the hospital and medical school would be guaranteed adequate clinical material. The board of the health-insurance organization would include representatives of the university, hospital, medical staff, community, and Metropolitan Life Insurance Company.

The Medical Board of the hospital, composed of the clinical chairmen, adamantly proclaimed that the medical services of the faculty were not for sale. The university's professional staff had been employed on the basis of education and research.[48] Patients cared for by the university staff should be available for teaching, and the physicians should be well compensated. There is no evidence in the minutes of the Yale Corporation that the health plan was ever considered formally. The New Haven Hospital, Saint Raphael's, and the Grace Hospital did cosponsor a hospital-insurance program, however. Families would be insured for twenty-one days of hospitalization at a cost of $1.50 per month.

In addition to the need to ensure an adequate supply of patients for medical-student teaching, there was the growing realization that the house staff of the New Haven Hospital should be thought of in educational terms. Samuel Clark Harvey, the chairman of surgery, noted that the time had come "when this graduate school in clinical medicine should be studied as a function of the school and hospital." The resident system had been initiated at Yale in 1916 by the professor of surgery, Joseph Marshall Flint, and was based on the Johns Hopkins model. The program had grown "without formal recognition as an educational enterprise of the School and Hospital and yet one of the greatest importance."[49]

Educational changes of course affected the hospital and dispensary and decreases in the hospital budget had an impact on the educational process of the medical school. The university was providing the hospital with $100,000 a year in financial support, which it could ill afford to do. Especially after the onset of the Depression, the university was under financial strain. Total university support for the medical school and hospital was $400,000, which meant that the medical school actually represented a bigger financial problem than the hospital. State and city appropriations for the hospital had increased only slightly over the years, and the mayor of New Haven, John W. Murphy, was using the city's financial contribution to the dispensary—which "the public regards as a Yale Institution"—as a bargaining chip to force the university to provide financial support to the city.[50] A request for an increase in the appropriation for the dispensary was turned down. "I do not think the city is in debt to Yale, for we are rendering a number of services to the university for which we get no compensation," said the mayor—an argument that has cropped up repeatedly in university-city relations. Bayne-Jones recommended to the corporation that the university make a five-year financial commitment that would be capped at $150,000 a year for the hospital and $350,000 a year for the medical school.[51] In 1938 the hospital raised patient fees and announced an inclusive ward rate—covering room, board, nursing services, and so forth—of $5.00 a day.[52] Although Mayor Murphy expressed surprise, the New Haven County Medical Association thought that the inclusive rate would benefit patients.

Bayne-Jones stepped down in 1940 after five years as dean, to be succeeded by Francis Blake, who also remained as chairman of medicine. The full-time program in clinical medicine was in place but required funding to remain viable. The growing hospital deficit demanded action. A temporary working agreement was reached, based on the medical school's 1945 estimate of a minimum of 350 teaching beds and eighty thousand outpatient visits a year to maintain its teaching program.[53] The university would provide $206,375 for the hospital and dispensary, a $50,000 increase, to offset teaching costs. To determine the university contribution for the support of education, the cost per day of ward patients and dispensary patients had to be established, as well as costs for such hospital services as clinical laboratory work and radiology. Blake could think of no immediate sources of a large endowment.

The deteriorating financial situation had finally brought the Grace Hospital to the point of merging with the New Haven Hospital in 1945. The Grace Hospital's facilities were obsolete and in danger of being condemned as a fire hazard. The New Haven Hospital needed to increase revenues, and adding the Grace physicians to its staff would bring more admissions. The new Grace–New Haven Community Hospital would have two medical services: a university service in the New Haven Hospital and a nonteaching service, primarily private and semiprivate wards, in the new hospital building.[54] The Advisory Medical Board of the Private Pavilion merged with the Grace Staff Executive Committee, bringing town and gown together. The Grace's board and medical staff were assured that the new hospital unit would be essentially self-contained, with separate operating rooms and radiology suite—which was in fact a very inefficient arrangement.[55]

There was also to be a new Veterans Administration hospital. To provide better medical care to veterans, Yale had been invited to recommend chiefs for the various medical services and to organize a residency program at a Veterans Administration hospital to be built in New Haven, and to develop a program at the existing Newington VA hospital. An earlier concerted effort had been made in 1929 to locate the veterans' hospital in New Haven rather than in the Hartford area. Proximity to the "well-nigh infinite resources of the new Yale University–New Haven Hospital plant" was touted as a compelling reason to situate the hospital in the New Haven area. Despite unbridled local enthusiasm and support, President Calvin Coolidge signed a recommendation that the hospital be located within a twenty-mile radius of

Hartford. Dean Winternitz graciously offered the resources of Yale to the new hospital but warned that the cost of cooperation increased the greater the distance from New Haven.[56]

Now there would be a veterans' hospital in the New Haven area with five hundred general medical and surgical beds and four hundred beds for tuberculosis. Yale wanted the general hospital located near the medical school and the tuberculosis hospital located on the site of the William Wirt Winchester Tuberculosis Hospital, three miles away in West Haven. Federal authorities were adamant that the entire VA hospital complex had to be in one location, which meant West Haven.

George Darling, Yale's director of medical affairs, who had a Ph.D. in public health, had been recruited in 1946 and been given responsibility for university-hospital relations. At the completion of his term in 1950, he came to the conclusion that the major problem with the relationship was the dominant role the university played in deciding hospital policy. The hospital administration objected to the imposition of programs by the medical school but was also aware that the university was paying for the programs.[57] Patient reimbursement from the state, city, and even insurance companies did not reflect the real costs, and the hospital had no incentive to adjust rates to its costs. Because ward beds were responsible for the financial deficit and teaching beds had to be ward beds, the hospital regarded the medical school as responsible for the loss. If the hospital closed the beds, the medical school could not support a clinical program, and the university could not afford to let this happen. So the deficit-financing agreement between hospital and university would have to continue.

The university and the hospital each considered the other responsible for providing service to the patients. If the university required more ward patients for teaching than the hospital could afford to subsidize, the university would have to provide additional financial support or the hospital would develop financial difficulties.[58] Darling concluded that in reality the patients—and appropriate third parties—were actually responsible for the cost of their illness. The concept that a teaching bed must be a ward bed changed only after much study and discussion, and it was agreed that semiprivate beds could be used for teaching.

Although the hospital clearly needed some form of subsidy, this had not always been the case. Addressing the University Council in 1950, Spencer Berger, president of the hospital board, commented that in 1926 Henry W. Farnam, then hospital president, had felt that closer affiliation with Yale University advantageous without affecting the character of the hospital as an independent institution. In 1950, however, when 70 percent of the hospital's beds were ward beds, the hospital could not operate without a subsidy. Furthermore, the hospital was regarded by the community as controlled by the medical school, and "all the unfortunate and unfair attitudes that usually develop in a 'town and gown' controversy were directed against it."[59]

The relationship between the medical school and the hospital certainly was mutually advantageous, and differences of opinion had to be clarified. The medical school was prepared to absorb costs of hospitalization resulting from teaching, but no other costs. Because clinical practice was vitally important to the hospital's future, Albert Snoke, the hospital director, wanted to be a member of the medical-school group practice and wanted the practice organized in a more businesslike manner. In a conciliatory gesture, Snoke had proposed that all the hospital laboratories be under the supervision of faculty, with full-time assistants, residents, and interns as needed, to allow time for research and teaching, and that a clinical-laboratory residency program be initiated. Accordingly, responsibility for quality remained with the medical school, while some of the costs were moved to the hospital, resulting in much improved laboratory service. Darling was pleased about the hospital's assuming some of the laboratory costs, but told Snokes he was "disappointed and puzzled by the hospital's failure to make a token reduction in the appropriation" and would have to resign from the hospital's board if a reduction were not made.[60]

Darling's words had the desired effect. Snoke commented at an October 1948 meeting of the Board of Permanent Officers that "it has been salutary to clarify the relationship. The function of the hospital is service, of the school, teaching and research."[61] Darling kept pushing for further reductions in university support for the hospital because the new president of Yale, Whitney Griswold, was "less enthusiastic or sympathetic to the mutual problems of the Medical School and the Hospital" than President Seymour had been.[62] Snoke thought that Griswold was under pressure from "certain members of the Yale family" to settle the university-hospital financial problem. University funding for the hospital decreased to $156,000 in 1949—it had been $206,900 in 1945—and the hospital began to assume more responsibility for services, like radiology, that had previously been supported by the university.[63]

The medical school and hospital were entering a period of intense change. In 1952 another new agreement with the hospital was in the offing.[64] Ever since 1913 the medical school's formal relationship with the hospital had been defined by a series of affiliation agreements. The new agreement, which contained four main provisions, was greeted with general approval. The university released any claim on buildings constructed on hospital land with funds secured by Yale. The hospital released land and buildings used for laboratories to the university. The medical school was guaranteed the use of the hospital for teaching and research programs, and, finally, the university would continue its financial subvention of $54,375 a year to the hospital for another three years, at which time financial support would end.[65]

Changes were afoot in Yale's nursing programs, too. In 1956 President Griswold, who believed strongly that any university program should be of high quality or cease to exist, announced that he intended to close down the Yale University School of Nursing, on the advice of the "President of Smith College and the Dean of Harvard Medical School, because the Yale School of Nursing was essentially a vocational school."[66] The hospital was home to three separate educational programs in nursing. With the formation of the Grace–New Haven Community Hospital, the hospital had acquired a nursing-diploma program. In addition, half the clinical program at the University of Connecticut School of Nursing was housed in the hospital, as was the Yale University School of Nursing. Still, Snoke thought a strong master of nursing program could be developed at Yale. He was supported by the former dean, Stanhope Bayne-Jones, who had been elected an alumni trustee of the Yale Corporation and is thought to have played a role in saving the nursing school. And so the Yale School of Nursing did not disappear. As a result of a growing preference among nursing students for a baccalaureate program, however, the Grace–New Haven Community Hospital diploma program, which was not connected with the university, closed in 1975.

As part of the change that was occurring, ambulatory-care services took on greater importance. The hospital and the medical school were looking for an individual to take charge of these services. At a meeting with the United Auto Workers to discuss the possibility of a medical center assuming responsibility for a major union's prepaid health-insurance group, Albert Snoke and Vernon Lippard were impressed by a Yale College graduate, Richard Weinerman.[67] Snoke wrote to a number of people for references, and they unanimously replied that Weinerman was an unacceptable risk. All agreed that he was extremely able but thought him a political risk.[68] Caldwell Esseltyn, a surgeon, wrote, "Whether he ever carried a card I am not in a position to say, but I am in a position to say that I feel very strongly Yale University cannot for one minute afford to consider Dick."[69] Despite these warnings, Richard Weinerman was appointed to Yale in medicine and public health and had a distinguished career, cut short by a tragic plane crash. As

I mentioned earlier, Weinerman foresaw the need for primary-care physicians and the advent of what was to become managed care.[70]

The Grace–New Haven Community Hospital remained in need of subsidizing. But financial support was not going to come from the local New Haven community. In an attempt to reach a wider audience, the Yale–New Haven Medical Center was organized for joint long-range planning, public relations, and—most important—fund-raising between the university and the hospital. Changes had to be made if the Yale–New Haven Medical Center were to be successful in its fund-raising efforts. George Stevenson, president of the Grace–New Haven Community Hospital, wrote a special article in *Connecticut Medicine* to allay the anxieties of community physicians, explaining that the function of the center was to "assist" and not to "administer."[71] Whether the doctors in the state were really comfortable or not, the university and the hospital had come together in a single although loose entity. The medical school now was affiliated with four hospitals, the Grace–New Haven Community Hospital, the West Haven Veterans Administration Hospital, the Yale Psychiatric Institute, and the Connecticut Mental Health Center.

President Whitney Griswold and Provost Kingman Brewster came to the conclusion that if the medical school and the hospital were to become a truly modern medical center, they would have to be better integrated. Vernon Lippard concurred, believing that relations with the hospital, satisfactory on the surface, were a constant source of irritation because of the difficulty in arriving at an equitable basis for division of financial responsibilities. Equally irritated, the hospital director, Albert Snoke, commented to Paul Zorn, the hospital president, that the major issues revolved around professional services and how to divide them equitably.[72] A committee of the hospital's board, however, had reached a different conclusion: "The method of determining the sharing of costs between the two institutions is effective and equitable."[73]

Funds were needed for hospital renovation, and the university was considered to be in a better position than the hospital to attract financial support. The hospital was also having a major problem in getting the City of New Haven to pay for patients on welfare.[74] Thus, the time was ripe for yet another affiliation agreement. Once again the university seriously considered assuming control of the hospital. In January 1963 Lippard told President Griswold that, with the available sources of insurance, "the operation of the hospital need not be a financial liability to the university. There would be enormous advantages to the school if we controlled the hospital." Lippard appreciated that community physicians and the hospital's board would not agree easily (an understatement!). The strongest leverage would be to threaten to build a university hospital. Lippard felt that "Yale would be foolish to procure large sums of money for the Grace–New Haven Community hospital without insisting on control of its administration and policy."[75] He conceded that Snoke had a "good national reputation" but was in a difficult situation in having to deal with two hostile medical staffs and a large, inefficient board. "I have always found him fair and easy to work with."[76]

University control of the hospital was evaluated in a long memorandum by John E. Ecklund, a lawyer. The "ideal" for the university was not complete university control but to have the hospital furnish from its own resources the environment required by the faculty. "Hospital Administration and even patient care are not direct goals of the University."[77] In his survey of medical centers, Ecklund noted that at the best medical schools, the schools themselves nominated the entire medical staff, and all patients were available for teaching. The issue for the hospital was whether there was an obligation to grant hospital privileges to physicians who were not interested in teaching.

To give Yale the power to nominate a majority of the directors of the hospital would require an amendment to the hospital charter and Yale would have to control two-thirds of the directors. Ecklund recommended the formation of a joint board that would act with the approval of the two parent boards. Equitable allocation of costs between the two organizations would be a problem, and it has continued to be a constant source of irritation between the medical school and the hospital. The university decided not to attempt to control the hospital—a wise decision in view of the present situation in which university-controlled hospitals lose tens of millions of dollars annually.

A Joint Committee on Affiliation, chaired by President Brewster and Paul Zorn, president of the hospital, was formed in 1964, with six members from the university and six members from the hospital. The committee recommended to the Yale Corporation and the Board of Directors of the hospital that there be university representation on the hospital's board and that a joint board be established to deal with planning, cross-payments, and use of facilities. The hospital should be the main university teaching hospital. Education and research should primarily be the responsibility of the university, while the hospital should be responsible for service and patient care. A single chief of service should be appointed, who would be the chairman of the department and would nominate an associate chief selected from the community.

The proposal was circulated among the medical staff for several months. The hospital appointed a committee from the Community Division of the staff to examine it, and the committee expressed "very serious reservations about the proposal." It cautioned the president of the hospital's board that the future welfare of the hospital and the medical school depended on relationships with the community. The committee believed that a large majority of the community physicians "completely opposed" the creation of a university hospital or a Grace–New Haven Community Hospital dominated by "University influence."[78]

Albert Snoke, the hospital director, attempted to weaken the Yale proposal by giving the community the power to nominate the chief of the private-practice division, to no avail. The most contentious issue clearly was the domination of the medical staff by the university chairmen, and Snoke thought this issue led to his downfall, because of his vigorous arguments about it with Kingman Brewster. Snoke demanded of Lippard, "How can you write into a bylaw that these chairmen must be the absolute boss, when you know as well as I do that they are either lushes or they are considered professionally less competent than community physicians—by their own colleagues."[79]

The affiliation agreement for the Yale–New Haven Hospital was ratified on March 22, 1965, and it essentially accepted the recommendations of the Brewster-Zorn committee.[80] Yale could nominate "not more than one-third and not less than one-fourth" of the hospital directorships. There would be a joint eight-member board, of which the dean of the medical school and the executive director of the hospital would be members. Ordinarily, members of the hospital's active staff would hold full-time or part-time faculty appointments. The Community Medical Service, in which community physicians operated independently, would be eliminated and the university and community wards would be consolidated under a single university chief, who would nominate an associate chief. The executive director of the hospital would serve on search committees for the clinical chairmen.

One of the most difficult parts of any affiliation agreement are the terms of the divorce. If several layers of arbitration failed, either party could terminate the agreement with a vote of two-thirds of the Yale Corporation or the Hospital Board at two meetings at least six months apart. The termination would take place five years later. The agreement was so written that once joined, the merger could not easily be torn asunder.

In view of the formation of the Yale–New Haven Hospital, Snoke had raised the question of whether the resident staff would represent a continuation of medical education or a straight hospital service program.[81] He was convinced that a survey would show that most of a resident's time was involved in educational pursuits, and that the costs should therefore be borne by the medical school. Lippard responded that only 16.5 percent of a resident's time was spent in either receiving instruction or teaching, and as his or her average work week was eighty hours, the service component dwarfed the educational component.

The house staff, reflecting the social unrest in the community during this period, organized a petition for increases in stipends and "full meal allowances" for house staff on duty at night. With previous increases in house-staff stipends, the hospital had withdrawn certain allowances, as for meals and laundry. The house staff petition had initially been supported by the clinical department heads, but when the house-staff organization threatened to write a letter to the *New York Times*, Paul Beeson forbade the Department of Medicine representative to do so.[82]

In December 1965 Snoke, in his capacity as executive director, warned Charles H. Costello, the president of the Yale–New Haven Hospital, that the hospital was in a serious financial condition. Charges were too high, and reimbursement for the medically indigent was inadequate, with the city and state in no hurry to correct the inadequacy. "Uncertainty, unrest, insecurity and contentiousness" were rampant among the medical staff, and especially among the full-time faculty, reflecting "a need for direction or cohesiveness." Furthermore, "there is gossip throughout the country," an indication that Vernon Lippard was nearing the end of his term.[83]

Snoke also cautioned that the joint Yale–New Haven Hospital Board was perceived as weak. The hospital and the university were not "really functioning as true partners." There was a danger of two hospital boards developing, one with sixteen community members and one with eight Yale members, rather than the single joint board spelled out in the affiliation agreement.

Vernon Lippard stepped down as dean of the medical school in 1967 after fifteen years and was succeeded by the chairman of psychiatry, Fritz Redlich, who came to consider hospital relations the most complex and least understood of organizational relationships.

Lippard was not the only person to have reached the end of his term. With strong university input, Albert Snoke's term as executive director also ended in 1967. Charles Costello sent a letter to the medical staff indicating that many of Snoke's decisions and attitudes had been "increasingly incompatible with those of the Board."[84] He went on to say that Snoke had been offered several alternatives, which were unacceptable to him, and the board had been forced to act. Charles B. Womer, who had been recruited from Cleveland to be the administrator of the hospital in 1965, was promoted to executive director.

As part of a national effort to increase medical standards, affiliations between the medical school and six community hospitals were formed as part of the Connecticut Regional Medical Program. Of particular importance was the affiliation with the Hospital of Saint Raphael in 1972, whose purpose was to facilitate coordination of health-care services in the New Haven area as well as to establish clinical clerkships for Yale medical students at Saint Raphael's. More and more Yale-trained physicians were joining the staff of Saint Raphael's, some of whom had spent several years on the full-time faculty and were interested in teaching. In 1968, amid the growing social unrest, *Sickness and Society*, by Yale's Raymond Duff and August Hollingshead, was published.[85] Focusing on the relationship between the care of hospitalized patients and the social environment of a hospital and medical school, and whether patients received optimal care, the authors were sympathetic to hospital administrators faced with dilemmas in dealing both with academic physicians and with community physicians.

The book occasioned a long article by Maya Pines in *McCalls* magazine, which said that "in the hospital jungle, all patients stand some chance of being misdiagnosed, inadequately treated. Lied to. Despair and frustration await many."[86] This assault on the quality of medical care at the Yale–New Haven Hospital could not have come at a worse time. The faculty and student body as well as the New Haven community were restive about social issues, and as unrest increased, the hospital and the medical school became more involved in community matters, both as health-care providers and as institutions located in the middle of the Hill neighborhood.

While the medical school and the hospital may have been viewed as a single entity from the outside, there was a real need to build better relations between the two. Accordingly, a decision was made to coordinate the clinical programs by appointing a single individual as both dean for clinical affairs in the medical school and chief of staff in the hospital. Robert Chase, a university surgeon, was offered the position, but he never assumed it, thanks to a change in deans. Fritz Redlich's five-year term was coming to an end, and he was succeeded by Lewis Thomas, chairman of pathology, who left after just one year, to be replaced by Robert Berliner, deputy director of the NIH. Decanal turnover made it difficult to define relations further between the medical school and the hospital during this period.

There will no doubt always be tensions—some creative, some not so creative—between the medical school and the hospital, because they differ in their primary responsibilities for teaching, research, and patient care. The medical school's primary mission involves learning and discovery, while the hospital's primary mission involves engagement in patient care. Although the two institutions have a symbiotic relationship, this fundamental difference has persisted over the past 150 years.

14

EPILOGUE

Although this account of the Yale University School of Medicine ends with Dean Fritz Redlich and the brief tenure of Dean Lewis Thomas, an understanding of its fortunes at the time of Yale's tercentenary allows the story to be put in context. It is generally recognized as one of the world's great medical schools. But what in particular makes it a preeminent medical institution? With some understanding of Yale's history, can the medical school's future be divined? Its future is closely associated with both the university and the hospital, but there are strong outside determinants, too. The direction of health care in the United States and the evolution of biomedical science will profoundly affect the future of the school.

Lewis Thomas was succeeded as dean by a distinguished researcher in renal physiology, Robert W. Berliner, deputy director of the NIH. His arrival in 1973 heralded an increased commitment to basic science, which catapulted the medical school into the top ranks of research-intensive medical institutions. Outstanding faculty burnished the school's image. George Palade was awarded the Nobel Prize in Medicine and Physiology soon after arriving at Yale. Gerhard Giebisch's recruitment as chairman of the Department of Physiology completed the transition from a traditional department into a world leader in the new cellular physiology. Murdock Ritchie replaced William Douglas as chair of pharmacology, and the department became a focal point for neuroscience, which burgeoned throughout the university. Samuel O. Thier succeeded Louis Welt as chairman of the megalithic Department of Medicine and set about replacing the subspecialty division directors with individuals interested in basic-science research. The new division directors in turn recruited young, laboratory-oriented investigators, which led to a level of research funding in the Department of Medicine now equal to that in all the preclinical basic-science departments.

With this basic-science orientation, the medical-curriculum revision that had condensed basic-science teaching into three semesters was no longer acceptable. The intention of the new curriculum was to have medical students return to basic science in their final elective year, after appreciating its importance in their clinical rotations. The students by and large remained entranced with the clinical experience, however, and elected to pursue clinical interests. Although a significant number of faculty members favored course examinations, a compromise was reached with anonymous qualifying examinations. The M.D./Ph.D. program became increasingly popular with the realization that academic medicine was going to require well-trained clinician-scientists.

At the same time, the medical school recognized an obligation to provide health care to the community and instituted a physicians' associate program within the Department of Surgery, after a prolonged debate whether the school should be involved in nondegree programs. In general, the focus never strayed far from scientific areas. Dean Berliner, convinced of their importance, created independent sections of neuroanatomy and immunology. In 1984 the focus on basic research continued with the appointment of Leon Rosenberg, chairman of human genetics, to succeed Berliner as dean. The Boyer Center for Molecular Biology opened in 1991 and provided space for twenty-three scientists, eight of them Howard Hughes investigators.

The primary mission of a medical school is to educate the next generation of physicians and other health professionals. Although the generation of new knowledge is a vital component, research institutes can accomplish that goal. Exemplary clinical care can be delivered in other venues, but education is unique to the medical school. There are twice as many full-time faculty members as medical students at Yale, one thousand responsible for about five hundred, with one hundred students in each class and a fifth "class" composed of students taking a year off to pursue research or other interests. In addition, there are public-health students, physician's associates, interns, residents, postdoctoral fellows, and Ph.D. graduate students.

Despite the primacy of medical education, promoting faculty members for their teaching abilities has been extremely difficult. The presumed commitment to education has more often been honored in the breach. Young faculty members have been advised to resist teaching commitments that will not foster their academic careers. Lack of objective criteria makes it difficult to evaluate educational excellence or clinical judgment, in contrast to research, where peer-reviewed publications and grants all provide objective evidence of excellence. As a consequence, a medical school's reputation is often linked to research prowess. At Yale, tenure appointments have been largely based on research accomplishments, reflecting the culture of Yale College and the Faculty of Arts and Sciences, which makes promotions on the basis of achievements in scholarship. Basing tenure primarily on research accomplishments is certainly a feature of other medical schools. But at Yale the school's close ties with the college have made this focus more apparent. The basic-science orientation of the medical school grew from its association with the college, dating back to Benjamin Silliman.

Tenure appointments are jealously guarded by the university, because they incur long-term financial obligation. At Yale, a faculty member must achieve tenure within ten years or leave. The "up or out" rule was intended to prevent faculty exploitation by the administration, but it works to the disadvantage of individuals who take time off (to, say, raise a family). A continuing-appointment track was instituted at the medical school to alleviate pressure on limited senior appointments. Associate professors on this track are not required to leave after ten years if they fail to be promoted, but the number of professorial slots in the track is limited. Professors on this track can be terminated only by eliminating the entire track for reasons of financial stringency, but the number of faculty qualified for promotion to professor increased faster than the number of positions the university was willing to make available. Recently, a third academic track has been added at the medical school, which offers less long-term security but allows attainment of professorial rank.

In addition to discovery and learning, an important part of a medical school's mission is engagement with the community through clinical practice. Medical schools play a significant role in setting the standard of practice in the surrounding community. The ability of New Haven to provide sufficient patients for the clinical program, compared to Boston or New York, was a concern during the Flexner era. The critics were partially correct, in that the relatively small size of New Haven makes it more difficult to attract faculty. Although the critics have been muted by the development of a strong program, clinical medicine at Yale has never achieved the same prominence as the research effort, nor has it been as well supported. Differences in the relative prominence of the clinical and research programs are also due in large measure to the strong influence of the Faculty of Arts and Sciences on the basic-science culture of the medical school.

The fact that the medical school accounts for approximately 44 percent of the total university operating budget and half the full-time faculty makes the tail capable of wagging the bulldog. Furthermore, 98 percent of the medical school's $541 million budget for the 1998–1999 fiscal year was dependent on outside funding—about 61 percent from research grants and 39 percent from clinical income. Yale University's endowment is almost $10 billion, but the medical school represents only about 8 percent of this endowment. "Every tub on its own bottom" is a phrase that makes medical-school deans cringe.

University accounting procedures have varied markedly during the medical school's existence, but comparisons are possible over the forty years from 1931 to 1971. More than a twentyfold increase in medical-school income in constant dollars occurred during this period. There was a correlation between significant increases in income and increasing federal support of research beginning in the 1950s and the advent of Medicare in the 1960s. If the sources of medical-school income as a percentage of total income are examined, university endowment and tuition became increasingly less important as research funding increased. Clinical income also began to rise. (See figures 41 and 42.)

The medical school grew rapidly in relation to the university following the introduction of Medicare in 1965. Increased research grants and reimbursement for patients who had previously been treated without charge provided funds for the recruitment of new faculty. The university benefited from the new sources of funding. While there was concern over the expansion of the medical school, no one wanted to kill the goose that laid the golden egg. Nevertheless, the recent growth of the medical school has been perceived as a threat to the integrity of the university. The Yale Corporation is uneasy about the financial risk to the university in having half of the full-time faculty at the medical school highly leveraged in terms of their salaries.

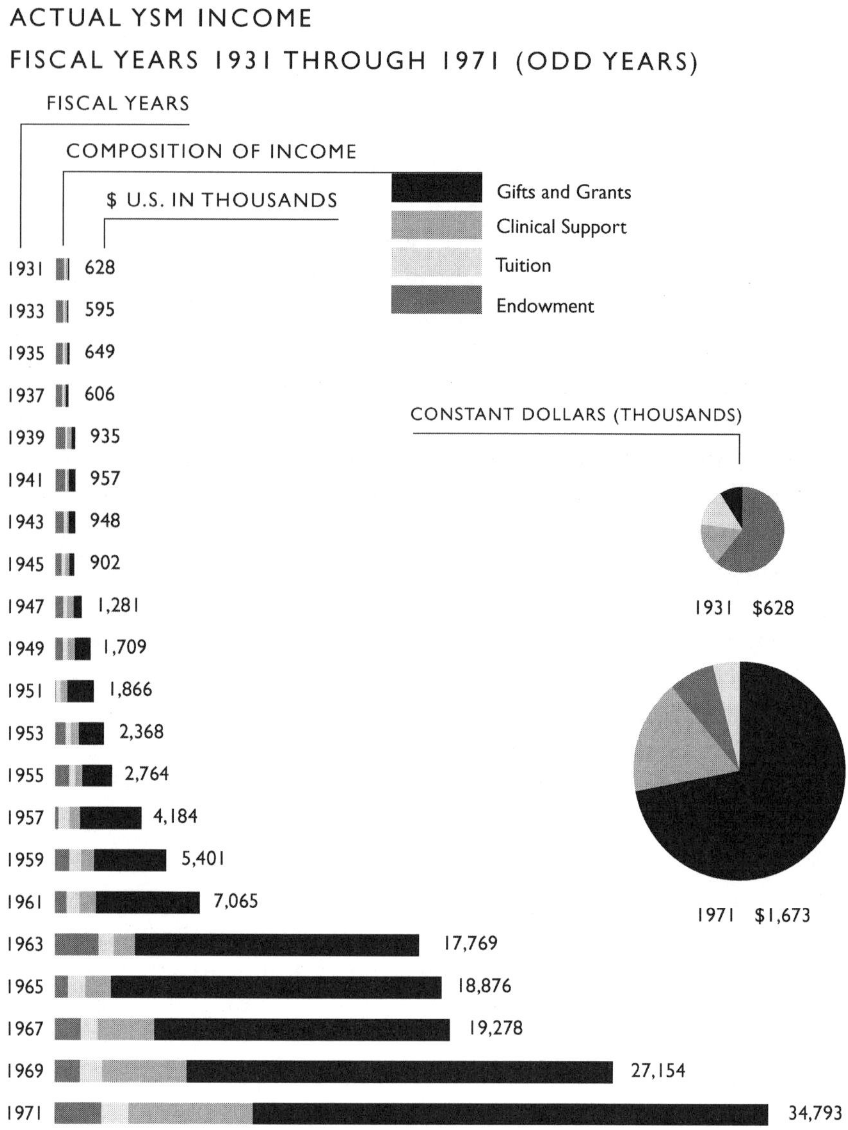

Figure 41. Yale School of Medicine income, 1931–1971

The medical school is also highly visible. It is said that American universities relate to the public through their football team and their medical school. At Yale, where the football team is not customarily the center of public attention, the medical school is all the more visible. On the academic side, the feeling that the medical school is a "trade school" and does not quite belong within the university still persists to some degree. It is not helpful that basic

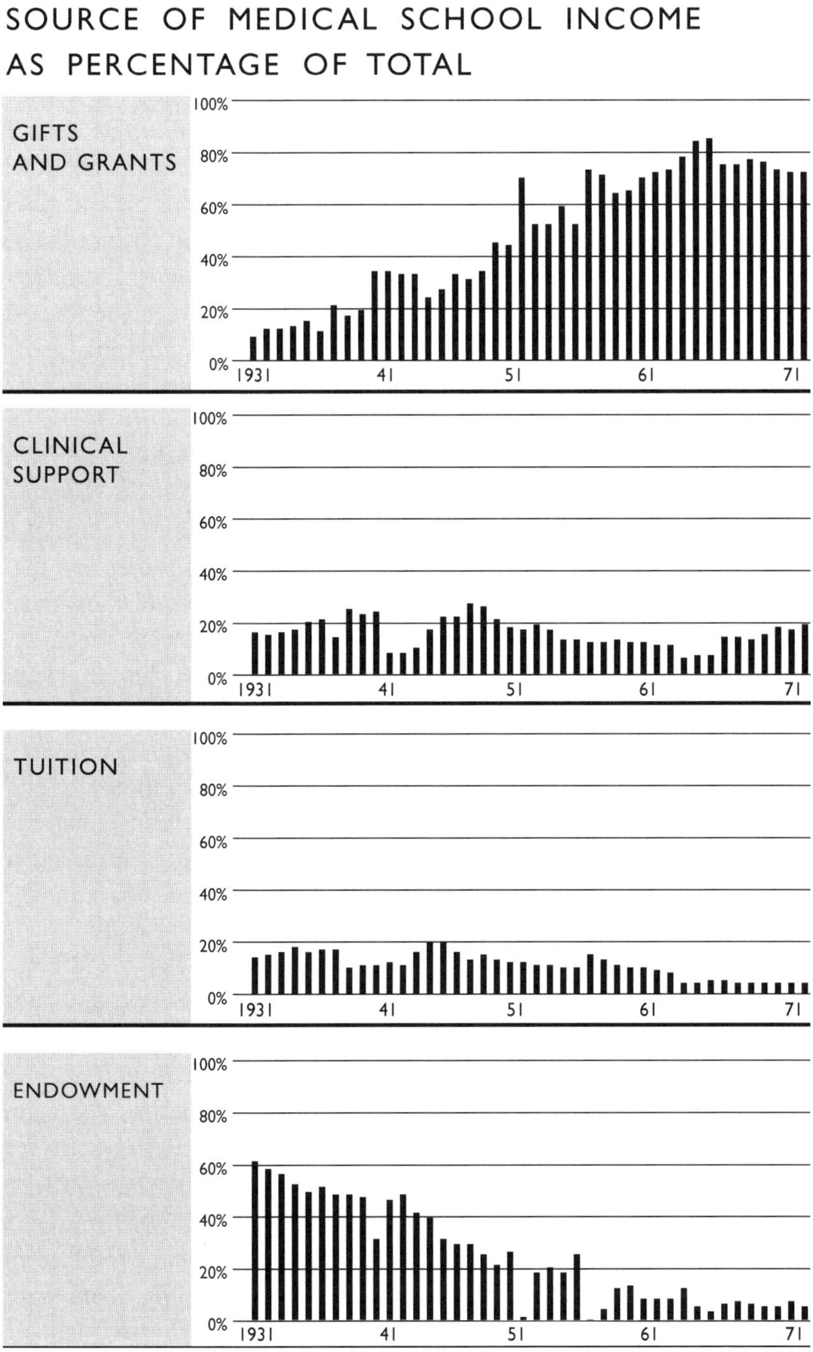

Figure 42. Sources of medical-school income, 1931–1971

scientists in the medical school may be paid more, and often have fewer teaching responsibilities, than comparable faculty in the arts and sciences.

The size and complexity of medical-school departments changed profoundly after the introduction of Medicare, creating tension between basic-science departments, who became have-nots but did much of the teaching, and the clinical departments, who felt they were supporting the school financially. The growth of specialization, which began at Yale in the 1920s, flourished with the increased availability of clinical revenue. Rosemary Stevens has argued that "specialization is the fundamental theme for the organization of medicine in the twentieth century."[1] The fourfold increase in the size of the faculty in the Department of Medicine during the past thirty-five years is directly attributable to increasing specialization.

Within clinical departments, tensions rose between faculty members primarily interested in clinical practice and those interested in investigation. The traditional triple-threat academic physician—a combination of clinician, scientist, and educator—became an endangered species, and the suggestion was made that the faculty be divided into a two-platoon system of clinicians and researchers. Tensions developed between commitment to education through research on the one hand, and through clinical practice on the other. Increasingly intense financial pressures make it easy to forget that education is what separates medical schools from research institutes and practice groups. Those financial pressures coupled with the fact that some clinical departments generate excess revenue result in strained relations between the dean and department chairs over allocation of resources, especially those from the faculty clinical-practice plan. Although members of the clinical faculty recognize that the academic program should benefit from clinical revenue, they would prefer that the revenue not be theirs.

Medical-school deans face particular challenges in governance. Universities and medical schools evolved from a collegial monastic life, and we must bear in mind that the word *collegial* means "a power or authority vested equally in a number of colleagues." The present organizational structure of the medical school is rather like having the dean as chief executive officer and the faculty members as hundreds of executive vice presidents with full voting rights. Faculty members revel in their independence. Tenure was instituted in universities to protect that independence, but as a result academic institutions often lack a common corporate vision. A 1987 Rand Corporation study of academic health centers concluded that their survival depended on integration of their departments and the ceding of some departmental autonomy—not an easy task.[2]

As managed health care has replaced traditional fee for service for physicians and generous reimbursement for hospitals, tensions between the medical school and the hospital medical center have increased. Perhaps the most complicated relationships are those between the dean and the hospital director. Although the hospital director may believe that teaching and research are important, he or she is acutely aware that the hospital director's job is to maintain a positive financial balance. The dean may recognize the importance of medical care, but academic accolades lie in teaching and research. Bright, entrepreneurial department chairs, aware of the schism, play the dean against the hospital director to gain departmental resources.

The teaching hospital and the medical school are often run as two entirely separate businesses, even though they represent a single entity or closely intertwined allies. There is a perception among the hospital directors that the medical-school deans regard the university hospital as a cash cow, while the deans feel that although the hospital may be a cash cow, it produces insufficient cash. So long as moneys received from patient care were sufficient to meet possible expenses and federal or state funds were available for health care, these financial disagreements were minor irritants. As efforts to control soaring health costs increased, patient reimbursement decreased to the point that teaching hospitals caring for large numbers of indigent patients developed desperate financial problems. At the same time, community hospitals started providing tertiary care in competition with teaching hospitals. As for the medical school, the decrease in federal and state support increased the need for remunerative clinical practice by the faculty.

In the current climate of managed care, university hospitals have difficulty being competitive in the marketplace. In times of financial constraint, collegial and entrepreneurial aspects of the academic physician easily come into conflict with the expansive bureaucracy needed to run a modern hospital. The overarching tension between the medical school and the hospital results from striving to balance the need to fulfill academic goals and the need to fill hospital beds in order to maintain financial solvency.[3]

In spite of its financial ups and downs over the past two hundred years, the Yale University School of Medicine ranks among the world's best. It is not easy to say why it does. The school has not produced more deans, researchers, or Nobel Prize winners than other schools. Certainly its connection with a great university greatly aids the perception of excellence, but there are other factors.

High among these factors is the quality of its students. Commitment to excellence and a liberal arts system of medical education brought an Emmy

Award-winning CBS News producer, a former vice president for Salomon Brothers, and a divinity-school graduate together as medical-school classmates. In a way, this unusual mix of individuals defines what is truly special about Yale. Medical students with such varied backgrounds bring a richness and diversity, which along with the emphasis on academic freedom results in a liberal-arts kind of medical school. Although the quality of students is difficult to quantify, a medical school can be judged in part by the students it admits as well as by the faculty it appoints and the faculty it promotes.

Approximately three thousand prospective medical students apply to Yale each year. About seven hundred are interviewed, and one hundred and fifty are accepted, to form a class of one hundred students. After initial winnowing to select students who will receive an interview, significant differences among the remaining applicants become difficult to discern. The class of 2002 was composed of forty-five women and fifty-five men with an average age of twenty-four. There were twenty-nine Asian-American students in the entering class, eleven black/African American, seven Hispanic/Latino, and four multiracial students. Eleven students already had a master's degree, and two students entered with a Ph.D. Ivy League students accounted for 51 percent of the entering class. Twenty-one graduates of Yale College chose to stay in New Haven for their medical-school education, and fifteen Harvard College graduates chose to join them. Eighty-three students had been science majors, and a number of students had multiple majors, with fifteen majoring in the humanities and twenty-seven in social science. Matriculating students had pursued multiple interests as well as being academically talented, with a grade-point average of 3.71 out of 4.0. Nine students elected to enter the M.D.-Ph.D. program.

The Yale system of medical education, characterized by the considerable academic freedom and individual responsibility of the student, a minimum of examinations, and a research-thesis requirement, has been in place for more than three-quarters of a century. In an anonymous survey, medical students mentioned the Yale system and the collegial atmosphere engendered by the lack of examination pressure as the "most significant" reasons for their attending Yale. In an era when there is pressure from accreditation bodies to homogenize the nation's 125 medical schools by requiring universal standards, Yale stands apart with its unique system of medical education and tends to attract exceptional students for that reason.

The rating of medical schools by magazines like *U.S. News and World Report* have become the center of a controversy over the rating criteria used.

Deans of medical and other professional schools universally decry the ratings as meaningless but are more comfortable doing so from the heights of the top ten schools listed rather than from the bottom ten. Yale has consistently ranked among the top ten medical schools and often among the top five. In 1995 the National Research Council published a ranking of various departments in the biological sciences, and Yale ranked among the very best.[4] The ratings give significant weight to research funding, one of Yale's great strengths.

Stringent criteria for NIH support result in only about 20 percent of acceptable grants being funded, and a ranking in the top 5 percent of schools provides a clear measure of excellence, at least in research. The basic-science culture of Yale College has strongly influenced and fostered the research attainments of the medical school ever since the days of Benjamin Silliman, perhaps the outstanding scientist of his time, who played such a prominent role in founding the Medical Institution of Yale College in 1810. By far the largest amount of the funding for research in the life sciences within the university now goes to the medical school. The Vannevar Bush Report in 1945, which had recommended federal support of basic research in universities, and the passage in 1965 of the Medicare Act, which reimbursed the costs of ward patients, resulted in rapid growth in the number of medical-school faculty members, many of whom engage in research. Because of Yale's basic-science orientation and limited clinical program, which permitted time for research, the medical school was able to capitalize on this increase in funds.

Where does the Yale University School of Medicine go from here? Based upon its past history, what form will the future medical school take? Although the crystal ball becomes cloudy, we can make some educated guesses about medicine over the next twenty-five years. Yale medical students graduating in the year 2002 will be reaching the peak of their professional life in 2025. Advances in cellular and molecular biology, sequencing the human genome, developments in neuroscience, and the computer age are causing a revolution in clinical medicine. While we are making great strides in the science that forms the basis of health care, however, the system that delivers health care in the United States is imploding. Both the scientific basis of medicine and the way that medicine is practiced will change dramatically over the next quarter century, and these changes will happen in a world very different from the world we know today. By 2025 the earth will contain a population of 8.5 billion people, compared to about six billion today, and

95 percent of the population increase will occur in developing countries. As a result, the global burden of disease will increase, and it will have direct effects on the population of the United States.

How will Yale prepare today's medical students to practice in a future health-care system that cannot be envisioned, on a scientific base that we cannot imagine? I believe that we need to produce physicians and other health-care professionals who are flexible and able to adapt to profound changes in medicine, physicians with a liberal education in the best Yale tradition.

Today's students study medicine in the same way envisioned by Dean Milton Winternitz some seventy-five years ago, when he instituted the Yale system of medical education. The amount of material to be mastered, however, has increased exponentially since then and is overwhelming. Lloyd H. Smith, a medical educator, commented, "Our students should be freed of the stupefying effects of fact engorgement which threatens to convert them into floppy disks encoded for our present ignorance."[5] Medical students need to acquire a core of basic information equivalent to the multiplication tables learned in primary school. The medical faculty needs to provide a conceptual framework into which students can integrate the acquired facts.

Information technology gives students instant access to enormous amounts of information. They need to learn how to formulate the critical questions needed to reach a clinical decision and then find the necessary information. Rapid growth of information technology along with access to the Internet makes long-distance learning completely feasible. The world's best teachers in any given field are now able to deliver a lecture that students can consult whenever convenient. Medical schools have yet to grapple seriously with the implications of information technology, but the impact will be profound.

The traditional medical-school curriculum demands four years of study. Medical-school deans are allotted four years in which to educate a physician to the level of an M.D. degree. Whether the time allotted is too little, too much, or just right is a matter for conjecture. Graduation is followed by three or four years in a postgraduate residency-training program, which could be viewed as part of the medical-education curriculum. Because of government reimbursement, residency training is supported by hospitals, and residents are considered hospital employees. If residency training were under the control of the medical schools, the seven or eight years of medical education and training could be combined into an integrated educational experience and probably be shortened.

How many physicians, and of what kind, are required for optimal medical care? This continues to be a subject for national debate. Whether or not the physician workforce in the United States is too large, its distribution is definitely uneven. American physicians are produced in a supply-side manner.[6] The individual physician decides whether he or she wishes to become a specialist in gastroenterology with little attention paid to whether gastroenterologists are needed on the demand side. Although there have been attempts in some specialties, particularly surgery, to limit the number of specialty-training positions, the medical profession has not paid sufficient attention to the problem.

Physician workforce issues are complicated by the large number of graduates of foreign medical schools who are in residency training in the United States. These foreign graduates equal half the graduating classes of American medical schools, and the great majority of them remain in the United States after training. The suggestion has been made that the number of residency-training positions be limited to 110 percent of the graduates of U.S. medical schools, but implementing this has been difficult. Whether the selection should be based on competition or location of medical-school education is a political issue.

The kind of physician emerging from an American medical school is a reflection of the school's values.[7] Education, research, and patient care form the core of mission statements in most of the nation's medical schools. The overwhelming majority of medical-school graduates are needed to provide patient care, not to become researchers. Yet medical-school ratings tend to focus on research funding and specialization, which encourages medical schools to become research intensive.

One of the great strengths of American medical schools has been the diversity of curricula, resulting in a wide variety of educational experiments. And diversity in American medical education is nowhere better illustrated than in the Yale system. There has recently been a trend to codify standards, which could homogenize medical education. Medical schools in the United States and Canada must be accredited by the Liaison Committee on Medical Education, composed of representatives from the Association of American Medical Colleges and the American Medical Association. The committee sets the minimum standards for a medical school to be accredited. It should focus on outcome rather than process. The problem is not limited to medical schools. The accreditation body for schools of public health has expressed increasing concern that the School of Epidemiology and Public Health at

Yale is located within the medical school. The health of the individual and the health of the public are inseparable, and the symbiotic relationship between the two disciplines has been further strengthened by globalization.

There are separate accrediting bodies for the various components of the academic health center, enormously complicating interdisciplinary education. Physicians need to be educated to work as members of a multidimensional health-care team, which includes public-health professionals. We should pay equal attention to the health of the public and the health of the individual. Within their areas of competency, nurses and physician's associates have been shown to be as effective as primary-care physicians. As much as three-quarters of a primary-care physician's practice can be successfully handled by a nurse practitioner. Socialization within the health-care team is vitally important, to ensure that everyone is comfortable with his or her abilities. Interdisciplinary education will become the norm in the future.

Against this background of issues in medical education, what will clinical medicine be like in 2025? With an understanding of the etiology of heart disease and cancer, specific treatment for the two leading causes of mortality will be available. With more knowledge of the immune system, we shall improve the prevention and treatment of autoimmune diseases like rheumatoid arthritis and shall develop—with difficulty—vaccines for AIDS and other retroviral diseases. With increased understanding of the genome, the likely future development of a disease could be predicted. Important ethical questions will be raised. Who should be tested, and who should have access to the information? Physicians will play a role in these decisions, and medical students need to be prepared accordingly.

Still, future developments remain unpredictable. One of the great medical advances of the twentieth century was the eradication of smallpox, a scourge that decimated populations over the centuries. The expectation was that tuberculosis would be eliminated in a similar manner, but it is now more virulent than ever, because of poor public-health practices. Although it was predicted that infectious disease would be eliminated, new and emerging infections appear to be with us for the foreseeable future.

An issue of major interest is whether aging can be arrested. Despite the incredibly exciting medical advances, the human body is not likely to become immortal and will simply keep on wearing out. Although there has been a significant change in life expectancy, there has been little change in the number of people living much past one hundred, and the increase in life expectancy has been due mostly to a decrease in childhood mortality. If the aging process is ineluctable, then the role of the physician is to compress morbidity into a short span between the onset of disability and death, at the oldest age possible. In other words, "Live old, die young!" The fastest-growing age group in North America is people older than eighty-five, a group increasing at a rate three times that of the population at large. Medical schools have taught that death is pathological and part of a disease process, with the implication that eradicating disease would eliminate death. How much health care is enough is one of the most significant questions that we shall have to answer over the next twenty-five years. Technology is available that can delay death considerably without prolonging meaningful life. Dealing with this issue is, and will be, an important facet of medical education. Medical schools have the clear responsibility to educate physicians who understand the difference between meaningful life and death delayed.

Solutions to the problems of aging will also have implications for the health-care system at large. Rising costs in health care have made hospitalization an increasingly undesirable option unless the patient is simply too ill to be managed in an outpatient setting. With the aging of the population, hospitals are gradually becoming geriatric intensive-care centers. Managed care as it is now constituted is not acceptable. Optimal medical care is cost-effective care, but what is currently being "managed" is cost, not care. Patients are unhappy, doctors are unhappy, and the payers are unhappy because the costs are rising.

There are more Americans without health insurance than ever before. The United States cannot continue to have one in every five citizens lack access to health care except on an emergency basis; the population must have access to health care other than through an emergency room. Health-care companies are ridding themselves of Medicare managed-care programs even as the elderly population continues to increase. Some form of universal health insurance appears inevitable, whether it is controlled by the government or by a consortium of insurance companies. Needless to say, the ultimate shape of the health-care system in the United States will have a profound influence on medical schools, as about half of the operating budget in most schools depends on clinical revenues.

Diminishing clinical income amid increasing costs of patient care and fluctuating research support are to a degree forcing medical schools like Yale to abandon the monastic life of the ivory tower for the secular world. But medical schools must remain true to the mission of teaching, research, and exemplary patient care, which is necessary to support the first two. Yale has a particular strength in translational research that takes a clinical observation to the laboratory or a laboratory observation to the bedside. A prime example was the clinical observation of a cluster of children with arthritis in the region of Lyme, Connecticut, that led to the laboratory identification of the infectious nature of Lyme Disease and definitive treatment of it.

In a lecture President Kingman Brewster delivered to the Association of American Medical Colleges during the social turbulence of 1969, he reminded us that "to extend ourselves way beyond our unique role of teaching and research . . . would be to do less well, that for which we are best fitted."[8] What the Yale School of Medicine does well is educate medical students to become future leaders, physicians of the highest quality who will be comfortable with the changes the future will bring. In 1960 Dean Vernon Lippard described the medical school and its objectives in a speech titled "The Yale School of Medicine in the Twentieth Century" that is equally applicable to the twenty-first century. "Our objective, however, remains perfectly clear—the maintenance and cultivation of a community of scholars who, at various levels of maturity, are learning together. In such an atmosphere, good physicians will be educated, and the frontiers of science and medicine will be advanced for the benefit of all mankind. This is an effort worthy of a great University."[9]

NOTES

CHAPTER 2: THE FOUNDING YEARS

1. "An Act in addition to and Alteration of an Act entitled An Act to incorporate the Medical Society." *Proceedings of the Connecticut Medical Society for 1811.*
2. Herbert Thoms, *The Doctors of Yale College, 1702–1815, and the Founding of the Medical Institution* (Hamden, Conn.: Shoe String Press, 1960).
3. William Welch, "The Relation of Yale to Medicine," *Yale Medical Journal* 8, no. 5 (1901): 130; Franklin B. Dexter, *Biographical Sketches of the Graduates of Yale College with Annals of the College History,* 6 vols. (New York: Henry Holt, 1885–1912).
4. *The Literary Diary of Ezra Stiles,* edited by Franklin B. Dexter, 3 vols. (New York: Charles Scribner's Sons, 1901), 2: 349.
5. Welch, "The Relation of Yale to Medicine," 129.
6. Cotton Mather, *Magnalia Christi Americana, or, The ecclesiastical history of New-England, from its first planting in the year 1620: unto the year of our Lord, 1698: in seven books* (London: T. Parkhurst, 1702), 151.

7. Martin Kaufman, *American Medical Education: The Formative Years, 1765–1910* (Westport, Conn.: Greenwood Press, 1976), 5.
8. T. J. Wertenbaker, *The Puritan Oligarchy: The Founding of American Civilization* (New York: Charles Scribner's Sons, 1947).
9. Edwin Oviatt, *The Beginnings of Yale, 1701–1726* (New Haven: Yale University Press, 1916), 347–48.
10. Jonathan Dickinson, *Observations on That Terrible Disease, Vulgarly Called the Throat-Distemper, With Advices as to the Method of Cure, In a Letter to a Friend* (Boston: S. Kneeland and T. Green, 1740).
11. James Thacher, *American Medical Biography or Memoirs of Eminent Physicians Who Have Flourished in America* (New York: Milford House, 1967).
12. H. B. Ferris, "Some Early Medical Teachers in Connecticut," *Bulletin of the Society of Medical History of Chicago* 3 (1923): 133–50.
13. Dexter, *Biographical Sketches.*
14. Welch, "The Relation of Yale to Medicince," 132.
15. Thoms, *The Doctors of Yale College.*
16. Minutes of the Yale Corporation, September 13, 1806, Yale University Library, Manuscripts and Archives.
17. Ebenezer K. Hunt, Presidential Address, "Public and Benevolent Institutions and Movements with which the Connecticut Medical Society has been prominently identified," *Proceedings of the Connecticut Medical Society* (Hartford, 1865).
18. Creighton Barker, *The Practice of Medicine in New Haven Following the Revolution* (New Haven: New Haven Medical Association, 1924).
19. Creighton Barker, "The Founding of the New Haven County Medical Association," Yale University Library, Manuscripts and Archives, Records of the President, YRG 2-A, box 138, folder 3043.
20. Noah Webster, *A Brief History of Epidemic and Pestilential Diseases: With the principal phenomena of the physical world, which precede and accompany them and observations deduced from the facts stated in the volumes* (Hartford: Hudson and Goodwin, 1799).
21. C. Barker, "The Origin of the Connecticut State Medical Society," in ed. H. Thoms, *The Heritage of Connecticut Medicine* (New Haven: Whaples-Bullis, 1942), 7.
22. Daniel Turner, *De morbis cutaneis: A Treatise of Diseases Incident to the Skin* (London: 1714).
23. Alan Lyell, "Daniel Turner (1667–1740), LRCP London (1711), M.D. Honorary, Yale (1723), Surgeon, Physician and Pioneer Dermatologist," *International Journal of Dermatology* 21 (1982): 162–70.
24. *The Yale University Library Gazette* 69 (1995).
25. Daniel Turner to Yale College, September 24, 1722, Yale University Library,

Manuscripts and Archives, Records of the Corporation, Prudential Committee Collection. Translation by C. Nockels Fabbri.

26. Dummer to Woodbridge, February 25, 1725; see F. B. Dexter, ed., *Documentary History of Yale University* (New Haven, 1916), 256–58.
27. *Annals of the Royal College of Physicians of London, 1518–1915,* 8 (December 22, 1721): 191–204. Microfiche.
28. *Annals of the Royal College of Physicians of London, 1518–1915,* 9 (November 5, 1725): 67–68. Microfiche.
29. Ibid., December 3, 68.
30. George P. Fisher, *Life of Benjamin Silliman,* 2 vols. (Philadelphia, 1866), 1:260.
31. Benjamin Silliman, *Origin and Progress I: Chemistry, Mineralogy, and Geology at Yale College and in Other Places with Personal Reminiscences,* 9 vols. (New Haven, 1857–1862). Silliman Family Papers, series 3, box 32, folder 33 A, B.
32. Silliman to Knight, January 4, 1812, and January 29, 1812, Yale Medical School Miscellaneous Papers, 1810–1884, Cushing/Whitney Medical Library, Yale University.
33. Silliman to Knight, May 18, 1812, Yale Medical School Miscellaneous Papers, 1810–1884, Cushing/Whitney Medical Library, Yale University.
34. Knight Sr. to Knight, December 9, 1812, Yale Medical School Miscellaneous Papers, 1810–1884, Cushing/Whitney Medical Library, Yale University.
35. Oliver S. Hayward and Constance E. Putnam, *Improve, Perfect, and Perpetuate: Dr. Nathan Smith and Early American Medical Education* (Hanover: University Press of New England, 1998).
36. Gridley to Knight, November 20, 1810, Yale Medical School Miscellaneous Papers, 1810–1884, Cushing/Whitney Medical Library, Yale University.
37. William Field, *The Good Doctor Smith: Life and Times of Dr. Nathan Smith, 1762–1829* (New Haven: Advocate Press, 1992), 113.
38. Emily A. Smith, *Life and Letters of Nathan Smith, M.B., M.D.* (New Haven, 1914), 79.
39. Hayward, "Nathan Smith (1762–1829), Politician," 1235–42.
40. Oviatt to Winternitz, February 5, 1930, Yale University Library, Manuscripts and Archives, Records of the Dean of the School of Medicine, YRG 2-A-14, RU 24, box 132, folder 1378.
41. Charles E. Cunningham, *Timothy Dwight, 1752–1817: A Biography* (New York: Macmillan, 1942), 218.
42. Silliman to Knight, December 22, 1812, Yale Medical School Miscellaneous Papers, 1810–1884, box 1, Cushing/Whitney Medical Library, Yale University.
43. Field, *The Good Doctor Smith.*
44. Welch, "The Relation of Yale to Medicine."
45. Minutes of the Yale Corporation, August 1813, Yale University Library, Manuscripts and Archives, Records of the Corporation.

46. *Laws of the Medical Institution of Yale College* (New Haven: Oliver Steele, 1815).
47. Timothy Dwight, "The Medical Institution," in *Catalogue of Yale College,* 1815 or 1816, Cushing/Whitney Medical Library, Yale University.
48. Nathan Smith, *A Practical Essay on Typhous Fever* (New York: Bliss and White, 1824).
49. Nathan Smith, "Observations on the Pathology and Treatment of Necrosis," *Philadelphia Journal of Medicine and Surgery* 1 (June 1827): 11–19 and 2 (July 1827): 66–75.
50. L. S. Wirthlin, "Nathan Smith (1762–1828)," *Brigham Young University Studies* 17 (1977): 319–37; L. S. Wirthlin, "Joseph Smith's Boyhood Operation: An 1813 Surgical Success," *Brigham Young University Studies* 21 (1981): 131–54.
51. Nathan Smith, "Case of Ovarian Dropsy, Successfully Removed by a Surgical Operation," *American Medical Recorder* 5 (1822): 124.
52. Howard Pearson, "Lectures on the Diseases of Children by Eli Ives, M.D., of Yale and New Haven: America's First Academic Pediatrician," *Pediatrics* 77 (1986): 680–86.
53. F. Bacon, "Some Account of the Medical Profession in New Haven," in ed. E. E. Atwater, *A History of the City of New Haven to the Present Time,* (New York: Munsell, 1887).
54. H. Pearson, "Lectures on the Diseases of Children," *Pediatrics* 77 (1986): 680–86.
55. Barker, "The Founding of the New Haven County Medical Association."
56. Barker, *The Practice of Medicine in New Haven,* 17–27.
57. Whitfield J. Bell, "The Medical Institution of Yale College, 1810–1885," *Yale Journal of Biology and Medicine* 33 (1960): 160–83.
58. Timothy Dwight, "The Medical Institution," in *Catalogue of Yale College,* 1815 or 1816, Cushing/Whitney Medical Library, Yale University.
59. J. Mirsky and Allan Nevins, *The World of Eli Whitney* (New York, 1952), 294–96.
60. Hannibal Hamlin, "The Dissection Riot of 1824 and the Connecticut Anatomical Law," *Yale Journal of Biology and Medicine* 7 (1934–1935): 275–89.
61. Ibid.
62. Wilcox to Humphreys, January 14, 1828, Connecticut Historical Society, Manuscripts, MS 73008.
63. Hamlin, "The Dissection Riot of 1824," 275–89.
64. Hayward, "Nathan Smith (1762–1829), Politician."
65. P. A. Jewett, *A Semi-Centennial History of the General Hospital Society of Connecticut* (New Haven: Tuttle Morehouse, 1876), 29.
66. Ibid., 4.
67. Welch, "The Relation of Yale to Medicine."

68. B. F. Corwin, "The Early Years of the Yale Medical School," *Yale Medical Journal* 1–2 (1894–1896): 210–13.
69. Thomas Cooper, *An Address Delivered before the Medical Board of South Carolina, at Columbia, December 1821* (Columbia: Gazette Office, 1821), 4.
70. H. Thoms, "Some Letters of Edmund Randolph Peaslee, B. A. Dartmouth 1836, M.D. Yale 1840," *Yale Journal of Biology and Medicine* 17 (1944–1945): 685–704.
71. Samuel Harvey, "Peter Parker: Initiator of Modern Medicine in China," *Yale Journal of Biology and Medicine* 8, no. 3 (1935): 225–52.
72. Peter Parker, letter to his mother and sister, November 25, 1831, cited in George B. Stevens, *The Life, Letters, and Journal of the Reverend and Hon. Peter Parker, M.D.* (Boston and Chicago: Congregational Sunday School and Publishing Society, 1896), 57.
73. Elizabeth H. Thomson, "Peter Parker," *Yale Medicine* (Summer 1979).
74. G. T. Lay, "Hospitals at Canton and Macao," *Boston Medical and Surgical Journal* 24 (1841): 137–39.
75. James Jackson et al., "Medical Missionary Society of China," *Boston Medical and Surgical Journal* 24 (1841): 176–78.
76. Stevens, *The Life, Letters, and Journals of Peter Parker,* 188.
77. Stevens, *The Life, Letters, and Journals of Peter Parker.*

CHAPTER 3: HARD TIMES

1. Silliman to Day, August 11, 1838, Yale Medical School Miscellaneous Papers, 1810–1884, Cushing/Whitney Medical Library, Yale University.
2. Whitfield Bell, "The Medical Institution of Yale College, 1810–1885," *Yale Journal of Biology and Medicine* 33 (1960): 160–83.
3. Francis Bacon, "The Practice of Medicine and Surgery," in *A History of the City of New Haven to the Present Time,* ed. E. E. Atwater (New York: Munsell, 1887).
4. H. Thoms, "Some Letters of Edmund Randolph Peaslee, B.A. Dartmouth, 1836, M.D. Yale 1840," *Yale Journal of Biology and Medicine* 17 (1944–1945): 685–704.
5. Howard Jones, *Mutiny on the Amistad* (New York and Oxford: Oxford University Press, 1987).
6. Toby Appel, personal communication. *Resolutions of the General Assembly incorporating the Connecticut Homeopathic Medical Society, the organization of said society, its officers, its bylaws, resolutions, and other proceedings with a list of homeopathic physicians and a sketch of the Conn. Homeopathic Society* (New Haven: Tuttle, Morehouse and Taylor, 1864).
7. *Catalogue of the Officers and Graduates of Yale University, 1701–1924* (New Haven: Yale University, 1924).
8. Editorial, "Yale and Medicine," *Yale Medical Journal* 2 (1904–1905): 259–60.
9. Bell, "The Medical Institution," 175.
10. *Medical Institution of Yale College,* February 1835 (leaflet).

11. *Yale College Catalogue,* 1865–1866.
12. Jerome Van Cortland Smith, editorial, *Boston Medical and Surgical Journal* 20 (1839): 16–17.
13. Frederick Rudolph, *The American College and University: A History* (Athens: University of Georgia Press, 1990), 231–32.
14. William P. Blake, ed., *History of the Town of Hamden, Connecticut* (New Haven: Price, Lee, 1888), 252–53.
15. William Beaumont, *Experiments and Observations on the Gastric Juice, and the Physiology of Digestion* (Plattsburgh: N.Y.: F. P. Allen, 1833), 7.
16. W. L. Kingsley, ed., *Yale College,* vol. 2: *The Sheffield Scientific School,* by T. R. Lounsbury (New Haven: 1879), 105–13.
17. C. R. Burns, "History of Medical Ethics," in *Encyclopedia of Bioethics,* ed. W. T. Reich, 4 vols. (New York: Free Press, 1978), 3: 966.
18. David F. Musto, "Worthington Hooker (1806–1867): Physician and Educator," *Connecticut Magazine* 48 (1994): 569–74.
19. Gardner to Lindsley, December 17, 1863, Yale Medical School Miscellaneous Papers, 1810–1884, Cushing/Whitney Medical Library, Yale University.
20. Bacon, "The Practice of Medicine and Surgery," 260–80.
21. Asa Hill to President and Faculty of Yale, November 2, 1865, Yale Medical School Miscellaneous Papers, 1810–1884, Cushing/Whitney Medical Library, Yale University.
22. Lindsley to Woolsey, July 20, 1868, Yale Medical School Miscellaneous Papers, 1810–1884, Cushing/Whitney Medical Library, Yale University.
23. Timothy Dwight, *Yale College: Some Thoughts Respecting Its Future* (New Haven: Tuttle, Morehouse and Taylor, 1871), 61.
24. A Memorial to the President and Fellows of Yale College in New Haven from the Faculty of the Medical Department, March 25, 1873, Yale Medical School Miscellaneous Papers, 1810–1884. Cushing/Whitney Medical Library, Yale University.
25. Henry Beecher and Mark Altschule, *Medicine at Harvard: The First 300 Years* (Hanover, N.H.: University Press of New England, 1977).
26. H. J. Bigelow, *Medical Education in America* (Cambridge, Mass.: Welch, Bigelow, 1871), 79.
27. A Memorial to the President and Fellows of Yale College in New Haven, June 24, 1873, Yale Medical School, Miscellaneous Papers, 1810–1884, Cushing/Whitney Medical Library, Yale University.
28. Rosemary Stevens, *American Medicine and the Public Interest: A History of Specialization* (Berkeley: University of California Press, 1998).
29. Memorial of the Medical Faculty, March 25, 1873, Yale Medical School Miscellaneous Papers, 1810–1884, Cushing/Whitney Medical Library, Yale University.
30. Lindsley to Porter, December 8, 1874, Yale Medical School Miscellaneous Papers, 1810–1884, Cushing/Whitney Medical Library, Yale University.

31. Lindsley to the Prudential Committee of Yale College, September 18, 1875, Yale Medical School Miscellaneous Papers, 1810–1884, Cushing/Whitney Medical Library, Yale University.
32. Smith to Porter, March 8, 1873, Yale Medical School Miscellaneous Papers 1810–1884, Cushing/Whitney Medical Library, Yale University.
33. S. C. Harvey, "Master Surgeons of America" *Surgery, Gynecology, and Obstetrics* 54 (1932): 254.
34. Dexter to Lindsley, June 27, 1878, Yale Corporation Letters, Yale Medical School Miscellaneous Papers, 1810–1884, Cushing/Whitney Medical Library, Yale University.
35. Report of General Assembly of the State Senate and House of Representatives, May 1866, Yale Medical School Miscellaneous Papers, 1810–1884, Cushing/Whitney Medical Library, Yale University.
36. By-laws for the Government of the Medical Department of Yale College, 1875, Yale Medical School Miscellaneous Papers, 1810–1884, Cushing/Whitney Medical Library, Yale University.
37. Connecticut State Legislature, House Bill no. 95, file 24, Yale Medical School Miscellaneous Papers, 1810–1884, Cushing/Whitney Medical Library, Yale University.
38. W. Welch, "The Relation of Yale to Medicine," *Yale Medical Journal* 8, no. 5 (1901): 143.
39. *Sixty-seventh Annual Announcement of the Medical Department of Yale College, 1879–1880* (New Haven: Tuttle, Morehouse and Taylor, 1879), 3.
40. H. Merkel, "The University of Michigan Medical School, 1850–2000," *JAMA* 283: 915–20.
41. Yandell Henderson, "The Medical School," *Yale Alumni Weekly,* February 13, 1907.
42. Ibid.
43. Medical Faculty Minutes, June 19 and July 21, 1877, Yale Medical School Miscellaneous Papers, 1810–1884, Cushing/Whitney Medical Library, Yale University.
44. Bronson et al., Letter to the Corporation, June 1879, Cushing/Whitney Medical Library, Yale University.
45. William H. Carmalt, "The Second Half Century of the General Hospital Society of Connecticut," in *General Hospital Society of Connecticut Centenary* (New Haven: Tuttle, Morehouse, and Taylor, 1926), 57–108.
46. Prudden to Dexter, July 6, 1880, Yale Medical School Miscellaneous Papers, 1810–1884, Cushing/Whitney Medical Library, Yale University.
47. Ibid.
48. White to Porter, Yale Medical School Miscellaneous Papers, 1810–1884, Cushing/Whitney Medical Library, Yale University.
49. White to Prudential Committee, June 21, 1882, Yale Medical School Miscellaneous Papers, 1810–1884. Cushing/Whitney Medical Library, Yale University.
50. Chamberlain to Porter, March 12, 1883, Yale Medical School Miscellaneous Papers, 1810–1884, Cushing/Whitney Medical Library.

51. Medical Faculty, Memorial to the President and Fellows of Yale College, a confidential printed memorandum, June 1882, Yale University Library, Manuscripts and Archives, Records of the President.
52. Porter to Faculty, December 17, 1885, Yale Medical School Miscellaneous Papers, Cushing/Whitney Medical Library, Yale University.
53. Medical Faculty, Memorial to the President and Fellows of Yale College, a confidential printed memorandum, June 1882, Yale University Library, Manuscripts and Archives, Records of the President.
54. William Osler, *Aphorisms from His Bedside Teachings and Writings,* ed. W. B. Bean (Springfield, Ill.: Thomas, 1961), 127.
55. Medical Faculty, Memorial to the President and Fellows of Yale College, June 1882, Yale University Library, Manuscripts and Archives, Records of the President.
56. Henderson, "The Medical School," *Yale Alumni Weekly,* February 13, 1907.
57. Timothy Dwight, *Yale College: Some Thoughts Respecting the Future* (New Haven, 1871).
58. Dwight, Report of the President, 1886–1887, Yale University Library, Manuscripts and Archives, Records of the President.
59. Ibid., 35.
60. Minute Book of the Yale Medical Society, 10th Anniversary, Cushing/Whitney Medical Library, Yale University.
61. Editorial, *Yale Medical Journal* 1–2 (1894): 31–34.
62. *Yale Medical Journal* 6 (1899–1900): 166–71.
63. *Yale Medical Journal* 12 (1905–1906): 953–55.
64. *Yale Medical Journal* 15 (1908–1909): 421–23, 232–34.
65. *Yale Medical Journal* 4 (1897–1898): 452–56.
66. R. H. Chittenden, "The Importance of Physiological Chemistry as a Part of Medical Education," *New York Medical Journal* 58 (1893): 370–74.
67. Dwight, Report of the President for Year Ending December 31, 1893, Yale University Library, Manuscripts and Archives, Records of the President.
68. Carmalt, "The Second Half Century," 66.
69. George Pierson, *Yale College, An Educational History, 1871–1921,* 2 vols. (New Haven: Yale University Press, 1952), 1: 106 and 1: 99.
70. Bacon, "The Practice of Medicine and Surgery."
71. Welch, "The Relation of Yale to Medicine," 127–58.
72. Smith to Welch, October 5, 1901, Yale University Library, Manuscripts and Archives, School of Medicine, Records of the Dean.
73. Welch to Emma Welch Walcott, June 15, 1901, Chesney Archives, Johns Hopkins Medical Institutions.
74. Welch, "The Relation of Yale to Medicine," 127–58.
75. George Blumer, "Reminiscences of an Old-Time Doctor," *Yale Journal of Biology and Medicine* 28 (1955–1956): 1–28.

76. John Spangler Nicholas, "Ross Granville Harrison, 1870–1959," *Yale Journal of Biology and Medicine* 32 (1960): 407–12.
77. Carmalt to Delavan, August 1906, Yale University Library, Manuscripts and Archives, School of Medicine, Records of the Dean, YRG 27-A, RU 285, box 102, folder 2410.
78. Blumer, "Reminiscences of an Old-Time Doctor," 1–28.
79. Cushing to Hadley, April 30, 1906, Yale University Library, Manuscripts and Archives, Records of the President, YRG 2-A-13, box 23, folder 469.
80. Ibid.
81. *Yale Medical Journal* 9 (1902): 247–48.
82. Cushing to Hadley, April 30, 1906.
83. Hadley to Cushing, February 7, 1907, Yale University Library, Manuscripts and Archives, Records of the President, YRG 2-A-13, box 23, folder 469.
84. Cushing to Hadley, March 21, 1907, Yale University Library, Manuscripts and Archives, Records of the President, YRG 2-A-13, box 23, folder 469.
85. *The New Haven Union,* October 5, 1913.
86. Address by the Rev. Edward Stone, Papers of Dr. William Verdi, Saint Raphael's Health Care System, Archives and Manuscripts, RG 420.
87. Newspaper clipping, origin unknown, February 2, 1907, Printed Material Scrapbook, 1905–1930, Saint Raphael's Health Care System, Archives and Manuscripts.
88. Report on Service of Attendings, New Haven Hospital Board of Directors Meeting, 1909–1910.
89. Herbert E. Smith, To the President and Fellows of Yale University, May 1905, Dean 285, box 103, folder 2410.
90. Herbert E. Smith, To the Committee of the Corporation, May 1906, Dean 285, box 103 folder 2410.
91. Carmalt, "The Second Half Century," 77.
92. Samuel C. Harvey, "Joseph Marshall Flint," *Yale Journal of Biology and Medicine* 17 (1945): 506.
93. Everett Gleason Hill, *A Modern History of New Haven* 2 vols. (New York: S. J. Clarke, 1918), 34–37.

CHAPTER 4: FLEXNER'S REPORT AND BLUMER'S DEANSHIP

1. Abraham Flexner did not have a doctoral degree.
2. Yale University Library, Manuscripts and Archives, Records of the Corporation, March 21, 1910.
3. Flexner's review was entitled *The American College: A Criticism* (New York: Century, 1908).

4. Abraham Flexner, *Medical Education in the United States and Canada: A Report to the Carnegie Foundation for the Advancement of Teaching* (New York: Century, 1910).
5. Flexner, *Medical Education in the United States and Canada.*
6. Hadley to Cushing, June 6, 1906, and Cushing to Hadley, June 16, 1906, Yale University Library, Manuscripts and Archives, Medical School Minutes, YRG 27-00, box 1, folder 4.
7. Blumer to Hadley, January 30, 1910, George Blumer Papers, Yale University Library, Manuscripts and Archives, MS 1274.
8. Smith to Stokes, June 30, 1910, Yale University Library, Manuscripts and Archives, Records of the Secretary, YRG 4-A, series 11, box 117, folder 1530.
9. Records of the Corporation, June 20, 1910, Yale University Library, Manuscripts and Archives.
10. Cushing to Hadley, April 30, 1906, Yale University Library, Manuscripts and Archives, YRG 2A-131, box 23, folder 469.
11. George Blumer, "Brief Recollections of the Yale Medical School (1906–1920)," *Yale Journal of Biology and Medicine* 21 (May 1946).
12. Stokes, Minutes of the Yale Corporation (Draft), Yale University Library, Manuscripts and Archives, Records of the Secretary, YRG 4-A (9–12), series 2, box 11, folder 158.
13. George Blumer, *Yale Alumni Weekly* 19, no. 39 (1913): 976.
14. Blumer to Stokes, March 4, 1911, Yale University Library, Manuscripts and Archives, Records of the Secretary, YRG 4-A (9–12), series 2, box 11, folder 158.
15. Blumer to Stokes, March 9, 1911, Yale University Library, Manuscripts and Archives, Records of the Secretary, YRG 4-A (9–12), series 2, box 2, folder 158.
16. Third- and fourth-year medical students on clinical rotations are still called "clinical clerks."
17. George Blumer, "The Relation of the Medical School to the Hospital," September 26, 1911, Stokes Papers, Yale University Library, Manuscripts and Archives, Records of the Secretary, YRG 4-A, series 2, box 11, folder 158.
18. Cushing to Hadley, April 30, 1906, Yale University Library, Manuscripts and Archives, Records of the President, YRG 2A-B, series 1, box 23, folder 469.
19. Minutes, General Hospital Society, January 26, 1912.
20. Blumer, Minutes, General Hospital Society, April 2, 1911.
21. Minutes, General Hospital Society, January 26, 1912.
22. Records of the Secretary, November 14, 1911, Yale University Library, Manuscripts and Archives, YRG 4-A (9–12), box 11, folder 158.
23. E. I. Kohorn, "The Department of Obstetrics and Gynecology at Yale: The First One Hundred Fifty Years, from Nathan Smith to Lee Buxton," *Yale Journal of Biology and Medicine* 66 (1993): 85–106.

24. Finance and Administration, March 3, 1894, Yale University Library, Manuscripts and Archives, Records of the Treasurer, YRG 5, series 6, box 378, folder 100.
25. Minutes, 1913, Yale University Library, Manuscripts and Archives, Records of the Corporation.
26. Flexner to Stokes, May 31, 1913, Yale University Library, Manuscripts and Archives, Records of the Secretary, YRG 4-A (9–12), series 2, box 50, folder 644.
27. Flexner to Stokes, June 14, 1914, Yale University Library, Manuscripts and Archives, Records of the Treasurer, YRG 5-B, series 2, box 332, folder 2170.
28. Blumer to Stokes, Yale University Library, Manuscripts and Archives, Records of the Treasurer, YRG 5-B, series 2, box 332, folder 2170.
29. Stokes to Rockefeller Foundation, April 22, 1914, General Education Board, box 635, folder 6661, Rockefeller Foundation Archives, Rockefeller Archive Center, North Tarrytown, New York (hereafter designated RAC).
30. GEB Refusal of Support 1914, Eben Sage GPD, January 23, 1914, General Education Board, box 635, Rockefeller Foundation Archives, RAC.
31. Jordan M. Prutkin, "Abraham Flexner and the Development of the School of Medicine," *Yale Journal of Biology and Medicine* 72 (1999): 269–79.
32. Cushing to Day, March 22, 1914, Yale University Library, Manuscripts and Archives, Records of the Treasurer.
33. Confidential Letter from Committee on Medical School Development appointed by Alumni Advisory Board, Yale University Library, Manuscripts and Archives, Records of the Treasurer, YRG 5-B, series 3, box 332, folder 2170.
34. Blumer to Stokes, April 7, 1914, Yale University Library, Manuscripts and Archives, Records of the Secretary, YRG 4, series 2, box 11, folder 160.
35. George P. Day, "A Statement in Regard to the Present Position of the Yale Medical School, and Its Great and Unique Opportunity," Treasurer's records YRG 5B, series 3, box 332, folder 2170.
36. AMA Council on Medical Education, *Third Classification of Medical Colleges,* AMA June 22, 1914.
37. A. E. Baue, "Joseph Marshall Flint and the Whole-Time System at Yale," *Yale Journal of Biology and Medicine* 51 (1978): 549–63.
38. Welch to Hadley, May 9, 1914, Yale University Library, Manuscripts and Archives, Records of the Treasurer, YRG-5-B, box 332, folder 2170.
39. Suggestions for Committee on Honorary Degrees, Yale University Library, Manuscripts and Archives, Records of the Secretary, YRG 4-A, series 2, box 64, folder 841.
40. *Memorial of the Centennial of the Yale Medical School, 1814–1914* (New Haven: Yale University Press, 1915).
41. Blumer to Stokes, January 13, 1915, Yale University Library, Manuscripts and Archives, Records of the Secretary, YRG 4, series 2, box 11, folder 161.

42. Blumer to Stokes, January 13, 1915, Yale University Library, Manuscripts and Archives, Records of the Secretary, YRG 4, box 11, folder 161.
43. Report of the Committee on the Full-time Professorship in Clinical Subjects, Yale University Library, Manuscripts and Archives, Records of the Secretary, YRG 4-1, series 2, box 11, folder 161.
44. Lewellys Barker, "Reforms in Medical Education," *Journal of the American Medical Association* 57 (1911): 613–621.
45. Cushing to Hadley, April 30, 1906, Yale University Library, Manuscripts and Archives, Records of the President, YRG 2A-13, series 1, box 23, folder 469.
46. The incursion of managed care and the continuing downward pressure on physician reimbursement has made it increasingly difficult for academic clinicians to generate sufficient clinical income and maintain their teaching and research commitments.
47. Stokes to Blumer, January 23, 1915, Yale University Library, Manuscripts and Archives, Records of the Secretary, YRG 4-A, series 2, box 12.
48. Blumer to Stokes, January 26, 1915, Yale University Library, Manuscripts and Archives, Records of the Secretary, YRG 4, box 11, folder 161.
49. Stokes to Flexner, January 26, 1915, Yale University Library, Manuscripts and Archives, Records of the Secretary, YRG 4-A, series 2, RU 49, box 11, folder 644.
50. Blumer to Stokes, February 10, 1915, Yale University Library, Manuscripts and Archives, Records of the Secretary, YRG 4, series 2, box 11, folder 161.
51. Yale Corporation Minutes, April 19, 1915, Yale University Library, Manuscripts and Archives, Records of the Corporation, YRG 1, p. 609.
52. Blumer to Flexner, March 20, 1915, General Education Board, box 635, Rockefeller Foundation Archives, RAC.
53. Smythe to Hadley, March 15, 1915, Yale University Library, Manuscripts and Archives, Records of the Secretary, YRG 4, box 11, folder 161.
54. Blumer to Stokes, April 19, 1915, Yale University Library, Manuscripts and Archives, Records of the Secretary.
55. "Limiting the Usefulness of College Professors," *Commercial and Financial Chronicle* 99, no. 2574, General Education Board, box 635, folder 6661, Rockefeller Foundation Archives, RAC.
56. Report of the Committee on a five-year medical course, October 20, 1914, Yale University Library, Manuscripts and Archives, School of Medicine, Records of the Dean, YRG 27-00, box 2, folder 6.
57. E. Blackwell, *Pioneer Work for Women* (New York: E. P. Dutton, 1914).
58. M. R. Walsh, *Doctors Wanted: No Woman Need Apply* (New Haven: Yale University Press, 1977).
59. W. Osler, "Harvard Medical Alumni Association," *Boston Medical and Surgical Journal* 131 (1894): 136.

60. Farnam to Hadley, March 31, 1916, Yale University Library, Manuscripts and Archives, Records of the President, YRG 2-A, box 31, folder 186.
61. S. J. Baserga, "The Early Years of Coeducation at the Yale University School of Medicine," *Yale Journal of Biology and Medicine* 53 (1980): 181–90.
62. S. J. Baserga, "Ella Clay Wakeman: Yale School of Medicine, 1921," *Yale Journal of Biology and Medicine* 68 (1995): 171–90.
63. *Yale Law Report* 34, no. 2 (Spring 1988): 26.
64. Detra MacDougall, Registrar, Yale Divinity School, personal communication, July 2000.
65. Hadley to Fisher, March 12 and 13, 1908, Yale University Library, Manuscripts and Archives, Records of the President.
66. *Yale Daily News,* September 29, 1916.
67. Blumer to Day, June 15, 1915, Yale University Library, Manuscripts and Archives, Records of the Treasurer, YRG 5-B, series 3, box 332, folder 2120.
68. Blumer to Hadley, February 28, 1917, Yale University Library, Manuscripts and Archives, Records of the President, YRG 2-A, RU 25, box 9, folder 164.
69. Blumer to Day, June 15, 1915.
70. Day, March 1, 1915, Yale University Library, Manuscripts and Archives, Records of the Treasurer, YRG 5-B, series 3, box 332, folder 2170.
71. Blumer to Stokes, December 16, 1916, Yale University Library, Manuscripts and Archives, Records of the Secretary, YRG 4, box 12, folder 162.
72. Ibid.
73. Ibid.
74. Blumer to Stokes, April 12, 1917, Yale University Library, Manuscripts and Archives, Records of the Secretary, YRG 4 series 2, box 12, folder 162.
75. Minutes of the Yale Corporation, April 16, 1917, Yale University Library, Manuscripts and Archives, Records of the Corporation, YRG 1, no. 879.
76. Stokes to Flexner, April 19, 1917, General Education Board, box 635, Rockefeller Foundation Archives, RAC.
77. *Yale Alumni Weekly* 27, no. 24, March 1, 1918.
78. Day to Blumer, November 24, 1917, Yale University Library, Manuscripts and Archives, Records of the Secretary, YRG 5B-3, box 352, folder 2430.
79. George Blumer, "The Yale School of Medicine," supplement to *Yale Alumni Weekly,* March 1, 1918.
80. Blumer to Hadley, February 28, 1917, Yale University Library, Manuscripts and Archives, Records of the President, YRG 2-A, RU 25, box 9, folder 164. Blumer to Hadley, March 1, 1917, Yale University Library, Manuscripts and Archives, Records of the President, YRG 2-A, RU 25, box 9, folder 184.
81. Stokes to Blumer, December 19, 1917, Yale University Library, Manuscripts and Archives, Records of the Secretary, YRG 4-A, series 1, box 27, folder 62.
82. Report to the Executive Committee of the New Haven Hospital, April 22,

1918, General Education Board, box 635, Dr. Winford H. Smith, Rockefeller Foundation Archives, RAC.

83. Samuel C. Harvey, "Joseph Marshall Flint," *Yale Journal of Biology and Medicine* 17 (1945): 503–15.
84. Joseph Marshall Flint, "The Yale Mobile Hospital Unit," in *Yale in the World War,* ed. George Henry Nettleton (New Haven: Yale University Press, 1925).
85. Report of the President and Secretary of Yale University, 1917.
86. Frank Pell Underhill, "The Army Chemical Unit," in *Yale in the World War,* ed. Nettleton.
87. Report of the President and Secretary of Yale University, 1917.
88. Hadley to Josephus Daniels, Yale University Library, Manuscripts and Archives, Records of the President, YRG 2A-13, box 32.
89. Snow to Blumer, December 28, 1919.
90. Report of the President and the Secretary of Yale University, 1920.
91. William H. Carmalt, "The Second Half Century of the General Hospital Society of Connecticut," in *General Hospital Society of Connecticut Centenary* (New Haven: Tuttle, Morehouse, and Taylor, 1926), 98.
92. Blumer to Fenn, November 20, 1918, New Haven Hospital Minutes.
93. Blumer to Stokes, January 11, 1919, Yale University Library, Manuscripts and Archives, Records of the Secretary, YRG 4, series 2, box 12, folder 163.
94. Blumer to Stokes, January 30, 1919, Yale University Library, Manuscripts and Archives, Records of the Secretary, YRG 4, series 2, box 12.
95. Stokes to Ullman, March 12, 1919, Yale University Library, Manuscripts and Archives, Records of the Treasurer, YRG 5-B, series 2, box 352, folder 2430.
96. Stokes to Ullman, April 23, 1919, Yale University Library, Manuscripts and Archives, Records of the Treasurer, YRG 5-B, series 3, box 352, folder 2430.
97. Memorandum to the Yale Corporation on the Development of the Yale Medical School, Yale University Library, Manuscripts and Archives, Records of the Secretary, YRG 4-A, series 2, box 88, folder 1141.
98. Memorandum to the Yale Corporation on the Development of the Yale Medical School, Yale University Library, Manuscripts and Archives, Records of the Secretary, YRG 4-A, series 2, box 88, folder 1141.
99. Blumer, Memorandum on the Meeting at Mr. Stokes, CC BPO, June 4, 1919, Yale University Library, Manuscripts and Archives, Records of the Secretary, YRG 4-A, series 2, box 12, folder 164.
100. Minutes, May 7, 1920, Records of the Hospital, Prudential Committee, YRG 37-Q-1.
101. Interview with George Parmly Day, Yale University Treasurer, April 6, 1920, General Education Board, box 635, Rockefeller Foundation Archives, RAC.
102. Blumer to Hadley, February 18, 1920, Yale University Library, Manuscripts

and Archives, Records of the President, YRG 2-A-13, series 1, box 9, folder 166.

103. Flexner to Stokes, April 17, 1919, General Education Board, box 635, folder 6662, Rockefeller Foundation Archives, RAC.
104. Flexner to Blumer, May 28, 1920, Yale University Library, Manuscripts and Archives, Records of the President, YRG 2-A-13, box 34, folder 657.
105. Meeting of the Administrative Subcommittee, July 9, 1920, Yale University Library, Manuscripts and Archives, Records of the Hospital, YRG 37-Q-1.
106. Blumer to Hadley, October 7, 1919, Yale University Library, Manuscripts and Archives, Records of the President, YRG 2-A, box 9, folder 166.
107. Blumer to Flexner, March 9, 1920, General Education Board, box 635, Rockefeller Foundation Archives, RAC.
108. Flexner to Flexner, March 12, 1920, General Education Board, box 635, folder 66630, Rockefeller Foundation Archives, RAC.
109. Report to the President and the Secretary of Yale University, 1920, School of Medicine, Report of the Dean.
110. News Release, March 1, 1920, Yale University Library, Manuscripts and Archives, Records of the Secretary, YRG 4-A-9-12, series 2, box 12, folder 167.

CHAPTER 5: "A STEAM ENGINE IN PANTS"

1. May 7, 1920, Minutes of the Board of Permanent Officers of the Yale University School of Medicine, Cushing/Whitney Medical Library, Historical Library, Archives.
2. A. A. Liebow and L. L. Waters, "Milton Charles Winternitz, February 19, 1885–October 3, 1959," *Yale Journal of Biology and Medicine* 32 (1959): 143–72.
3. Ibid.
4. John F. Fulton, "Some Notes on the Yale University School of Medicine with Special Reference to Milton Winternitz," *Yale Journal of Biology and Medicine* 22 (1950): 590.
5. J. R. Paul, "Dean Winternitz and the Rebirth at Yale Medical School in the 1920's," *Yale Journal of Biology and Medicine* 43 (1970): 110.
6. Susan Cheever, *Treetops* (New York: Bantam Books, 1991).
7. Liebow and Waters, "Milton Charles Winternitz."
8. Paul, "Dean Winternitz," 110–19.
9. Cheever, *Treetops.*
10. R. Yesner, "A Century of Pathology at Yale: Personal Reflections," *Yale Journal of Biology and Medicine* 71 (1998): 397–408.
11. Watson to Winternitz, March 28, 1917, Yale University Library, Manuscripts and Archives, Milton C. Winternitz Papers, manuscript group 859, box 2.

12. Abraham Flexner, *I Remember: The Autobiography of Abraham Flexner* (New York: Simon and Schuster, 1940), 258.
13. Dan A. Oren, *Joining the Club: A History of Jews and Yale* (New Haven: Yale University Press, 1985), 144.
14. Joseph S. Fruton, *Eighty Years* (New Haven: Epikouros Press, 1994).
15. Seymour to Taft, December 16, 1920, Yale University Library, Manuscripts and Archives, George Dudley Seymour Papers, manuscript group 442, box 29, folder 287.
16. M. G. Synott, *The Half-Opened Door* (Westport, Conn.: Greenwood Press, 1979).
17. M. C. Winternitz, *Collected Studies on the Pathology of War Gas Poisoning* (New Haven: Yale University Press, 1920).
18. M. C. Winternitz, Isabel M. Wason, and Frank P. McNamara, *The Pathology of Influenza* (New Haven: Yale University Press, 1920).
19. Angell, Report of the President of Yale University, 1934–1935, 15.
20. Arthur J. Viseltear, "Milton C. Winternitz and the Yale Institute of Human Relations: A Brief Chapter in the History of Social Medicine," *Yale Journal of Biology and Medicine* 57 (1984): 869–89.
21. Angell to Henderson, Yale University Library, Manuscripts and Archives, Records of the Office of the President, James R. Angell, YRG 2-A-14, RU 24, box 101, folder 1025.
22. George W. Pierson, *Yale: The University College, 1921–1937* (New Haven: Yale University Press, 1955), 260.
23. M. C. Winternitz, *The Past, Present, and Future of the Yale University School of Medicine and Affiliated Clinical Institutions, Including the New Haven Hospital, the New Haven Dispensary, and the Connecticut Training School for Nurses* (New Haven: Printed for the University, 1922).
24. George Pierson, *Yale College: An Educational History, 1871–1937* (New Haven: Yale University Press, 1952).
25. *Yale Alumni Weekly* 21, February 28, 1919.
26. Pierson, *Yale College,* 490.
27. Seymour to Fisher, March 19, 1920, Alumni Committee, Yale University Library, Manuscripts and Archives, Samuel H. Fisher Papers, manuscript group 213.
28. Pierson, *Yale College,* 5.
29. Ibid., 13. Pierson's footnote reads: "Conversations of G. W. P. with S. H. Fisher, 15 July 1940 and 14 October 1942." He notes that "whether these discussions took place at a formal or informal meeting of the Fellows I am not clear."
30. Ibid., 14.
31. Rosemary Stevens, *American Medicine and the Public Interest* (Berkeley: University of California Press, 1998).
32. Max Taffel, "Samuel Clark Harvey, 1886–1953," *Yale Journal of Biology and Medicine* 26 (1953): 261–67.

33. Liebow and Waters, "Milton Charles Winternitz."
34. Park to Angell, March 8, 1927, Yale University Library, Manuscripts and Archives, Records of the Office of the President, James R. Angell, YRG 2-A-14, RU 24, box 132, folder 1376.
35. Park to Angell, March 8, 1927.
36. Marion Hunt, "Extraordinarily Interesting and Happy Years: Martha M. Eliot and Pediatrics at Yale, 1921–1935," *Yale Journal of Biology and Medicine* 68 (1995): 159–70.
37. Murphy to Angell, May 5, 1927, Yale University Library, Manuscripts and Archives, Records of the President, James R. Angell, YRG 2-A-14, RU 24, box 132, folder 1376.
38. Angell to Murphy, Yale University Library, Manuscripts and Archives, Records of the Office of the President, James R. Angell, YRG 2-A-14, RU 24, box 132, folder 1376.
39. Winternitz, *The Past, Present, and Future,* 7.
40. Flexner to Winternitz, February 24, 1920, General Education Board, box 635, folder 6633, Rockefeller Foundation Archives, RAC.
41. Winternitz, *The Past, Present, and Future,* 2.
42. Table, November 1922, General Education Board, box 635, folder 6668, Rockefeller Foundation Archives, RAC.
43. Oren, *Joining the Club,* 148.
44. Winternitz to Postal, December 4, 1934, Yale University Library, Manuscripts and Archives, Records of the Dean of the School of Medicine, YRG 27-A-[5–9], RU 285, box 100, folder 2367.
45. Miriam K. Dasey, "Selection of Students for Admission to the Yale School of Medicine: Procedure," October 13, 1934, and February 1, 1935, Yale University Library, Manuscripts and Archives, Records of the Dean of the School of Medicine, YRG 27-A, RU 285, box 4, folders 55–58.
46. Winternitz, Yale University School of Medicine, Report of the Dean, 1921–1922.
47. Winternitz, Yale University School of Medicine, Report of the Dean, 1924–1925.
48. Raymond Hussey, "The Study of Medicine at Yale," *Yale Journal of Biology and Medicine* 1 (October 1928): 18–21.
49. Milton C. Winternitz, "The Relationship of the Medical School and Nursing School in the University," Yale University Library, Manuscripts and Archives, Records of the Dean of the School of Medicine, YRG 27-A, RU 285, box 99, folder 2362.
50. Report to Board of Permanent Officers on a University School of Nursing, 1921–1922, Cushing/Whitney Medical Library, Historical Library, Archives.
51. Minutes, November 20, 1920, Yale University Library, Manuscripts and Archives, Minutes of the Yale University Corporation and the Prudential Committee, ca. 1701-1999, RU 307.

52. C.-E. A. Winslow, *Dean Winternitz and the Yale School of Medicine: An Address before the Association of Yale Alumni in Medicine on 17 June 1935* (New Haven: Yale University Press, 1935).
53. Hadley to Flexner, Yale University Library, Manuscripts and Archives, Records of the Office of the President, Arthur T. Hadley, YRG 2-A-13, RU 25, series 2, box 134.
54. May 27, 1921, Yale University Library, Manuscripts and Archives, Records of the Office of the President, Arthur T. Hadley, YRG 2-A-13, RU 25, series 1, box 34, folder 657.
55. Flexner, *I Remember,* 259.
56. Minutes of the New Haven Hospital Executive Committee, September 13, 1920, Yale University Library, Manuscripts and Archives, Records of Yale–New Haven Hospital (and earlier organizations), YRG 37-Q-1, RU 480.
57. Flexner to Wilbur, July 24, 1924, General Education Board, box 635, folder 6664, Rockefeller Foundation Archives, RAC.
58. Winternitz to Flexner, January 28, 1925, Yale University Library, Manuscripts and Archives, Milton C. Winternitz Papers, manuscript group 859.
59. Flexner to Winternitz, November 23, 1926, Yale University Library, Manuscripts and Archives, Milton C. Winternitz Papers, manuscript group 859.
60. Harvey Cushing, "Experimentum Periculosum; Judicium Difficile," *Science* 61 (April 10, 1925): 373–79.
61. Cushing, "Experimentum Periculosum."
62. John F. Fulton, *Harvey Cushing: A Biography* (Springfield, Ill.: C. C. Thomas, 1946).
63. Ibid.
64. Angell, Sterling Hall of Medicine Dedication 1925, Records of the President, Yale University Library, Manuscripts and Archives, YRG 2A, RU 24, box 135, folder 1425.
65. "Dedicate Sterling Hall of Medicine. Pres. Angell Accepts for University," *Yale Medicine* (Spring 1975): 16.
66. Liebow and Waters, "Milton Charles Winternitz," 151.
67. C.-E. A. Winslow, *Dean Winternitz and the School of Medicine.*
68. Winternitz, Report of the Dean, 1928–1929.
69. Viseltear, "Milton C. Winternitz and the Yale Institute of Human Relations," *Yale Journal of Biology and Medicine* 57 (1984): 869–89.
70. J. R. Angell, "Yale's Institute of Human Relations," *Yale Alumni Weekly,* April 1929.
71. Pierson, *Yale College, 1921–1937.*
72. Winternitz, Report of the Dean, 1927–1928.
73. R. H. Granger, "Yale Child Study Center, 1911–1999," Report of the Director of the Child Study Center, 1998–1999.

74. Arnold Gesell, *History of Psychology in Autobiography,* ed. E. G. Boring et al., vol. 4 (Worcester Mass.: Clark University Press, 1952), 126.
75. Abraham Flexner, *Universities: American, English, German* (New York: Oxford University Press, 1930).
76. Flexner to Angell, January 23, 1930, Yale University Library, Manuscripts and Archives, Records of the Office of the President, James R. Angell, YRG 2-A-14, RU 234, box 84, folder 835.
77. Flexner, *Universities: American, English, German.*
78. Flexner to Winternitz, February 12, 1929, Yale University Library, Manuscripts and Archives, Records of the Office of the Dean of the School of Medicine, Yale University Library, Manuscripts and Archives, YRG 27-A, RU 285, folders 1855–1856.
79. Flexner to Winternitz, April 10, 1930, Yale University Library, Manuscripts and Archives, Records of the Office of the Dean of the School of Medicine, Yale University Library, Manuscripts and Archives, YRG 27-A, RU 285, folders 1855–1856.
80. Flexner to Winternitz, May 12, 1930, Yale University Library, Manuscripts and Archives, Records of the Office of the Dean of the School of Medicine, Yale University Library, Manuscripts and Archives, YRG 27-A, RU 285, folders 1855–1856.
81. Winternitz to Flexner, January 20, 1931, Yale University Library, Manuscripts and Archives, Records of the Office of the Dean of the School of Medicine, Yale University Library, Manuscripts and Archives, YRG 27-A, RU 285, folders 1855–1856.
82. Angell to Vincent, March 21, 1930, Yale University Library, Manuscripts and Archives, Records of the Office of the President, James R. Angell, YRG 2-A-14, RU 24, box 114, folder 1169.
83. Flexner to Stokes, June 25, 1931, Library of Congress, Manuscripts Division, Abraham Flexner Papers, box 14.
84. Stokes to Flexner, June 29, 1931, Library of Congress, Manuscripts Division, Abraham Flexner Papers, box 14.
85. Flexner to Stokes, July 7, 1931, Records of the Office of the Secretary, Yale University Library, Manuscripts and Archives, YRG 4-A, RU 49, series 2, box 50, folders 644–46.
86. Flexner to Stokes, July 7, 1931, Records of the Office of the Secretary, Yale University Library, Manuscripts and Archives, YRG 4-A, RU 49, series 2, box 50, folders 644–46. See also Flexner to Winternitz, April 30, 1930, Records of the Office of the Dean of the School of Medicine, Yale University Library, Manuscripts and Archives, YRG 27-A, RU 285, folders 1855–1856. Flexner's letter states that "[Pearce] made recommendation as a means of helping psychiatry."
87. Stokes to Flexner, July 10, 1931, Abraham Flexner Papers, Manuscript Division, Library of Congress.

88. *Yale Alumni Weekly* 39, no. 25 (March 17, 1930).
89. "Buildings of the Yale School of Medicine," *Science* 71 (February 28, 1930): 235–36.
90. *Yale Alumni Weekly* 39, no. 25 (March 7, 1930).
91. Ibid., 683.
92. Winternitz, "Practical Study of Social Relations: Plan for a Graduate Department of Clinical Sociology at Yale," 1930, Yale University Library, Manuscripts and Archives, Records of the Dean of the School of Medicine, YRG 27-A, RU 285.
93. Winternitz, Yale University School of Medicine, Report of the Dean, 1927–1928.
94. Ibid.
95. Angell to Winternitz, December 3, 1930, Yale University Library, Manuscripts and Archives, Records of the Dean of the School of Medicine, YRG 27-A, RU 285, box 90, folder 1917.
96. Winternitz, Yale University School of Medicine, Report of the Dean, 1932–1933.
97. *Yale Daily News,* April 1, 1927.
98. Winternitz, Yale University School of Medicine, Report of the Dean, 1930–1931.
99. L. Davey, "John Farquhar Fulton," *Neurosurgery* 43 (1998): 185–87.
100. Liebow and Waters, "Milton Charles Winternitz," 150.
101. Cushing to Angell, June 13, 1932, Yale University Library, Manuscripts and Archives, Records of the Office of the President, James R. Angell, YRG 2-A-14, RU 24, box 56, folder 574.
102. Angell to Cushing, June 16, 1932, Yale University Library, Manuscripts and Archives, Records of the Office of the President, James R. Angell, YRG 2 A, RU 24, box 56, folder 574.
103. Lafayette B. Mendel Anniversary Issue, *Yale Journal of Biology and Medicine,* 1932.
104. M. W. Rossiter, "Mendel the Mentor," *Journal of Chemical Education* 71 (1994): 215–19.
105. Winternitz, Yale University School of Medicine, Report of the Dean, 1929–1930.
106. Murphy to Day, December 4, 1929, Yale University Library, Manuscripts and Archives, Records of the Dean of the School of Medicine, YRG 27-A, RU 285, box 94, folder 2138.
107. Cheever, *Treetops.*
108. Winternitz, Yale University School of Medicine, Report of the Dean, 1932–1933.
109. Winternitz, Yale University School of Medicine, Report of the Dean, 1931–1932.
110. *The Harkness Hoot* 1, nos. 5–6 (April–May, 1931).

111. "Joint Committee of the Connecticut State Medical Society and Yale University School of Medicine," Yale University Library, Manuscripts and Archives, Records of the Dean of the School of Medicine, YRG 27-A-[5–9], RU 285, box 136, folder 2992.
112. Winternitz, Yale University School of Medicine, Report of the Dean, 1929–1930.
113. Winternitz to Rice, March 26, 1934, Yale University Library, Manuscripts and Archives, Records of the Dean of the School of Medicine, YRG 27-A, RU 285, box 99, folder 2361.
114. National Conference on the Costs of Medical Care, New York Academy of Medicine, 1932.
115. Winternitz, "Medicine and the People," 1933, Yale University Library, Manuscripts and Archives, Records of the Dean of the School of Medicine, YRG 27-A, RU 285, box 99, folder 2326.
116. *New Haven Register,* June 4, 1934.
117. Winternitz, "Medicine and the People."
118. Winternitz, Memorandum, December 1, 1933, Yale University School of Medicine, 27 A, RU 285, box 99, folder 2363.
119. Winternitz, "A Study of General Practice," Yale University Library, Manuscripts and Archives, Records of the Dean of the School of Medicine, YRG 27-A, RU 285, box 99, folder 2363.
120. Gregg to Winternitz, December 27, 1933, Yale University Library, Manuscripts and Archives, Records of the Dean of the School of Medicine YRG 27-A-[5–9], RU 285, box 118, folder 2693.
121. Buckner to Buckner, January 23, 1934, Yale University Library, Manuscripts and Archives, Records of the Dean of the School of Medicine, YRG 27-A-[5–9], RU 285, box 118, folder 2693.
122. Report of the Committee on Clinical Subjects, Yale University Library, Manuscripts and Archives, Records of the Dean of the School of Medicine, YRG 27-A-[5–9], RU 285, box 90, folder 1187.
123. Angell, Report of the President of Yale University, 1933–1934.
124. Winternitz, Yale University School of Medicine, Report of the Dean, 1933–1934.
125. *Bulletin of Yale University,* no. 24 (September 1935).
126. Cushing to Angell, November 1, 1932, Yale University Library, Manuscripts and Archives, Records of the Office of the President, James R. Angell, YRG 2-A-14, RU 24, box 132, folder 1375.
127. Harvey to Angell, November 1, 1932, Yale University Library, Manuscripts and Archives, Samuel Clark Harvey papers, manuscript group 1244, series 1, box 1.
128. Angell, Memorandum, December 24, 1934, Yale University Library, Manuscripts and Archives, Records of the Office of the President, James R. Angell, YRG 2-A-14, RU 24, box 133, folder 1393.

129. Angell, Memorandum, December 24, 1934, Yale University Library, Manuscripts and Archives, Records of the Office of the President, James R. Angell, YRG 2 A, RU 24, box 133, folder 1393.
130. Angell, Memorandum, December 24, 1934, Yale University Library, Manuscripts and Archives, Records of the Office of the President, James R. Angell, YRG 2-A-14, RU 24, box 133, folder 1393.
131. Winternitz to Angell, January 4, 1935, Yale University Library, Manuscripts and Archives, Records of the Office of the President, James R. Angell, YRG 2-A-14, RU 24, box 194, folder 2119.
132. Cheever, *Treetops*, 58.
133. Flexner to Winternitz, January 16, 1935, Yale University Library, Manuscripts and Archives, Milton C. Winternitz Papers, manuscript group 859, box 5.
134. Angell, Report of the President of Yale University, 1934–1935.

CHAPTER 6: THE BUBBLE BURSTS

1. Winternitz to Angell, May 23, 1930, Yale University Library, Manuscripts and Archives, Records of the Office of the President, James R. Angell, YRG 2-A-14, RU 24, box 194, folder 2119.
2. Winternitz to Lohmann, June 8, 1931, Yale University Library, Manuscripts and Archives, Records of the Office of the President, James R. Angell, YRG 2-A-14, RU 24, box 133, folder 1384.
3. S. Bayne-Jones, Oral History, 1966, Yale University Library, Manuscripts and Archives, Stanhope Bayne-Jones Papers, manuscript group 1271, box 1, typescript vol. 3, 382.
4. Susan Cheever, *Treetops* (New York: Bantam Books, 1991), 55.
5. Bayne-Jones, Oral History, 383.
6. M. C. Leikind, "Stanhope Bayne-Jones: Physician, Teacher, Soldier, Scientist-Administrator, Friend of Medical Libraries," *Bulletin of New York Academic Medicine* 48, no. 3 (April 1972): 584–95.
7. Bayne-Jones, Oral History, 367.
8. Bayne-Jones, Yale University School of Medicine, Report of the Dean, 1935–1936.
9. Bayne-Jones, Yale University School of Medicine, Report of the Dean, 1935–1936.
10. Day to Fosdick, July 28, 1936, General Education Board, box 636, folder 6676, Rockefeller Foundation Archives, RAC.
11. Bayne-Jones, Yale University School of Medicine, Report of the Dean, 1935–1936.
12. Ibid.
13. January 18, 1936, Yale University Library, Manuscripts and Archives, Records of the Dean of the School of Medicine, YRG 27-A-[5–9], RU 285, box 14, folder 192.

14. Bayne-Jones, Yale University School of Medicine, Report of the Dean, 1935–1936.
15. In the 1935–1936 academic year, a total of 217 students were enrolled in the M.D. program, including eighteen women.
16. Bayne-Jones, Yale University School of Medicine, Report of the Dean, 1939–1940.
17. Enrollment figures compiled from *Bulletins of Yale University,* September 1935 to 1941.
18. Bayne-Jones, Yale University School of Medicine, Report of the Dean, 1935–1936.
19. Bayne-Jones, Yale University School of Medicine, Report of the Dean, 1936–1937.
20. The onslaught of managed care is dismantling the role of the physician in determining health care in the United States.
21. Bayne-Jones, Yale University School of Medicine, Report of the Dean, 1936–1937.
22. Angell to Winslow, July 9, 1937, Yale University Library, Manuscripts and Archives, C.-E. A. Winslow Papers, YMG 749, box 2, folder 39.
23. Bayne-Jones, Yale University School of Medicine, Report of the Dean, 1936–1937.
24. Schoolcraft to Bayne-Jones, July 8, 1938, Yale University Library, Manuscripts and Archives, Records of the Dean of the School of Medicine, YRG 27-A, RU 285, box 106, folder 2472.
25. Report of the New Haven Dispensary, November 19, 1931, Yale University Library, Manuscripts and Archives, Records of the Dean of the School of Medicine, YRG 27-A, RU 285, box 102, folder 2419.
26. Knight to Seymour, April 8, 1937, Yale University Library, Manuscripts and Archives, Records of the Office of the President, Charles Seymour, YRG 2-A-15, RU 23, box 109, folder 926.
27. The President's Committee on University Development, "Doctors for America," November 1938, Yale University Library, Manuscripts and Archives, Records of the Office of the President, Charles Seymour, YRG 2-A-15, RU 23, box 130, folder 1096.
28. Bayne-Jones to Seymour, January 7, 1938, Yale University Library, Manuscripts and Archives, Records of the Office of the President, Charles Seymour, YRG 2-A-15, RU 23, box 104, folder 882.
29. Bayne-Jones, Yale University School of Medicine, Report of the Dean, 1936–1937.
30. Bayne-Jones, Yale University School of Medicine, Report of the Dean, 1937–1938.
31. Stanhope Bayne-Jones Papers, Yale University Library, Manuscripts and Archives, manuscript group 1271, box 1, 1966.
32. Cheney to Bayne-Jones, October 15, 1937, Yale University Library,

Manuscripts and Archives, Records of the Dean of the School of Medicine, YRG 27-A-[5–9], RU 285, box 25, folder 350.

33. Bayne-Jones, Yale University School of Medicine, Report of the Dean.
34. Winternitz to Bayne-Jones, October 5, 1939, Yale University Library, Manuscripts and Archives, Records of the Dean of the Medical School, YRG 27-A-[5–9], RU 285, box 100, folder 7364.
35. January 19, 1938, Yale University Library, Manuscripts and Archives, Records of the Office of the President, Charles Seymour, YRG 2-A-15, RU 23, box 197, folder 907.
36. August 26, 1939, Yale University Library, Manuscripts and Archives, Records of the Office of the President, Charles Seymour, YRG 2-A-15, RU 23, box 107, folder 907.
37. *Time,* February 26, 1940, 70–71.
38. Bayne-Jones, Oral History, Yale University Library, Manuscripts and Archives, Stanhope Bayne-Jones Papers, YMG 1271, typescript vol. 4, 505.
39. M. Stanton, *The Making of a Library* (New Haven: Yale University Press, 1959).
40. Lewis, W. S., "Dedication of the Yale Medical Library," *Yale Journal of Biology and Medicine* 13 (1940–41): 865–68.
41. "Proposal for an Institute of Nutrition," November 15, 1939, Yale University Library, Manuscripts and Archives, Records of the Office of the President, Charles Seymour, YRG 2-A-15, RU 23, box 110, folder 935.
42. "Proposal for an Institute of Nutrition," November 15, 1939, Yale University Library, Manuscripts and Archives, Records of the Office of the President, Charles Seymour, YRG 2 A, RU 223, box 110, folder 935.
43. Seymour to Francis, May 29, 1939, Yale University Library, Manuscripts and Archives, Records of the Dean of the School of Medicine, YRG 27-A, RU 285, box 137, folder 3017.
44. Ibid.
45. Stanhope Bayne-Jones Papers, Yale University Library, Manuscripts and Archives, manuscript group 1271, box 1, 1966.
46. Ibid.
47. Dunn to Day, January 3, 1940, Yale University Library, Manuscripts and Archives, Records of the Dean of the School of Medicine, YRG 27A-[5–9], RU 285, box 137 folder 3007.
48. Bayne-Jones to Seymour, June 5, 1940, Yale University Library, Manuscripts and Archives, Records of the Dean of the School of Medicine, YRG 27-A-[5–9], RU 285, box 137, folder 3006.
49. Walderman Kaempffert, "Research in Nutrition," *New York Times,* January 4, 1942.
50. Bayne-Jones to Seymour, July 19, 1940, Yale University Library, Manuscripts and Archives, Records of the Office of the President, Charles Seymour, YRG 2-A-15, RU 23, box 104, folder 884.

51. Seymour to Gregg, February 15, 1940, Yale University Library, Manuscripts and Archives, Records of the Office of the President, Charles Seymour, YRG 2-A-15, RU 23, box 106, folder 904.
52. Winslow to Seymour, March 13, 1940, Yale University Library, Manuscripts and Archives, Records of the Office of the President, Charles Seymour, YRG 2-A-15, RU 23, box 106, folder 904.
53. Gregg to Seymour, March 19, 1940, Yale University Library, Manuscripts and Archives, C.-E. A. Winslow Papers, YMG 749, box 26, folder 664.

CHAPTER 7: THE MEDICAL SCHOOL GOES TO WAR

1. L. Pickett, Oral History, December 10, 1991, Yale University Library, Manuscripts and Archives, Oral History Tapes and Transcripts of the Griswold-Brewster Oral History Project, Yale University, 1990–1993, RU 217.
2. Pickett, Oral History, December 10, 1991, 29.
3. Bayne-Jones to Long, April 24, 1940, Yale University Library, Manuscripts and Archives, Records of the Office of the President, Charles Seymour, YRG 2-A-15, RU 23, box 130, folder 197.
4. Bayne-Jones to Gilman, Yale University Library, Manuscripts and Archives, Records of the Office of the President, Charles Seymour, YRG 2-A-15, RU 23, box 130, folder 937.
5. Blake, Yale University School of Medicine, Report of the Dean, 1940–1941.
6. Blake, Yale University School of Medicine, Report of the Dean, 1940–1941.
7. Yale University Library, Manuscripts and Archives, Records of the Office of the President, Charles Seymour, YRG 2-A-15, RU 23, box 106, folder 895.
8. Taylor to Seymour, May 5, 1941, Yale University Library, Manuscripts and Archives, Records of the Office of the President, Charles Seymour, YRG 2-A-15, RU 23, box 23, folder 117.
9. Taylor to Staupers, April 18, 1941, Yale University Library, Manuscripts and Archives, Records of the Office of the President, Charles Seymour, YRG 2-A-15, RU 23, box 23, folder 117.
10. Seymour to Stokes, May 8, 1941, Yale University Library, Manuscripts and Archives, Records of the Office of the President, Charles Seymour, YRG 2-A, RU 23, box 23, folder 117.
11. Blake, Yale University School of Medicine, Report of the Dean, 1940–1941.
12. Blake, Yale University School of Medicine, Report of the Dean, 1941–1942.
13. Blake, Yale University School of Medicine, Report of the Dean, 1941–1942.
14. Minutes of the Board of Permanent Officers of the Yale University School of Medicine, October 21, 1942, Cushing/Whitney Medical Library, Historical Library, Archives.
15. Minutes of the Board of Permanent Officers of the Yale University School of Medicine, June 2, 1942, Cushing/Whitney Medical Library, Historical Library, Archives.

16. Blake, Yale University School of Medicine, Report of the Dean, 1941–1942, 11.
17. Program of the 54th Annual Meeting of the Association of American Medical Colleges, October 25–27, 1943, Cleveland, Ohio.
18. Minutes of the Board of Permanent Officers of the Yale University School of Medicine, November 6, 1943, Cushing/Whitney Medical Library, Historical Library, Archives.
19. Blake, Yale University School of Medicine, Report of the Dean, 1942–1943, 2.
20. Ibid, 8.
21. A. A. Liebow, "Reunion: Yale Medical Unit of World War II," *Yale Medicine* 2, no. 3 (Fall 1967).
22. A. A. Liebow, "Encounter with Disaster—A Medical Diary of Hiroshima, 1945," *Yale Journal of Biology and Medicine* 38 (1965): 161–239.
23. Yale University School of Medicine, Report of the Institute of Human Relations, 1942–1943, 2.
24. Blake, Yale University School of Medicine, Report of the Dean, 1944–1945, 2.
25. Minutes of the Board of Permanent Officers of the Yale University School of Medicine, May 1, 1944, Cushing/Whitney Medical Library, Historical Library, Archives.
26. Minutes of the Board of Permanent Officers of the Yale University School of Medicine, July 17, 1944, Cushing/Whitney Medical Library, Historical Library, Archives.
27. Blake, Yale University School of Medicine, Report of the Dean, 1941–1942.
28. Blake, Yale University School of Medicine, Report of the Dean, 1944–1945.
29. Ibid.
30. *Supplement to the Bulletin of Yale University* 38, no. 13 (December 7, 1944).
31. Blake, Yale University School of Medicine, Report of the Dean, 1944–1945.
32. Toby A. Appel, *Shaping Biology: The National Science Foundation and American Biological Research, 1945–1975* (Baltimore: Johns Hopkins University Press, 2000).
33. Report of the Subcommittee on the Bush Report to the Committee on Postwar Medical Service, September 21, 1945, Yale University Library, Manuscripts and Archives, Records of the Dean of the Medical School, YRG 27-A-[5–9], box 85, folder 1689.
34. Editorial, *JAMA* 128 (August 11, 1945): 1100–1101.
35. United States, Office of Scientific Research and Development, *Science, the Endless Frontier: A Report to the President by Vannevar Bush, Director of the Office of Scientific Research and Development* (Washington, D.C.: U.S. Government Printing Office, 1945).
36. Report of the Committee on Readjustment of the Medical School Program following the Accelerated Schedule, Yale University Library, Manuscripts and

Archives, Records of the Office of the President, Charles Seymour, YRG 2-A-15, RU 23, box 105, folder 888.

37. Ibid.
38. Blake, Yale University School of Medicine, Report of the Dean, 1946–1947.
39. Committee upon the Deanship and the Study of the Administrative Organization of the School of Medicine, November 19, 1945, Yale University Library, Manuscripts and Archives, Records of the Office of the President, Charles Seymour, YRG 2-A-15, RU 23, box 106, folder 895.
40. Grover Powers, December 20, 1945, Yale University Library, Manuscripts and Archives, Records of the Office of the President, Charles Seymour, YRG 2-A-15, RU 23, box 106, folder 895.
41. Minutes of the Corporation, February 9, 1946, Yale University Library, Manuscripts and Archives, Minutes of the Yale University Corporation and the Prudential Committee, ca. 1701–1999, RU 307.
42. January 14, 1946, Yale University Library, Manuscripts and Archives, Records of the Office of the President, Charles Seymour, YRG 2-A-15, RU 23, box 106, folder 895.
43. Minutes of the Board of Permanent Officers of the Yale University School of Medicine, January 9, 1946, Cushing/Whitney Medical Library, Historical Library, Archives.

CHAPTER 8: PEACE AND READJUSTMENT

1. Seymour to Board of Permanent Officers, December 18, 1946, Minutes of the Board of Permanent Officers of the Yale University School of Medicine, Cushing/Whitney Medical Library, Historical Library, Archives.
2. Minutes of the Yale Corporation, January 7, 1946, Yale University Library, Manuscripts and Archives, Minutes of the Yale University Corporation and the Prudential Committee, ca. 1701–1999, RU 307.
3. Minutes of the Yale Corporation, November 6, 1948, Yale University Library, Manuscripts and Archives, Minutes of the Yale University Corporation and the Prudential Committee, ca. 1701–1999, RU 307.
4. May 15, 1948, Yale University Library, Manuscripts and Archives, Records of the Office of the President, A. Whitney Griswold, YRG 2-A, RU 22, box 218, folder 2015.
5. University Council, Medical Affairs Committee, December 7, 1948, Yale University Library, Manuscripts and Archives, Records of the Office of the President, A. Whitney Griswold, YRG 2-A, RU 22, box 218, folder 2015.
6. Minutes of the Board of Permanent Officers of the Yale University School of Medicine, January 5, 1949, Cushing/Whitney Medical Library, Historical Library, Archives.
7. C. N. H. Long, Yale University School of Medicine, Report of the Dean, 1947–1948, 57.

8. Ibid., 30.
9. Seymour to McConaughey, February 11, 1947, Yale University Library, Manuscripts and Archives, Records of the Office of the President, Charles Seymour, YRG 2-A-15, RU 23, box 108, folder 922.
10. McConaughey to Seymour, February 13, 1947, Yale University Library, Manuscripts and Archives, Records of the Office of the President, Charles Seymour, YRG 2-A-15, RU 23, box 108, folder 922.
11. *New Haven Register,* October 19, 1949.
12. Darling to Griswold, July 12, 1950, Yale University Library, Manuscripts and Archives, Records of the Office of the President, A. Whitney Griswold, YRG 2-A-16, RU 22, box 152, folder 1390.
13. Long, Yale University School of Medicine, Report of the Dean, 1948–1949.
14. Committee on Pre-clinical Sciences, June 15, 1950, Yale University Library, Manuscripts and Archives, Records of the Office of the President, A. Whitney Griswold, YRG 2-A-16, RU 22, box 152, folder 1393.
15. Hearings on Medical Research, May 14, 1948, Yale University Library, Manuscripts and Archives, Records of the Office of the President, Charles Seymour, YRG 2-A-15, RU 23, box 108, folder 925.
16. George B. Darling, Report of the Director of Medical Affairs, 1946–1947 to 1949–1950.
17. Darling, Report of the Director of Medical Affairs, 1946–1947 to 1949–1950, appendix A, University-Hospital Relations.
18. Stevenson to Canniffe, June 2, 1951, Yale University Library, Manuscripts and Archives, Records of the Office of the President, Charles Seymour, YRG 2-A-15, RU 23, box 154, folder 1399.
19. *Yale Daily News,* about May 8, 1951.
20. Seymour, Alumni Day Address, Records of the Office of the President, Charles Seymour, YRG 2-A-15, RU 23, series 1, box 7, folders 65–67.
21. Darling to Seymour, March 1, 1948; Minutes of the Board of Permanent Officers of the Yale University School of Medicine, March 20, 1948, Cushing/Whitney Medical Library, Historical Library, Archives.
22. Minutes of the Board of Permanent Officers of the Yale University School of Medicine, October 11, 1950, Cushing/Whitney Medical Library, Historical Library, Archives.
23. Long to Lawrence, July 6, 1948, Yale University Library, Manuscripts and Archives, Records of the Dean, YRG 27-A, RU 285, box 1, folder 11.
24. Milton J. E. Senn, *Insights on the Child Development Movement in the United States* (Chicago: University of Chicago Press, 1975).
25. Minutes of the Yale Corporation, October 6, 1950, Yale University Library, Manuscripts and Archives, Minutes of the Yale University Corporation and the Prudential Committee, ca. 1701–1999, RU 307.
26. Furniss to Griswold, October 31, 1950, Yale University Library, Manuscripts

and Archives, Records of the Office of the President, A. Whitney Griswold, YRG 2-A, RU 22, box 152, folder 1393.

27. Minutes of the Yale Corporation, November 11, 1950, Yale University Library, Manuscripts and Archives, Minutes of the Yale University Corporation and the Prudential Committee, ca. 1701–1999, RU 307.
28. Griswold, November 15, 1950, Yale University Library, Manuscripts and Archives, Records of the Office of the President, A. Whitney Griswold, YRG 2-A-16, RU 22, box 152, folder 393.
29. Darling to Winchell, July 12, 1951, Yale University Library, Manuscripts and Archives, Records of the Office of the President, A. Whitney Griswold, YRG 2-A, RU 22, box 152, folder 1390.
30. Minutes of the Board of Permanent Officers of the Yale University School of Medicine, November 29, 1951, Cushing/Whitney Medical Library, Historical Library, Archives.
31. Long to Hall, July 6, 1948, Yale University Library, Manuscripts and Archives, Records of the Dean of the Medical School, RU 285, YRG 27-A, box 1, folder 7.
32. Sinnott to Fruton, February 24, 1950, Yale University Library, Manuscripts and Archives, Records of the Office of the President, Charles Seymour, YRG 2-A-15, RU 23, box 111, folder 937.
33. Joseph S. Fruton, *Eighty Years* (New Haven: Epikouros, 1994).
34. January 14, 1951; December 28, 1950; January 10, 1951; January 14, 1951, Yale University Library, Manuscripts and Archives, Records of the Office of the President, A. Whitney Griswold, YRG 2-A-16, RU 22, box 154, folder 1410.

CHAPTER 9: EXPANSION YEARS

1. Arthur Ebbert Jr., "Vernon W. Lippard," *Yale Journal of Biology and Medicine* 39 (1967): 343–45.
2. Minutes of the Board of Permanent Officers, April 22, 1952, Report of the ad hoc Committee on the Functions of the Deanship, Cushing/Whitney Medical Library, Historical Library Archives.
3. Griswold to Dyde, February 2, 1953, Yale University Library, Manuscripts and Archives, Records of the Office of the President, A. Whitney Griswold, YRG 2-A-16, RU 22, box 152, folder 1390.
4. Ibid.
5. Darling to Griswold, February 14, 1953, Yale University Library, Manuscripts and Archives, Records of the President, A. Whitney Griswold, YRG 2-A, RU 22, box 152, folder 1390.
6. Snoke to Griswold, June 3, 1952, Yale University Library, Manuscripts and Archives, Office of the President, A. Whitney Griswold, YRG 2-A-16, RU 22, box 152, folder 138.
7. Lippard to Griswold, October 17, 1952, Yale University Library, Manuscripts

and Archives, Records of the Office of the President, A. Whitney Griswold, YRG 2-A-16, RU 22, box 152, folder 138.

8. Griswold, Report of the President of Yale University, 1952–1953, 13 A.
9. Lippard, Yale University School of Medicine, Report of the Dean, 1952–1953.
10. Arthur Ebbert Jr., "The Yale School of Medicine in the 1950s: Personal Reminiscences and Observations on Then and Now," Lucia P. Fulton Fellow's Lecture, Nathan Smith Club, 1968.
11. Minutes of the Board of Permanent Officers of the Yale University School of Medicine, February 17, 1954, Cushing/Whitney Medical Library, Historical Library, Archives.
12. Paul B. Beeson, Yale University School of Medicine, Report of the Department of Medicine, 1953–1954.
13. Veterans Administration Cooperative Study Group on Antihypertensive Agents, "Comparative Effects of Ticrynafen and Hydrochlorothiazide in the Treatment of Hypertension," *New England Journal of Medicine* 301 (1979): 293–97.
14. Beeson, Report of the Department of Medicine, 1954–1955.
15. Lippard, Yale University School of Medicine, Report of the Dean, 1955–1956.
16. Vernon W. Lippard, "The Medical School—Janus of the University," *Journal of Medical Education* 30, no. 12 (1955): 698–706.
17. Ebbert, "Vernon W. Lippard."
18. L. J. Evans, *The Crisis in Medical Education* (Ann Arbor: University of Michigan Press, 1964), 25.
19. C. Arden Miller, "The Medical School and the University," *Yale Journal of Biology and Medicine* 39 (1967): 374–82.
20. Visitation report, Yale University School of Medicine, November 10–13, 1958, Association of American Medical Colleges Archives, Programs Medical Education (LCME) Accreditation Survey Reports, box 1.
21. Light to Griswold, February 12, 1957, Yale University Library, Manuscripts and Archives, Records of the Office of the President, A. Whitney Griswold, YRG 2-A-16, RU 22, box 218, folder 2015.
22. Committee on Medical Affairs, May 8, 1959, Yale University Library, Manuscripts and Archives, Records of the Office of the President, A. Whitney Griswold, YRG 2-A-16, RU 22, box 218, folder 2015.
23. Ibid.
24. Minutes of the Board of Permanent Officers of the Yale University School of Medicine, April 16, 1959, Cushing/Whitney Medical Library, Historical Library, Archives.
25. Minutes, Committee on Medical Affairs of the University Council, October 16, 1953, Yale University Library, Manuscripts and Archives, Records of the

Office of the President, A. Whitney Griswold, YRG 2-A-16, RU 22, box 218, folder 2016.

26. Proposed Citizens' Committee for a Connecticut Medical-Dental School, September 1960, Yale University Library, Manuscripts and Archives, Yale–New Haven Hospital Records, YMG 835, box 4.
27. Minutes of the Board of Permanent Officers of the Yale University School of Medicine, March 5, 1959, Cushing/Whitney Medical Library, Historical Library, Archives.
28. Minutes of the Board of Permanent Officers of the Yale University School of Medicine, March 16, 1966, Cushing/Whitney Medical Library, Historical Library, Archives.
29. Minutes of the Board of Permanent Officers of the Yale University School of Medicine, February 3, 1956, Cushing/Whitney Medical Library, Historical Library, Archives.
30. Minutes of the Board of Permanent Officers of the Yale University School of Medicine, December 3, 1959, Cushing/Whitney Medical Library, Historical Library, Archives.
31. Minutes of the Board of Permanent Officers of the Yale University School of Medicine, November 23, 1960, Cushing/Whitney Medical Library, Historical Library, Archives.
32. Minutes of the Board of Permanent Officers of the Yale University School of Medicine, November 21, 1962, Cushing/Whitney Medical Library, Historical Library, Archives.
33. Report of the Committee on Medical Affairs of the University Council, November 30, 1956, Yale University Library, Manuscripts and Archives, Records of the Office of the President, A. Whitney Griswold, YRG 2-A-16, RU 22, box 218, folder 2015.
34. Forbes to Furniss, April 16, 1952, Yale University Library, Manuscripts and Archives, Records of the Office of the President, YRG 2-A, RU 22, box 152, folder 1392.
35. Minutes of the Board of Permanent Officers of the Yale University School of Medicine, June 8, 1949, Cushing/Whitney Medical Library, Historical Library, Archives.
36. Ebbert, "The Yale School of Medicine in the 1950s."
37. Lippard, Yale University School of Medicine, Report of the Dean, 1956–1957, 2.
38. Report of the Committee on Medical Affairs of the University Council, November 30, 1956, Yale University Library, Manuscripts and Archives, Records of the Office of the President, A. Whitney Griswold, YRG 2-A-16, RU 22, box 218, folder 2015.
39. Joseph S. Fruton, *Eighty Years* (New Haven: Epikouros Press, 1994).
40. Lippard to Ribicoff, January 15, 1957, Yale University Library, Manuscripts

and Archives, Records of the Office of the President, A. Whitney Griswold, YRG 2-A-16, RU 22, box 153, folder 1396.

41. Edgar Furniss, "Proposal Regarding the Institute of Human Relations," December 17, 1951, Yale University Library, Manuscripts and Archives, Records of the Office of the President, A. Whitney Griswold, YRG 2-A-16, RU 22, box 125, folder 1148.
42. Furniss to Griswold, February 14, 1957, Yale University Library, Manuscripts and Archives, Records of the Office of the President, A. Whitney Gridwold, YRG 2-A-16, RU 22, box 125, folder 1148.
43. Lippard to Griswold, July 17, 1961, Yale University Library, Manuscripts and Archives, Records of the Office of the President, A. Whitney Griswold, YRG 2-A-16, RU 22, box 153, folder 1398.
44. Lippard to Brewster, October 30, 1961, Yale University Library, Manuscripts and Archives, Records of the Office of the President, A. Whitney Griswold, YRG 2-A-16, RU 22, box 153, folder 1398.
45. Lippard, Yale University School of Medicine, Report of the Dean, 1961–1962.
46. Lippard to Brewster, December 20, 1963, Yale University Library, Manuscripts and Archives, Records of the Office of the President, Kingman Brewster, YRG 2-A-17, RU 11, box 143, folder 15.
47. Cook to Brewster, July 23, 1964, Yale University Library, Manuscripts and Archives, Records of the Office of the President, Kingman Brewster, YRG 2-A-17, RU 11, box 143, folder 15.
48. Beeson, Yale University School of Medicine, Report of the Department of Medicine, 1960–1961, 115.
49. Kazerian to Lippard, November 17, 1964, Yale University Library, Manuscripts and Archives, Records of the Office of the President, Kingman Brewster, YRG 2-A-17, RU 11, box 143, folder 15.
50. Kerr to Brewster, June 22, 1966, Yale University Library, Manuscripts and Archives, Records of the Office of the President, Kingman Brewster, YRG 2-A-17, RU 11, box 144, folder 8.
51. Lippard to Griswold, January 10, 1963, Yale University Library, Manuscripts and Archives, Records of the Office of the President, A. Whitney Griswold, YRG 2-A-16, RU 22, box 153, folder 1398.
52. Lippard, Yale University School of Medicine, Report of the Dean, 1965–1966, 15.
53. Mary Griswold, Oral History, April 10, 1990, 15, Yale University Library, Manuscripts and Archives, Oral History Tapes and Transcripts of the Griswold-Brewster Oral History Project, Yale University, 1990–1993, RU 217, box 5.
54. Minutes of the Board of Permanent Officers of the Yale University School of Medicine, April 25, 1963, Cushing/Whitney Medical Library, Historical Library, Archives.

55. Fruton, *Eighty Years.*
56. Minutes of the Board of Permanent Officers of the Yale University School of Medicine, November 9, 1966, Cushing/Whitney Medical Library, Historical Library, Archives.
57. Minutes of the Board of Permanent Officers of the Yale University School of Medicine, December 7, 1966, Cushing/Whitney Medical Library, Historical Library, Archives.
58. Galston to Taylor, October 7, 1965, Yale University Library, Manuscripts and Archives, Records of the Office of the President, Kingman Brewster, YRG 2-A-17, RU 11, box 143, folder 18.
59. Hunt to Brewster, November 18, 1965, Yale University Library, Manuscripts and Archives, Records of the Office of the President, Kingman Brewster, YRG 2-A-17, RU 11, box 143, folder 18.
60. Welch to Taylor, February 16, 1966, Yale University Library, Manuscripts and Archives, Records of the Office of the President, Kingman Brewster, YRG 2-A-17, RU 11, box 144, folder 1.
61. Bondy to Taylor, February 22, 1966, Yale University Library, Manuscripts and Archives, Records of the Office of the President, Kingman Brewster, YRG 2-A-17, RU 11, box 144, folder 1; Ebbert to Taylor, March 29, 1966, Yale University Library, Manuscripts and Archives, Records of the Office of the President, Kingman Brewster, YRG 2-A-17, RU 11, box 144, folder 2.
62. Buxton to Brewster, July 22, 1965, Yale University Library, Manuscripts and Archives, Records of the Office of the President, Kingman Brewster, YRG 2-A-17, RU 11, box 143, folder 17.
63. Weinerman to Brewster, March 16, 1966, Yale University Library, Manuscripts and Archives, Records of the Office of the President, Kingman Brewster, YRG 2-A-17, RU 11, box 144, folder 1.
64. L. Lasagna, "The Mind and Morality of the Doctor," *Yale Journal of Biology and Medicine* 37 (1965): 361–77.
65. Williams to Brewster, June 30, 1965, Yale University Library, Manuscripts and Archives, Records of the Office of the President, Kingman Brewster, YRG 2-A-127, RU 11, box 143, folder 17.
66. Robert Q. Marston, letter to the editor, *Yale Journal of Biology and Medicine* 38 (August 1965): 47–48.
67. Kingman Brewster, [1969], Yale University Library, Manuscripts and Archives, Records of the Office of the President, Kingman Brewster, YRG 2-A-17, RU 11, box 72, folder 7.

CHAPTER 10: SOCIAL UNREST

1. Beeson to Brewster, July 14, 1966, Yale University Library, Manuscripts and Archives, Records of the President, Kingman Brewster, YRG 2-A, RU 11, box 145, folder 8.
2. Wagner to Waxman, July 20, 1966, Yale University Library, Manuscripts and

Archives, Records of the President, Kingman Brewster, YRG 2-A, RU 11, box 145, folder 8.

3. Epstein to Brewster, November 7, 1966, Yale University Library, Manuscripts and Archives, Records of the President, Kingman Brewster, YRG 2-A, RU11, box 145, folder 10.
4. Brewster to Hickam, January 16, 1967, Yale University Library, Manuscripts and Archives, Records of the President, Kingman Brewster, YRG 2-A-7, RU 11, box 145, folder 11.
5. Bondy to Brewster, February 23, 1967, Yale University Library, Manuscripts and Archives, Records of the President, Kingman Brewster, YRG 2-A-7, RU 11, box 145, folder 11.
6. Redlich to Brewster, May 9, 1967, Yale University Library, Manuscripts and Archives, Records of the President, Kingman Brewster, YRG 2-A7, RU 11, box 145, folder 111.
7. *Time,* March 24, 1967, 46.
8. Redlich, Yale University School of Medicine, Report of the Dean, 1966–1968.
9. Cook to Brewster, November 21, 1968, Yale University Library, Manuscripts and Archives, Records of the President, Kingman Brewster, YRG 2-A RU 11, box 144, folder 5.
10. Redlich to Cook, December 2, 1970, Yale University Library, Manuscripts and Archives, Records of the President, Kingman Brewster, YRG 2-A, RU 11, box 145, folder 7.
11. Snoke to Redlich and Lippard, May 24, 1967, Yale University Library, Manuscripts and Archives, Records of the President, Kingman Brewster, YRG 2-A RU 11, box 144, folder 4.
12. Redlich to Brewster, September 9, 1968, Yale University Library, Manuscripts and Archives, Records of the President, Kingman Brewster, YRG 2-A-7 RU 11, box 146, folder 1.
13. Bondy, School of Medicine, Report of the Department of Medicine, 1967–1968, 210.
14. Redlich, Yale University School of Medicine, Report of the Dean, 1967–1968.
15. Daryl K. Daniels, "African-Americans at the Yale University School of Medicine: 1810–1960," unpublished M.D. thesis, Yale University, 1991.
16. M. G. Synott, *The Half-Opened Door* (Westport, Conn.: Greenwood Press, 1979).
17. Redlich, Yale University School of Medicine, Report of the Dean, 1967–1968, 13.
18. Weinerman to Brewster, September 30, 1969, Yale University Library, Manuscripts and Archives, Records of the President, Kingman Brewster, YRG 2-A, RU 11, box 144, folder 5.
19. E. R. Weinerman, "Social Demands upon the Health Care Delivery System," Workshop on Medical School Curriculum, AAMC, September 19, 1968.

20. Redlich, Yale University School of Medicine, Report of the Dean, 1968–1969, 10.
21. A. K. Rice, Yale–New Haven Medical Center, March 6, 1969, Yale University Library, Manuscripts and Archives, Records of the President, Kingman Brewster, YRG 2A RU 11, box 294, folder 6.
22. *Yale Medical Center Newsletter* 1, no. 16.
23. Redlich, Yale University School of Medicine, Report of the Dean, 1968–1969, 14.
24. Redlich, Yale University School of Medicine, Report of the Dean, 1968–1969.
25. Redlich, Yale University School of Medicine, Report of the Dean, 1969–1970, 1 and 2.
26. Committee for Change, "Proposals for Change," Yale University Library, Manuscripts and Archives, Records of the President, Kingman Brewster, YRG 2-A, RU 11, box 144, folder 6.
27. Raymond S. Duff and August B. Hollingshead, *Sickness and Society* (New York: Harper and Row, 1968), foreword.
28. Ibid.
29. Samuel Shem, *The House of God* (New York: R. Marek, 1978).
30. Redlich to Brewster, September 8, 1969, Yale University Library, Manuscripts and Archives, Records of the President, Kingman Brewster, YRG 2-A RU 11, box 145, folder 7.
31. School of Medicine, Yale University Reports, 1969–1970, 22.
32. Redlich to Brewster, February 12, 1970, Yale University Library, Manuscripts and Archives, Records of the President, Kingman Brewster, YRG 2-A, RU 11, box 145, folder 7.
33. Davis to Novack, October 29, 1970, Yale University Library, Manuscripts and Archives, Records of the President, Kingman Brewster, YRG 2-A, RU 11, box 145, folder 7.
34. Redlich to Brewster, January 27, 1971, Yale University Library, Manuscripts and Archives, Records of the President, Kingman Brewster, YRG 2-A-17, box 297, folder 7.
35. Redlich to Glaser, March 30, 1971, Yale University Library, Manuscripts and Archives, Records of the President, Kingman Brewster, YRG 2-A, RU 11, box 145, folder 7.
36. A. M. Sadler Jr., B. L. Sadler, and A. A. Bliss, *The Physician's Assistant: Today and Tomorrow* (New Haven: Yale University Press, 1972).
37. *Yale School of Medicine Diagnostic Review,* March 13, 1972.
38. Minutes of the Board of Permanent Officers, December 20, 1972.
39. McCollum to Brewster, May 28, 1971, Yale University Library, Manuscripts and Archives, Records of the President, Kingman Brewster, YRG 2-A, RU 11, box 294, folder 7.
40. Memorandum from Kingman Brewster, June 1971, Yale University Library,

Manuscripts and Archives, Records of the President, Kingman Brewster, YRG 2A-17, box 294, folder 7.

CHAPTER 11: THE DEPARTMENT OF MEDICINE

1. Oliver S. Hayward and Elizabeth H. Thomson, eds., *The Journal of William Tully, Medical Student at Dartmouth, 1808–1809* (New York: Science History Publications, 1977).
2. William W. Field, *The Good Doctor Smith: Life and Times of Dr. Nathan Smith, 1762–1829* (New Haven: Advocate Press, 1992).
3. *New England Medical and Surgical Journal* 13 (1824): 324.
4. Smith to Porter, March 8, 1873, Cushing/Whitney Medical Library, Yale Medical School Miscellaneous Papers, 1810–1884, box 1.
5. *Catalogue of the Medical Department of Yale College,* 1887–1888.
6. Ibid.
7. Ibid.
8. Ibid.
9. Charles A. Lindsley, "Abstract of a Lecture before the Medical Class, June 7th, 1897," *Yale Medical Journal* 3 (1897): 379–85.
10. *Yale Medical Journal* 12 (1906): 841.
11. Ibid., 23–24.
12. Blumer to Stokes, "Relation of a Medical School to a Hospital," September 26, 1911, Yale University Library, Manuscripts and Archives, Records of the Secretary, YRG 4-A, series 2, box 11, folder 158.
13. Blumer to Flexner, March 9, 1920, General Education Board, Rockefeller Foundation Archives, RAC.
14. Alan Gregg, "Addenda to the Agenda for the Decade 1940–1950," *Journal of the American Medical Association* 114, no. 13 (1940): 1139–41.
15. John R. Paul, "Francis Gilman Blake," *Yale Journal of Biology and Medicine* 24 (1951–1952): 434–41.
16. John P. Peters, "Dean Francis Gilman Blake," Cushing/Whitney Medical Library, Obituary File.
17. Paul, "Francis Gilman Blake."
18. Paul H. Lavietes, "John Punnett Peters: An Appreciation," *Yale Journal of Biology and Medicine* 30 (1957): 175–82.
19. John R. Paul and Cyril N. H. Long, "John Punnett Peters," in *Biographical Memoirs,* vol. 31 (New York: National Academy of Sciences, 1958), 347–60.
20. Winternitz to Flexner, March 30, 1924, Yale University Library, Manuscripts and Archives, Winternitz Papers, YMG 859.
21. John P. Peters and D. D. Van Slyke, *Quantitative Clinical Chemistry* (Baltimore: William and Wilkins, 1932).
22. D. D. Van Slyke, "John Punnett Peters," *Clinical Chemistry* 3, no. 4, suppl. (1957): 287–92.

23. Paul and Long, "John Punnett Peters."
24. Martin Miller, "John P. Peters," *Diabetes* 6 (1957): 99.
25. "Mencken Calls Hospitals Worst Anti-Social Agencies in U.S.; He Would Sterilize Unfit to Solve Medical Care Problems; Drs. Peters and Fishbein Give Views on Medical Economics," *Wire Story by Mail* (Science Service: October 10, 1938).
26. John P. Peters, "The Social Responsibilities of Medicine," *Annals of Internal Medicine* 12, no. 4 (1938): 536–43.
27. J. P. Peters, Yale University Library, Manuscripts and Archives, Records of the President, Charles Seymour, YRG 2A, RU 23, box 109, folder 929.
28. Federal Security Agency to Peters, February 18, 1949, Yale University Library, Manuscripts and Archives, Records of the President, Charles Seymour, YRG 2-A, RU22, box 153, folder 1394.
29. Griswold to Peters, September 18, 1953, Yale University Library, Manuscripts and Archives, Records of the President, A. Whitney Griswold, YRG 2-A, RU22, box 153, folder 1394.
30. Griswold to Peters, June 6, 1955, Yale University Library, Manuscripts and Archives, Records of the President, A. Whitney Griswold, YRG 2-A, RU 22, box 153, folder 1395.
31. Richard Rapport, *Physician: The Life of Paul Beeson* (Fort Lee, N.J.: Barricade Books, 2001).
32. William Hollingsworth, *Taking Care: The Legacy of Soma Weiss, Eugene Stead, and Paul Beeson* (San Diego: Medical Education and Research Foundation, 1994).
33. Ibid.
34. Beeson, Report of the Department of Medicine, 1955–1956, 198.
35. Ibid.
36. Paul Beeson, "Changing Times: Reflections on a Professional Lifetime: An Interview with Paul Beeson," interview by R. V. Lee, *Annals of Internal Medicine* 132, no. 1 (2000): 71–79.
37. Spiro to Redlich, March 19, 1971, Yale University Library, Manuscripts and Archives, Records of the President, Kingman Brewster, YRG 2-A, RU 11, box 294, folder 7.

CHAPTER 12: PUBLIC HEALTH AND THE GREATER GOOD

1. Committee on Preventive Medicine and Public Health, 1907–1908 (New Haven, 1908).
2. Arthur J. Viseltear, "C.-E. A. Winslow and the Early Years of Public Health at Yale, 1915–1925," *Yale Journal of Biology and Medicine* 55 (1982): 137–51.
3. Fisher to Blumer, August 24, 1907, Yale University Library, Manuscripts and Archives, Records of the Dean of the School of Medicine, YRG 27-A, RU 285.

4. Blumer to Yale Community, February 11, 1908, Yale University Library, Manuscripts and Archives, Records of the Dean of the School of Medicine, YRG 27-A, RU 285.
5. Henderson to Blumer, November 1, 1907, Yale University Library, Manuscripts and Archives, Records of the Dean of the School of Medicine, YRG 27-A, RU 285, box 90, folder 1939.
6. Elizabeth Fee, "Competition for the First School of Public Health," *Bulletin of the History of Medicine* 57 (1983): 339–63.
7. Blumer to Flexner, October 28, 1914, and November 2, 1914, Rockefeller Foundation Archives, RG 1.1, S.200.
8. John F. Fulton, "C.-E. A. Winslow, Leader in Public Health," *Science* 125 (June 21, 1957): 1236.
9. Winslow to Bristol, April 30, 1915, Yale University Library, Manuscripts and Archives, C.-E. A. Winslow Papers, manuscript group 749, box 5, folder 102.
10. Blumer to Hadley, April 3, 1915, Yale University Library, Manuscripts and Archives, Records of the Office of the President, Arthur T. Hadley, YRG 2-A-13, RU 25, series 1, box 9, folder 163.
11. Fee, "Competition."
12. Hadley to Fisher, March 12 and 13, 1908, Yale University Library, Manuscripts and Archives, Records of the Office of the President, Arthur T. Hadley, YRG 2-A-13, RU 25, series 2, box 112.
13. Winslow to Hadley, February 5, 1919, Yale University Library, Manuscripts and Archives, Records of the Office of the President, Arthur T. Hadley, YRG 2-A-13, RU 25, box 94, folder 1851.
14. Winslow to Hadley, March 13, 1919, Yale University Library, Manuscripts and Archives, Records of the Office of the President, Arthur T. Hadley, YRG 2-A-13, RU 25, box 94, folder 1851.
15. Viseltear, "C.-E. A. Winslow and the Early Years."
16. Winslow to Hadley, October 8, 1919, Yale University Library, Manuscripts and Archives, Records of the Office of the President, Arthur T. Hadley, YRG 2-A-13, RU 25, box 94, folder 1851.
17. Winslow to Blumer, December 10, 1919, Yale University Library, Manuscripts and Archives, Records of the Office of the President, Arthur T. Hadley, YRG 2-A-13, RU 25, box 94, folder 1851.
18. Winslow to Hadley, December 1919, Yale University Library, Manuscripts and Archives, Records of the Office of the President, Arthur T. Hadley, YRG 2-A-13, RU 25, box 94, folder 1851.
19. C.-E. A. Winslow, "The Place of Public Health in a University," *Science* 62 (1925): 335–38.
20. Viseltear, "C.-E. A. Winslow and the Early Years."
21. Winslow to Hadley, June 11 and December 18, 1919, Yale University Library, Manuscripts and Archives, Records of the Office of the President, Arthur T. Hadley, YRG 2-A-13, RU 25, series 1, box 9, folder 166.

22. H. F. Vaughan, "Local Health Services in the United States: The Story of CAP," *American Journal of Public Health* 62 (January 1972): 95–111.
23. Winslow to Angell, February 12, 1929, Yale University Library, Manuscripts and Archives, C.-E. A. Winslow Papers, manuscript group 749, box 2, folder 38.
24. "C.-E. A. Winslow: First Chairman of the Department of Public Health at Yale," *Yale Medicine* (Spring 1977): 1–8.
25. C.-E. A. Winslow, "The Recommendations of the Committee on the Costs of Medical Care," *New England Journal of Medicine* 207 (1932): 1138–42.
26. Committee on the Costs of Medical Care, *Medical Care for the American People: The Final Report* (Chicago: University of Chicago Press, 1932); J. F. Jekel, "Health Departments in the U.S., 1920–1988: Statements of Mission with Special Reference to the Role of C.-E. A. Winslow," *Yale Journal of Biology and Medicine* 64 (1991): 467–69.
27. C.-E. A. Winslow, "A Program for Medical Care in the United States," *Science* 77 (1933): 102–07.
28. Bayne-Jones, Yale University School of Medicine, Report of the Dean, 1936–1937, 2.
29. Arnold to Winslow, August 5, 1938, Yale University Library, Manuscripts and Archives, C.-E. A. Winslow Papers, manuscript group 749, box 2, folder 41; "Right of Corporation to Practice Medicine," *Yale Law Journal* 48 (1938): 346–51.
30. Angell to Winslow, November 22, 1927, Yale University Library, Manuscripts and Archives, C.-E. A. Winslow Papers, manuscript group 749, box 2, folder 38.
31. Winslow to Angell, September 25, 1935, Yale University Library, Manuscripts and Archives, C.-E. A. Winslow Papers, manuscript group 749, box 2, folder 39.
32. C.-E. A. Winslow, *The Evolution and Significance of the Modern Public Health Campaign* (New Haven: Yale University Press, 1923).
33. C.-E. A. Winslow, "The University and Public Health Statesmanship," 1940, Yale University Library, Manuscripts and Archives, Records of the Office of the President, Charles Seymour, YRG 2-A-15, RU 23, box 104, folder 884.
34. Winslow to Seymour, October 29, 1935, Yale University Library, Manuscripts and Archives, C.-E. A. Winslow Papers, manuscript group 749, box 26, folder 664.
35. Winslow to Seymour, October 6, 1939, Yale University Library, Manuscripts and Archives, C.-E. A. Winslow Papers, manuscript group 749, box 26, folder 664.
36. A. J. Viseltear, "C.-E. A. Winslow and the Later Years of Public Health at Yale, 1940–1945," *Yale Journal of Biology and Medicine* 60 (1987): 447–70.
37. Minutes of the Prudential Committee of the Yale University School of

Medicine, April 24, 1940, Cushing/Whitney Medical Library, Historical Library, Archives.

38. Minutes of the Board of Permanent Officers of the Yale University School of Medicine, April 24, 1940, Cushing/Whitney Medical Library, Historical Library, Archives.
39. John R. Paul, "Preventive Medicine at the Yale University School of Medicine, 1940–49," *Yale Journal of Biology and Medicine* 22 (1950): 199–211.
40. Minutes of the Board of Permanent Officers of the Yale University School of Medicine, March 15, 1944, Cushing/Whitney Medical Library, Historical Library, Archives.
41. Minutes of the Board of Permanent Officers of the Yale University School of Medicine, May 1, 1944, Cushing/Whitney Medical Library, Historical Library, Archives.
42. Winslow to Seymour, May 27, 1944, Yale University Library, Manuscripts and Archives, Records of the Office of the President, Charles Seymour, YRG 2-A-15, RU 23, box 106, folder 899.
43. Paul to Seymour, Preliminary and Basic Plans for the Future Development of Public Health at Yale University, June 7, 1944, Yale University Library, Manuscripts and Archives, Records of the Office of the President, Charles Seymour, YRG 2-A-15, RU 23, box 106, folder 899.
44. Furniss to Seymour, June 21, 1944, Yale University Library, Manuscripts and Archives, Records of the Office of the President, Charles Seymour, YRG 2-A-15, RU 23, box 106, folder 899.
45. Paul to Seymour, July 17, 1944, Yale University Library, Manuscripts and Archives, Records of the Office of the President, Charles Seymour, YRG 2-A-15, RU 23, box 106, folder 899.
46. [Winslow] to Paul, July 19, 1944, Yale University Library, Manuscripts and Archives, Records of the Office of the President, Charles Seymour, YRG 2-A-15, RU 23, box 106, folder 899.
47. Paul to Seymour, August 24, 1944, Yale University Library, Manuscripts and Archives, Records of the Office of the President, Charles Seymour, YRG 2-A-15, RU 23, box 106, folder 899.
48. Minutes of the Board of Permanent Officers of the Yale University School of Medicine, September 14, 1944, Cushing/Whitney Medical Library, Historical Library, Archives.
49. Peters to Blake, November 3, 1944, Yale University Library, Manuscripts and Archives, Records of the Dean of the School of Medicine, YRG 27-A, RU 285, box 42, folder 710.
50. Yale University School of Medicine, Minutes of the Committee on Program and Policy, October 31, 1944, Cushing/Whitney Medical Library, Historical Library, Archives.
51. Seymour to Blake, November 7, 1944, Yale University Library, Manuscripts

and Archives, Records of the Dean of the School of Medicine, YRG 27-A, RU 295, box 42, folder 710.

52. Paul to Blake, June 20, 1944, Yale University Library, Manuscripts and Archives, Records of the Dean of the School of Medicine, YRG 27-A, RU 285, box 42, folder 710.
53. Jekel, "Health Departments in the U.S., 1920–1988," 467–79.
54. Olsen and Nicklas to Griswold, September 4, 1954, Yale University Library, Manuscripts and Archives, Records of the Office of the President, A. Whitney Griswold, YRG 2-A-16, RU 22, box 153, folder 1395.
55. "A Proposal for Reorganization of the Program in the Field of Public Health in Yale University," Minutes of the Board of Permanent Officers, April 7, 1959, Cushing/Whitney Medical Library, Historical Library, Archives.
56. Ibid.
57. Lippard to Schmehl, June 14, 1962, Yale University Library, Manuscripts and Archives, Records of the Office of the President, Kingman Brewster, YRG 2-A-17, RU 11, box 145, folder 5.
58. Committee on Medical Affairs, January 19, 1962, Yale University Library, Manuscripts and Archives, Records of the Office of the President, Kingman Brewster, YRG 2-A-17, RU 11, box 218, folder 2015.
59. Blumer to Hadley, April 3, 1915, Yale University Library, Manuscripts and Archives, Records of the Office of the President, Arthur T. Hadley, YRG 2-A-13, RU 25, box 9, folder 163.
60. M. I. Roemer and L. S. Falk, "The Committee on Costs of Medical Care, and the Drive for National Health Insurance," *American Journal of Public Health* 75 (1985): 841–48.
61. Yale University School of Medicine, Report of the Department of Epidemiology and Public Health, 1967–1968, Cushing/Whitney Medical Library, Historical Library, Archives.

CHAPTER 13: THE STATE HOSPITAL

1. P. A. Jewett, *Semi-Centennial History of the General Hospital Society of Connecticut* (New Haven: Tuttle, Morehouse and Taylor, 1876), 29.
2. Francis Bacon, "The Practice of Medicine and Surgery," in *The History of the City of New Haven to the Present Time,* ed. Edward Atwater (New York: W. W. Munsal, 1887).
3. Henry Farnam, "Salutory," in *General Hospital of Connecticut Centenary* (New Haven: Tuttle, Morehouse, and Taylor, 1926).
4. Ibid.
5. Charter of the General Hospital Society of Connecticut (New Haven: May 26, 1826), Cushing/Whitney Medical Library, Historical Library, Archives.
6. *Knight Hospital Record,* 1862–1865.
7. W. C. Minor, *Post Mortem Examinations Made at Knight U.S.A. General Hospital* (New Haven: Knight Hospital Printer, 1864).

8. Simon Winchester, *The Professor and the Madman* (New York: Harper Collins, 1998).
9. *General Hospital Society of Connecticut Centenary.*
10. William H. Carmalt, "The Second Half Century of the General Hospital Society of Connecticut," in *General Hospital Society of Connecticut Centenary.*
11. Bishop to George Farnam, June 12, 1933, Yale University Library, Manuscripts and Archives, Records of the Secretary of the University, YRG 4-A-12, box 222, folder 889.
12. W. H. Carmalt, *General Hospital Society of Connecticut Centenary* (New Haven: Tuttle, Morehouse and Taylor, 1926).
13. *The Spirit of Gaylord: A History, 1902–1997* (New Haven: Gaylord Hospital Publications, 1997).
14. July 1905, Yale University Library, Manuscripts and Archives, Yale–New Haven Hospital Records, manuscript group 835, box 2.
15. Ibid.
16. *Dr. Skinner's Sanatorium, 1st Semi-Annual Report,* December 1912 (New Haven, 1912).
17. Minutes of the Prudential Committee, July 1905, Yale University Library, Manuscripts and Archives, Yale–New Haven Hospital Records, manuscript group 835, box 2.
18. Memorandum Concerning Reorganization of the New Haven Dispensary, Yale University Library, Manuscripts and Archives, Records of the Medical School Dean, YRG 27-A, RU 285, box 105, folder 2467.
19. Cushing to Hadley, April 30, 1907, Yale University Library, Manuscripts and Archives, Office of the President, Arthur T. Hadley, YRG 2-A-13, RU 25, series 1, box 23, folder 469.
20. *New Haven Hospital, 81st Annual Report* (New Haven, 1908).
21. S. B. Nuland, "An Informal History of Our School," transcript of presentation to YMS Council, May 4, 1995.
22. Abraham Flexner, *Medical Education in the United States and Canada: A Report to the Carnegie Foundation for the Advancement of Teaching* (New York, 1910).
23. Blumer to Stokes, March 9, 1911, Yale University Library, Manuscripts and Archives, Records of the Office of the Secretary, YRG 4-A-[9–12], RU 49, series 2, box 11, folder 158.
24. George Blumer, Memorandum, "The Relation of the Medical School to the Hospital," Yale University Library, Manuscripts and Archives, Records of the Office of the Secretary, YRG 4-A-[9–12], RU 49, series 2, box 11, folder 158.
25. Minutes of the General Hospital Society, January 26, 1912, Yale University Library, Manuscripts and Archives, Records of the General Hospital Society, YRG 37-AA, RU 473.

26. Minutes of the General Hospital Society, April 19, 1912, Yale University Library, Manuscripts and Archives, Records of the General Hospital Society, YRG 37-AA, RU 473.
27. Winford Smith, April 22, 1918, Yale University Library, Manuscripts and Archives, Yale–New Haven Hospital Records, manuscript group 835, box 2.
28. Memorandum for the Directors of the New Haven Hospital, 1919, Yale University Library, Manuscripts and Archives, Yale–New Haven Hospital Records, manuscript group 835, box 2.
29. Blumer to Stokes, Yale University Library, Manuscripts and Archives, Records of the Office of the Secretary, YRG 4-A-[9–12], RU 49, series 2, box 12, folder 163.
30. Carmalt, "The Second Half Century."
31. Blumer to Stokes, January 11, 1919, Yale University Library, Manuscripts and Archives, Records of the Office of the Secretary, YRG 4-A-[9–12], RU 49, series 2, box 12, folder 163.
32. Report of the Committee on the Relationship between the Hospital, the Dispensary, and the Medical School, Yale University Library, Manuscripts and Archives, Records of the Dean of the School of Medicine, YRG 27-A-[5–9], RU 285, box 21, folder 293.
33. Minutes of the Prudential Committee of the Hospital, May 7, 1920, Yale University Library, Manuscripts and Archives, Records of the Yale–New Haven Hospital Prudential Committee, YRG 37-Q-1, RU 480.
34. Interview with George Parmly Day, Treasurer of Yale University, April 6, 1920, General Education Board, Rockefeller Foundation Archives, RAC.
35. Flexner to Blumer, May 28, 1920, Yale University Library, Manuscripts and Archives, Records of the Office of the President, Arthur T. Hadley, YRG 2-A-13, RU 25, box 34, series 1, folder 657.
36. Meeting of the Administrative Subcommittee, July 9, 1920, Yale University Library, Manuscripts and Archives, Yale–New Haven Hospital Records and Earlier Organizations, YRG 37-Q-1, RU 480.
37. Carmalt, "The Second Half Century."
38. Vincent to Farnam, August 21, 1922, Yale University Library, Manuscripts and Archives, Records of the President, YRG 2-A, RU 24, box 134, folder 1411.
39. Rappeleye to Angell, November 12, 1923, Yale University Library, Manuscripts and Archives, Records of the President, YRG 2-A, RU 24, box 134, folder 1411.
40. Flexner to Angell on teaching-hospital costs, 1924, Yale University Library, Manuscripts and Archives, Records of the Office of the President, James R. Angell, YRG 2-A, RU 24, box 84, folder 835.
41. Winternitz, Yale University School of Medicine, Report of the Dean, 1924–1925.

42. Dinner invitation, Farnam to Angell, 1925, Yale University Library, Manuscripts and Archives, Records of the Office of the President, James R. Angell, YRG 2-A, RU 24, box 77, folder 789.
43. Winternitz to Angell, October 5, 1928, Yale University Library, Manuscripts and Archives, Records of the Office of the President, James R. Angell, YRG 2-A-14, RU 24, box 112, folder 1141.
44. Memorandum Concerning the Development of Further Clinical Facilities in Association with the Yale University School of Medicine, January 30, 1928, Yale University Library, Manuscripts and Archives, Records of the Office of the President, James R. Angell, YRG 2-A-14, RU 24, box 112, folder 1141.
45. Yale University Library, Manuscripts and Archives, Records of the Dean of the School of Medicine, YRG 27-A, RU 285, box 99, folder 2358.
46. *New Haven Journal-Courier,* March 25, 1927, 1.
47. Lund to Angell, April 7, 1930, Yale University Library, Manuscripts and Archives, Records of the Office of the President, James R. Angell, YRG 2-A-14, RU 24, box 110, folder 1124.
48. "A Project for Health and Sickness Insurance," Yale University Library, Manuscripts and Archives, Records of the Office of the President, James R. Angell, YRG 2-A-14, RU 24, box 110, folder 1124.
49. Bayne-Jones, Yale University School of Medicine, Report of the Dean, 1939–1940.
50. "Yale-City Aid Problem before Finance Board," *New Haven Journal-Courier,* July 24, 1937, 1.
51. Bayne-Jones to Seymour, January 7, 1938, Yale University Library, Manuscripts and Archives, Records of the Office of the President, Charles Seymour, YRG 2-A-15, RU 23, box 104, folder 882.
52. "N. H. Hospital Boosts Rate to $5 per Day," *New Haven Evening Register,* December 16, 1938, 1.
53. Blake, Yale University School of Medicine, Report of the Dean, 1944–1945, 40.
54. Memorandum of Agreement, Yale University Library, Manuscripts and Archives, Records of the Office of the President, Charles Seymour, YRG 2-A-15, RU 23, box 1110, folder 932.
55. Albert W. Snoke, Oral History, Yale University Library, Manuscripts and Archives, Albert W. Snoke Papers, manuscript group 1471, box 1, folder 13.
56. *New Haven Journal-Courier,* March 16 and May 21, 1929.
57. George B. Darling, Appendix A, Report of the Director of Medical Affairs, 1946–1947 to 1949–1950, Yale University Library, Records of the Office of the President, Charles Seymour, YRG 2-A-15, RU 23, box 108, folder 925.
58. Snoke, Oral History, Yale University Library, Manuscripts and Archives, Albert W. Snoke Papers, manuscript group 1471, box 1, folder 11.

59. Memorandum to Members of the Committee on Medical Affairs, June 2, 1950, Yale University Library, Manuscripts and Archives, Records of the Office of the President, Charles Seymour, YRG 2-A-15, RU 23, box 218, folder 2015.
60. Darling to Snoke, June 11, 1948, Yale University Library, Manuscripts and Archives, Records of the Office of the President, Charles Seymour, YRG 2-A-15, RU 23, box 108, folder 924.
61. Minutes of the Board of Permanent Officers of the Yale University School of Medicine, October 7, 1948, Yale Medical Library, Archives.
62. Snoke to Berger, March 30, 1950, Yale University Library, Manuscripts and Archives, Records of the Yale–New Haven Hospital, manuscript group 835, box 3.
63. Snoke to Berger, May 10, 1950, Yale University Library, Manuscripts and Archives, Records of the Yale–New Haven Hospital, manuscript group 835, box 3.
64. Galpin to Griswold, October 8, 1952, Yale University Library, Manuscripts and Archives, Records of the Office of the President, A. Whitney Griswold, YRG 2-A-16, RU 22, box 154, folder 1399.
65. Joint Declaration of Policy, Yale University Library, Manuscripts and Archives, Records of the Office of the President, A. Whitney Griswold, YRG 2-A-16, RU 22, box 154, folder 1399.
66. Snoke, Yale Medical School Philosophy, Yale University Library, Manuscripts and Archives, Albert W. Snoke Papers, manuscript group 1471, box 1, folder 1.
67. Snoke, April 12, 1961, Yale University Library, Manuscripts and Archives, Albert W. Snoke Papers, manuscript group 1471, box 1, folder 11.
68. Masur to Snoke, June 8, 1961, Yale University Library, Manuscripts and Archives, Albert W. Snoke Papers, manuscript group 1741, box 1.
69. Esseltyn to Snoke, May 31, 1961, Yale University Library, Manuscripts and Archives, Albert W. Snoke Papers, manuscript group 1741, box 1.
70. E. R. Weinerman, A Comment upon the Educational Policy and Program of the School of Medicine, February 8, 1965, Yale University Library, Manuscripts and Archives, Albert W. Snoke Papers, manuscript group 1741, box 1, folder 7.
71. George S. Stevenson, *Connecticut Medicine* 23 (1959): 476–80.
72. Snoke to Zorn, July 22, 1960, Yale University Library, Manuscripts and Archives, Yale–New Haven Hospital Records, manuscript group 835, box 1.
73. Lippard to Buck, February 22, 1960, Yale University Library, Manuscripts and Archives, Records of the Office of the President, A. Whitney Griswold, YRG 2-A, RU 22, box 155, folder 1411.
74. Snoke, Memorandum, September 1, 1963, Yale University Library, Manuscripts and Archives, Yale–New Haven Hospital Records, manuscript group 835, box 3.
75. “File on medical school, to be discussed with Mr. Brewster at the earliest”

[January 10, 1963], Yale University Library, Manuscripts and Archives, Records of the Office of the President, A. Whitney Griswold, YRG 2-A-16, RU 22, box 153, folder 1398.

76. Lippard to Griswold, January 10, 1963, Yale University Library, Manuscripts and Archives, Records of the Office of the President, A. Whitney Griswold, YRG 2-A-16, RU 16, box 153, folder 1398.
77. J. E. Ecklund, Memorandum on Yale University School of Medicine and Grace–New Haven Community Hospital, January 9, 1964, Yale University Library, Manuscripts and Archives, Records of the Office of the President, YRG 2-A-17, RU 11, box 145, folder 13.
78. Rilance to Ramsay, April 8, 1964, Yale University Library, Manuscripts and Archives, Records of the Office of the President, Kingman Brewster, YRG 2-A-17, RU 11, series 1, box 231, folder 2.
79. Yale Hospital Relations, Yale University Library, Manuscripts and Archives, Albert W. Snoke Papers, manuscript group 1471, box 1, folder 11.
80. Ecklund to Brewster, March 24, 1965, Yale University Library, Manuscripts and Archives, Records of the Office of the President, Kingman Brewster, YRG 2-A-17, RU 11, series 1, box 231, folder 2.
81. Snoke to Lippard, December 23, 1964, Yale University Library, Manuscripts and Archives, Albert W. Snoke Papers, manuscript group 1741, box 1.
82. House Staff Petition, Yale University Library, Manuscripts and Archives, Albert W. Snoke Papers, manuscript group 1471, box 1, folder 4.
83. Snoke to Costello, December 27, 1965, Yale University Library, Manuscripts and Archives, Records of the Office of the President, Kingman Brewster, YRG 2-A-17, RU 11, box 146, folder 3.
84. Costello, Letter to Medical Staff Meeting, January 16, 1968, Yale University Library, Manuscripts and Archives, Records of the Office of the President, Kingman Brewster, YRG 2-A-17, RU 11, box 144, folder 5.
85. Raymond S. Duff and August B. Hollingshead, *Sickness and Society* (New York: Harper and Row, 1968), 381.
86. Maya Pines, "Hospital. Enter at your own risk," *McCalls* 79 (May 1968): 138–42.

CHAPTER 14: EPILOGUE

1. Rosemary Stevens, *American Medicine and the Public Interest: A History of Specialization* (Berkeley: University of California Press, 1998).
2. L. Williams, G. M. Carter, G. T. Hammons, and D. Poenter, *Managing for Survival: How Successful Academic Medical Centers Cope with Harsh Environments* (Santa Monica: Rand Publication Series, 1987).
3. Kenneth M. Ludmerer, *Time to Heal* (Oxford: Oxford University Press, 1999).
4. *New York Times,* September 13, 1995.
5. L. H. Smith, "Medical Education for the 21st Century," *Journal of Medical Education* 60 (1985): 106–12.

6. John R. Evans, "The 'Health of the Public' Approach to Medical Education," *Academic Medicine* 67, no. 11 (1992): 719–23.
7. Ludmerer, *Time to Heal.*
8. Kingman Brewster, "The Alan Gregg Memorial Lecture," *Journal of Medical Education* 45 (1970): 5–10.
9. Vernon W. Lippard, "The Yale School of Medicine in the Twentieth Century," *Yale Journal of Biology and Medicine* 33 (1960): 162–70.

SELECTED BIBLIOGRAPHY

PRIMARY SOURCES

Archives and Manuscripts

New Haven, Connecticut. Connecticut Historical Society. Manuscripts.
MS 73008. Letter. Wilcox to Humphreys. January 14, 1828.

New Haven, Connecticut. Saint Raphael's Health Care System. Archives and Manuscripts.
Papers of Dr. William Verdi.
Printed Material Scrapbook. 1905–1930.

New Haven, Connecticut. Yale University. Harvey Cushing / John Hay Whitney Medical Library, Historical Library.
Broadside. Timothy Dwight. [1815 or 1816.]
Letter. Nathan Smith to Mills Olcott. May 1819. Copy of letter kept at Dartmouth College Library.
Minute Book of the Yale Medical Society, 10th Anniversary.

Minutes of the Board of Permanent Officers of the Yale University School of Medicine.

Minutes of the Committee on Program and Policy.

Miscellaneous Papers, 1810–1884.

Proceedings of the Connecticut Medical Society for 1811.

Reports of the Dean of the School of Medicine.

Reports of the Department of Epidemiology and Public Health, 1967–1968.

Reports of the Department of Medicine.

Reports of the Director of Medical Affairs.

Reports of the Institute of Human Relations.

Report to Board of Permanent Officers on a University School of Nursing, 1921–1922.

Minutes of the Yale Medical Alumni Association.

New Haven, Connecticut. Yale University. Yale University Library. Manuscripts and Archives. Stanhope Bayne-Jones Papers. Manuscript Group 1271.

Minutes of the Yale University Corporation and the Prudential Committee, ca. 1701–1999. Record Unit 307.

Records of the Yale University Corporation, ca. 1714–1990. Record Unit 164.

Records of the Dean of the School of Medicine. Record Unit 285.

Samuel H. Fisher Papers. Manuscript Group 213.

Records of the General Hospital Society. Record Unit 473.

Oral History Tapes and Transcripts of the Griswold-Brewster Oral History Project, Yale University, 1990–1993. Record Unit 217.

Samuel Clark Harvey Papers. Manuscript Group 1244.

Records of Thomas Clap as President of Yale College, ca. 1720–1765. Record Unit 130.

Records of Theodore Dwight Woolsey as President of Yale College, ca. 1855–1859. Record Unit 337.

Records of Arthur Twining Hadley as President of Yale University, 1899–1921. Record Unit 25.

Records of James Rowland Angell as President of Yale University, 1921–1937. Record Unit 24.

Records of Charles Seymour as President of Yale University, 1917–1956. Record Unit 23.

Records of Alfred Whitney Griswold as President of Yale University, 1950–1963. Record Unit 22.

Records of Kingman Brewster Jr. as President of Yale University, 1941–1977. Record Unit 11.

Records of the Yale Secretary's Office, 1899–1953. Record Unit 49.

Records of the Yale Secretary's Office, 1860–1899. Record Unit 52.

Records of Franklin B. Dexter as Secretary of Yale University, 1833–1910. Record Unit 51.

Records of Reuben A. Holden as Secretary of Yale University, 1833–1910. Record Unit 19.
George Dudley Seymour Papers. Manuscript Group 442.
Albert W. Snoke Papers. Manuscript Group 1471.
Records of the Treasurer of Yale University. Record Unit 151.
C.-E. A. Winslow Papers. Manuscript Group 749.
Milton C. Winternitz Papers. Manuscript Group 859.
Yale–New Haven Hospital Records. Manuscript Group 835.
Records of Yale–New Haven Hospital (and Earlier Organizations). Record Unit 480.

North Tarrytown, New York. Rockefeller Foundation Archives. Rockefeller Archive Center.
Records of the General Education Board.

Washington, D.C. American Association of Medical Colleges. Archives.
Programs Medical Education (LCME) Accreditation Survey Reports.

Washington, D.C. Library of Congress. Manuscript Division.
Abraham Flexner Papers.

Periodicals

Boston Medical and Surgical Journal 20 (1839): 16–17.
Bulletin of Yale University.
Harkness Hoot. 1930–1934.
Knight Hospital Record. 1862–1865.
New Haven Journal-Courier. 1927–1937.
New Haven Register. 1934–1949.
New Haven Union. 1913.
Yale Alumni Weekly. 1907–1930.
Yale Daily News. 1927–1951.
Yale Law Report 34, no. 2 (Spring 1988): 26.
Yale Medical Journal. 1894–1909.

SECONDARY SOURCES

AMA Council on Medical Education. *Third Classification of Medical Colleges.* AMA, June 22, 1914.
Annals of the Royal College of Physicians of London, 1518–1915, 8 (Dec. 22, 1721): 191–204.
Annual Circular of the Medical Institution of Yale College. New Haven, 1839.
Appel, Toby A. *Shaping Biology: The National Science Foundation on American Biological Research, 1945–1975.* Baltimore: Johns Hopkins University Press, 2000.
Atwater, Edward, ed. *The History of the City of New Haven to the Present Time.* New York: W. W. Munsall, 1887.

Bacon, Francis. "The Practice of Medicine and Surgery." In *The History of the City of New Haven to the Present Time.* Edited by E. E. Atwater. New York: W. W. Munsall, 1887.

Barker, Creighton. *The Practice of Medicine in New Haven Following the Revolution.* New Haven: New Haven Medical Association, 1924.

———. "The Founding of the New Haven County Medical Association," Yale University Library, Manuscripts and Archives, Records of the President, YRG 2-A, box 138, folder 3043.

Barker, Lewellys. "Reforms in Medical Education." *Journal of the American Medical Association* 57 (1911): 613–21.

Baue, A. E. "Joseph Marshall Flint and the Whole-Time System at Yale." *Yale Journal of Biology and Medicine* 51 (1978): 549–63.

Beaumont, William. *Experiments and Observations on the Gastric Juice, and the Physiology of Digestion.* Plattsburgh, N.Y.: F. P. Allen, 1833.

Beecher, Henry, and Mark Altschule. *Medicine at Harvard: The First 300 Years.* Hanover, N.H.: University Press of New England, 1977.

Beeson, Paul. "Changing Times: Reflections on a Professional Lifetime: An Interview with Paul Beeson." Interview by R. V. Lee. *Annals of Internal Medicine* 132, no. 1 (2000): 71–79.

Bell, Whitfield J. "The Medical Institution of Yale College, 1810–1885." *Yale Journal of Biology and Medicine* 33 (1960): 169–83.

Bigelow, H. J. *Medical Education in America.* Cambridge, Mass.: Welch, Bigelow, 1871.

Blackwell, E. *Pioneer Work for Women.* New York: E. P. Dutton, 1914.

Blake, W. P., ed. *History of the Town of Hamden, Connecticut.* New Haven: Price, Lee, 1888.

Blumer, George. "Brief Recollections of the Yale Medical School (1906–1920)." *Yale Journal of Biology and Medicine* 21 (May 1946).

———. "Reminiscences of an Old-Time Doctor." *Yale Journal of Biology and Medicine* 28 (1955–1956): 1–28.

Burns, C. R. "History of Medical Ethics." In *Encyclopedia of Bioethics.* Edited by W. T. Reich. New York: Free Press, 1975.

Carmalt, William H. "The Second Half Century of the General Hospital Society of Connecticut." In *General Hospital Society of Connecticut Centenary.* New Haven: Tuttle, Morehouse and Taylor, 1926.

Catalogue of the Officers and Graduates of Yale University, 1701–1924. New Haven: Yale University, 1924.

"C.-E. A. Winslow: First Chairman of the Department of Public Health at Yale." *Yale Medicine* (Spring 1977): 1–8.

Cheever, Susan. *Treetops.* New York: Bantam Books, 1991.

Chittenden, R. H. "The Importance of Physiological Chemistry as a Part of Medical Education." *New York Medical Journal* 58 (1893): 370–74.

Committee on the Cost of Medical Care. *Medical Care for the American People: The Final Report.* Chicago: University of Chicago Press, 1932.

Cooper, Thomas. *An Address Delivered before the Medical Board of South Carolina, at Columbia, December 1821.* Columbia, S.C.: Gazette Office, 1821.

Corwin, B. F. "The Early Years of the Yale Medical School." *Yale Medical Journal* 1–2 (1894–1896): 210–13.

Cunningham, E. S. *Timothy Dwight.* New York: Macmillan, 1942.

Cushing, Harvey. "Experimentum Periculosum: Judicium Difficile." *Science* 61 (April 10, 1925): 373–79.

Daniels, Daryl K. "African-Americans at the Yale University School of Medicine: 1810–1960." Yale University School of Medicine. Unpublished M.D. thesis, 1991.

Davey, L. "John Farquhar Fulton." *Neurosurgery* 43 (1998): 185–87.

Dexter, Franklin B. *Biographical Sketches of the Graduates of Yale College with Annals of the College History.* 6 vols. New York: Henry Holt, 1885–1912.

———, ed. *Documentary History of Yale University.* New Haven, 1916.

Dickinson, Jonathan. *Observations on that disease vulgarly called the throat-distemper, With advices as to the method of cure, In a letter to a friend.* Boston: S. Kneeland and T. Green, 1740.

Dr. Skinner's Sanatorium, 1st Semi-Annual Report, December 1912. New Haven, 1912.

Duff, Raymond S., and August B. Hollingshead. *Sickness and Society.* New York: Harper and Row, 1968.

Dwight, Timothy. "The Medical Institution." In *Catalogue of Yale College,* 1815 or 1816, Cushing/Whitney Medical Library, Yale University.

———. *Yale College: Some Thoughts Respecting Its Future.* New Haven, 1871.

Ebbert, Arthur Jr. "Vernon W. Lippard." *Yale Journal of Biology and Medicine* 39 (1967): 343–45.

———. "The Yale School of Medicine in the 1950s: Personal Reminiscences and Observations on Then and Now." Lucia P. Fulton Fellow's Lecture. Nathan Smith Club, 1968.

Eliot, Ellsworth Jr. *Yale in the Civil War.* New Haven: Yale University Press, 1932.

Evans, John R. "The 'Health of the Public' Approach to Medical Education." *Academic Medicine* 67, no. 11 (1992): 719–23.

Evans, L. J. *The Crisis in Medical Education.* Ann Arbor: University of Michigan Press, 1964.

Fee, Elizabeth. "Competition for the First School of Public Health." *Bulletin of the History of Medicine* 57 (1983): 339–63.

Ferris, H. B. "Some Early Medical Teachers in Connecticut." *Bulletin of the Society of Medical History of Chicago* 3 (1923): 133–50.

Field, William W. *The Good Doctor Smith: Life and Times of Dr. Nathan Smith, 1762–1829.* New Haven: Advocate Press, 1992.

Fisher, George P. *Life of Benjamin Silliman, M.D., LL.D., Late Professor of Chemistry, Mineralogy, and Geology in Yale College.* 2 vols. Philadelphia: Charles Scribner, 1866.

Flexner, Abraham. *The American College: A Criticism.* New York: Century, 1908.

———. *Medical Education in the United States and Canada: A Report to the Carnegie Foundation for the Advancement of Teaching.* New York, 1910.

———. *I Remember: The Autobiography of Abraham Flexner.* New York: Simon and Schuster, 1940.

———. *Universities: American, English, German.* Oxford: Oxford University Press, 1930.

Flint, Joseph Marshall. "The Yale Mobile Hospital Unit." In *Yale in the World War.* Edited by George Henry Nettleton. New Haven: Yale University Press, 1925.

Fruton, Joseph S. *Eighty Years.* New Haven: Epikouros Press, 1994.

Fulton, John F. "C.-E. A. Winslow, Leader in Public Health." *Science* 125 (June 21, 1957): 1236.

———. *Harvey Cushing: A Biography.* Springfield, Ill.: C. C. Thomas, 1946.

———. "Some Notes on the Yale University School of Medicine with Special Reference to Milton Winternitz." *Yale Journal of Biology and Medicine* 22 (1950): 590.

General Assembly. *Resolutions of the General Assembly Incorporating the Connecticut Homeopathic Medical Society, the Organization of Said Society, Its Officers, Its Bylaws, Resolutions and Other Proceedings with a List of Homeopathic Physicians and a Sketch of the Conn. Homeopathic Society.* New Haven: Tuttle, Morehouse, and Taylor, 1864.

General Hospital Society of Connecticut Centenary. New Haven: Tuttle, Morehouse and Taylor, 1926.

Gesell, Arnold. *History of Psychology in Autobiography.* Volume 4. Edited by E. G. Boring et al. Worcester, Mass.: Clark University Press, 1952.

Gregg, Alan. "Addenda to the Agenda for the Decade 1940–1950." *Journal of the American Medical Association* 114, no. 13 (1940): 1139–41.

Hamlin, Hannibal. "The Dissection Riot of 1824 and the Connecticut Anatomical Law." *Yale Journal of Biology and Medicine* 7 (1934–1935): 275–89.

Harvey, Samuel C. "Joseph Marshall Flint." *Yale Journal of Biology and Medicine* 17 (1945): 503–15.

———. "Master Surgeons of America." *Surgery, Gynecology, and Obstetrics* 54 (1932).

———. "Peter Parker: Initiator of Modern Medicine in China." *Yale Journal of Biology and Medicine* 8, no. 3 (1935): 225–52.

Hayward, Oliver S. "Nathan Smith (1762–1829), Politician." *New England Journal of Medicine* 263 (1960): 1235–42.

———, and Constance E. Putnam. *Improve, Perfect and Perpetuate: Dr. Nathan*

Smith and Early American Medical Education. Hanover, N.H.: University Press of New England, 1998.

———, and Elizabeth H. Thomson, eds. *The Journal of William Tully, Medical Student at Dartmouth, 1808–1809.* New York: Science History Publications, 1977.

Hill, E. G. *A Modern History of New Haven.* New York: S. J. Clarke, 1918.

Hollingsworth, William. *Taking Care: The Legacy of Soma Weiss, Eugene Stead, and Paul Beeson.* San Diego: Medical Education and Research Foundation, 1994.

Hunt, Ebenezer. Presidential Address, "Public and Benevolent Institutions and Movements with which the Connecticut Medical Society has been prominently identified." Hartford: Proceedings of the Connecticut Medical Society 1865.

Hunt, Marion. "Extraordinarily Interesting and Happy Years: Martha M. Eliot and Pediatrics at Yale, 1921–1935. *Yale Journal of Biology and Medicine* 68 (1995): 159–70.

Hussey, Raymond. "The Study of Medicine at Yale." *Yale Journal of Biology and Medicine* 1 (October 1928): 18–21.

Jackson, James, et al. "Medical Missionary Society of China." *Boston Medical and Surgical Journal* 24 (1941): 176–78.

Jacobson, Wendy Nan. "American Medicine in Transition: The Case of the Yale Medical School, 1900–1920." Wesleyan University. Unpublished B.A. Honors thesis, 1976.

Jekel, J. F. "Health Departments in the U.S., 1920–1988: Statements of Mission with Special Reference to C.-E. A. Winslow." *Yale Journal of Biology and Medicine* 64 (1991): 467–69.

Jewett, P. A. *A Semi-Centennial History of the General Hospital Society of Connecticut.* New Haven: Tuttle, Morehouse, and Taylor, 1876.

Jones, Howard. *Mutiny on the Amistad.* New York: Oxford University Press, 1987.

Kaufman, Martin. *American Medical Education: The Formative Years, 1765–1910.* Westport, Conn.: Greenwood Press, 1976.

Kingsley, William, ed. *Yale College: A Sketch of Its History.* 2 vols. New York: Henry Holt, 1879.

Kohorn, E. I. "The Department of Obstetrics and Gynecology at Yale: The First One Hundred Fifty Years, from Nathan Smith to Lee Buxton." *Yale Journal of Biology and Medicine* 66 (1993): 85–106.

Lasagna, L. "The Mind and Morality of the Doctor." *Yale Journal of Biology and Medicine* 37 (1965): 361–77.

Lavietes, Paul H. "John Punnett Peters: An Appreciation." *Yale Journal of Biology and Medicine* 30 (1957): 175–82.

Laws of the Medical Institution of Yale College. New Haven: Oliver Steele, 1815.

Lay, G. T. "Hospitals at Canton and Macao." *Boston Medical and Surgical Journal* 23 (1840): 137–39.

Leikind, M. C. "Stanhope Bayne-Jones: Physician, Teacher, Soldier, Scientist-

Administrator, Friend of Medical Libraries." *Bulletin of New York Academic Medicine* 48, no. 3 (April 1972): 584–95.

Liebow, A. A. "Encounter with Disaster—A Medical Diary of Hiroshima, 1945." *Yale Journal of Biology and Medicine* 38 (1965): 161–239.

———. "Reunion: Yale Medical Unit of World War II." *Yale Medicine* 2, no. 3 (Fall 1967).

———, and L. L. Waters. "Milton Charles Winternitz, February 19, 1885–October 3, 1959." *Yale Journal of Biology and Medicine* 32 (1959): 143–72.

Lindsley, Charles A. "Abstract of a Lecture before the Medical Class, June 7th, 1897." *Yale Medical Journal* 3 (1897): 379–85.

Lippard, Vernon W. "The Medical School—Janus of the University." *Journal of Medical Education* 30, no. 12 (1955): 698–706.

———. "The Yale School of Medicine in the Twentieth Century." *Yale Journal of Biology and Medicine* 33 (1960): 184–92.

Lounsbury, T. R. *The Sheffield Scientific School.* Volume 2 of *Yale College,* edited by W. L. Kingsley. New Haven, 1879.

Ludmerer, Kenneth M. *Learning to Heal.* New York: Basic Books, 1985.

———. *Time to Heal.* Oxford: Oxford University Press, 1999.

Lyell, Alan. "Daniel Turner (1667–1740), LRCP London (1711), M.D. Honorary, Yale (1723), Surgeon, Physician and Pioneer Dermatologist." *International Journal of Dermatology* 21 (1982): 162–70.

Mather, Cotton. *Magnalia Christi Americana, or, The ecclesiastical history of New-England, from its first planting in the year 1620: unto the year of our Lord, 1698: in seven books.* London: T. Parkhurst, 1702.

Memorial of the Centennial of the Yale Medical School, 1814–1914. New Haven: Yale University Press, 1915.

"Mencken Calls Hospitals Worst Anti-Social Agencies in U.S.; He Would Sterilize Unfit to Solve Medical Care Problems; Drs. Peters and Fishbein Give Views on Medical Economics." *Wire Story by Mail.* Science Service. October 10, 1938.

Merkel, H. "The University of Michigan Medical School, 1850–2000." *JAMA* 283: 915–20.

Miller, C. Arden. "The Medical School and the University." *Yale Journal of Biology and Medicine* 39 (1967): 374–82.

Miller, Martin. "John P. Peters." *Diabetes* 6 (1957): 99.

Minor, W. C., and A. A. Surgeon. *Post Mortem Examinations made at Knight U.S.A. General Hospital.* New Haven: Knight Hospital Printer, 1864.

Mirsky, J., and A. Nevins. *The World of Eli Whitney.* New York, 1952.

Musto, David F. "Worthington Hooker (1806–1867): Physician and Educator." *Connecticut Magazine* 48 (1994): 569–74.

National Conference on the Costs of Medical Care. New York: New York Academy of Medicine, 1932.

Nettleton, G. H., ed. *Yale in the World War.* New Haven: Yale University Press, 1925.

Nuland, S. B. "An Informal History of Our School." Transcript of presentation to YMS Council, May 4, 1995.

Oren, Dan A. *Joining the Club: A History of Jews and Yale.* New Haven: Yale University Press, 1985.

Osler, William. *Aphorisms from His Bedside Teachings and Writings,* edited by W. B. Bean. Springfield, Mass., 1951.

Oviatt, Edwin. *The Beginnings of Yale, 1701–1726.* New Haven: Yale University Press, 1916.

Paul, J. R. "Dean Winternitz and the Rebirth at Yale Medical School in the 1920's." *Yale Journal of Biology and Medicine* 43 (1970): 110–19.

———. "Francis Gilman Blake," *Yale Journal of Biology and Medicine* 24 (1951–1952): 434–41.

———. "Preventive Medicine at the Yale University School of Medicine, 1940–49." *Yale Journal of Biology and Medicine* 22 (1950): 199–211.

———, and Cyril N. H. Long. "John Punnett Peters." *Biographical Memoirs.* Vol. 31. New York: National Academy of Sciences, 1958, 347–60.

Pearson, Howard. "Lectures on Diseases of Children by Eli Ives, M.D., of Yale and New Haven: America's First Academic Pediatrician." *Pediatrics* 77 (1986): 680–86.

Peters, John P., "The Social Responsibilities of Medicine." *Annals of Internal Medicine* 12, no. 4 (1938): 536–43.

———, and D. D. Van Slyke. *Quantitative Clinical Chemistry.* Baltimore: Williams and Wilkins, 1932.

Pierson, George W. *Yale College: An Educational History, 1871–1921.* New Haven: Yale University Press, 1952.

———. *Yale: The University College, 1921–1937.* New Haven: Yale University Press, 1955.

Pines, Maya. "Hospital. Enter at Your Own Risk." *McCalls* (May 1968): 138–42.

Program of the 54th Annual Meeting of the Association of American Medical Colleges, October 25–27, 1943. Cleveland, Ohio, 1943.

Prutkin, Jordan M. "Abraham Flexner and the Development of the School of Medicine." *Yale Journal of Biology and Medicine* 72 (1999): 269–79.

Rapport, Richard. *Physician: The Life of Paul Beeson.* Fort Lee: Barricade Books, 2001.

"Right of Corporations to Practice Medicine." *Yale Law Journal* 48 (1938): 346–51.

Roemer, M. I., and L. S. Falk. "The Committee on Costs of Medical Care, and the Drive for National Health Insurance." *American Journal of Public Health* 75 (1985): 841–48.

Rossiter, M. W. "Mendel the Mentor." *Journal of Chemical Education* 71 (1994): 215–19.

Rudolph, F. *The American College and University: A History.* Athens: University of Georgia Press, 1990.

Sadler, A. M., B. L. Sadler, and A. A. Bliss. *The Physician's Assistant: Today and Tomorrow.* New Haven: Yale University Press, 1972.

Senn, Milton J. E. *Insights on the Child Development Movement in the United States.* Chicago: University of Chicago Press, 1975.

Shem, Samuel. *The House of God.* New York: R. Marek, 1978.

Silliman, Benjamin. *Origin and Progress. I. Chemistry, Mineralogy, and Geology at Yale College and in Other Places with Personal Reminiscences.* 9 vols. New Haven, 1857–1862. Silliman Family Papers, series III, box 32, folder 33A,B.

Sixty-seventh Annual Announcement of the Medical Department of Yale College, 1879–1880. New Haven: Tuttle, Morehouse, and Taylor, 1879.

Smith, Arthur H., and Frank P. Underhill. Lafayette B. Mendel Anniversary Issue. *Yale Journal of Biology and Medicine* (March 1932).

Smith, Emily A. *Life and Letters of Nathan Smith, M.B., M.D.* New Haven, 1914.

Smith, L. H. "Medical Education for the 21st Century." *Journal of Medical Education* 60 (1985): 106–12.

Smith, Nathan. "Case of Ovarian Dropsy, Successfully Removed by a Surgical Operation." *American Medical Recorder* 5 (1822): 124–27.

———. "Observations on the Pathology and Treatment of Necrosis." *Philadelphia Journal of Medicine and Surgery* 1 (June 1827): 11–19 and 2 (July 1827): 66–75.

———. *A Practical Essay on Typhous Fever.* New York: Bliss and White, 1824.

The Spirit of Gaylord: A History, 1902–1997. New Haven: Gaylord Hospital Publications, 1997.

Stanton, M. *The Making of a Library.* New Haven: Yale University Press, 1959.

Stevens, George B. *The Life, Letters, and Journals of the Reverend and Hon. Peter Parker, M.D.* Boston: Congregational Sunday-School and Publishing Society, 1896.

Stevens, Rosemary. *American Medicine and the Public Interest.* Berkeley: University of California Press, 1998.

Stevenson, George S. *Connecticut Medicine* 23 (1959): 476–80.

Stiles, Ezra. *The Literary Diary of Ezra Stiles.* Edited by Franklin B. Dexter. 3 vols. New York: Charles Scribner's Sons, 1901.

Synott, M. G. *The Half-Opened Door.* Westport, Conn.: Greenwood Press, 1979.

Taffel, Max. "Samuel Clark Harvey, 1886–1953." *Yale Journal of Biology and Medicine* 26 (1953): 261–67.

Thacher, James. *American Medical Biography, or Memoirs of Eminent Physicians Who Have Flourished in America.* New York: Milford House, 1967.

Thoms, H. "Some Letters of Edmund Randolph Peaslee, B.B. Dartmouth, 1836, M.D. Yale 1840." *Yale Journal of Biology and Medicine* 17 (1945): 685–704.

Thoms, Herbert. *The Doctors of Yale College, 1702–1815, and the Founding of the Medical Institution.* Hamden, Conn.: Shoe String Press, 1960.

Thomson, Elizabeth H. "Peter Parker." *Yale Medicine* (Summer 1979).

Turner, Daniel. *De morbis cutaneis: A Treatise of Diseases Incident to the Skin.* London, 1714.

United States, Office of Scientific Research and Development. *Science, the Endless Frontier: A Report to the President by Vannevar Bush, Director of the Office of Scientific Research and Development.* Washington, D.C.: U.S. Government Printing Office, 1945.

Underhill, Frank Pell. "The Army Chemical Unit." In *Yale in the World War.* Edited by George Henry Nettleton. New Haven: Yale University Press, 1925.

Van Slyke, D. D. "John Punnett Peters." *Clinical Chemistry* 3, no. 4, suppl. (1957): 287–92.

Vaughan, H. F. "Local Health Services in the United States: The Story of CAP." *American Journal of Public Health* 62 (January 1972): 95–111.

Viseltear, Arthur J. "C.-E. A. Winslow and the Early Years of Public Health at Yale, 1915–1925." *Yale Journal of Biology and Medicine* 55 (1982): 137–51.

———. "C.-E. A. Winslow and the Later Years of Public Health at Yale, 1940–1945." *Yale Journal of Biology and Medicine* 60 (1987): 447–70.

———. "Milton C. Winternitz and the Yale Institute of Human Relations: A Brief Chapter in the History of Social Medicine." *Yale Journal of Biology and Medicine* 57 (1984): 869–89.

Walsh, M. R. *Doctors Wanted: No Woman Need Apply.* New Haven: Yale University Press, 1977.

Webster, Noah. *A Brief History of Epidemic and Pestilential Diseases: With the principal phenomena of the physical world, which precede and accompany them and observations deduced from the facts stated in the volumes.* Hartford: Hudson and Goodwin, 1799.

Welch, William. "The Relation of Yale to Medicine." *Yale Medical Journal* 8, no. 5 (1901).

Wertenbaker, T. J. *The Puritan Oligarchy: The Founding of American Civilization.* New York: Charles Scribner's Sons, 1947.

Williams, L., G. M. Carter, G. T. Hammons, and D. Poenter. *Managing for Survival: How Successful Academic Medical Centers Cope with Harsh Environments.* Santa Monica: Rand Publication Series, 1987.

Winchester, Simon. *The Professor and the Madman.* New York: Harper Collins, 1998.

Winslow, C.-E. A. *The Evolution and Significance of the Modern Public Health Campaign.* New Haven: Yale University Press, 1923.

———. "The Place of Public Health in a University." *Science* 62 (1925): 335–38.

———. "A Program for Medical Care in the United States." *Science* 77 (1933): 102–07.

———. "The Recommendations of the Committee on the Costs of Medical Care." *New England Journal of Medicine* 207 (1932): 1138–42.

Winternitz, M. C. *Collected Studies on the Pathology of War Gas Poisoning.* New Haven, 1920.

———. *The Past, Present, and Future of the Yale University School of Medicine and Affiliated Clinical Institutions, Including the New Haven Hospital, the New Haven Dispensary, and the Connecticut Training School for Nurses.* New Haven: Printed for the University, 1922.

———, Isabel M. Wason, and Frank P. McNamara. *The Pathology of Influenza.* New Haven: Yale University Press, 1920.

Wirthlin, L. S. "Joseph Smith's Boyhood Operation: An 1813 Surgical Success." *Brigham Young University Studies* 21 (1981): 131–54.

———. "Nathan Smith (1762–1828)." *Brigham Young University Studies* 17 (1977): 319–37.

Yesner, R. "A Century of Pathology at Yale: Personal Reflections." *Yale Journal of Biology and Medicine* 71 (1998): 397–408.

INDEX

Page numbers in *italics* refer to illustrations.